Notes

on

Anatomy
and
Physiology

by

William L. Traxel, M.D.

Booklocker.com, Inc.
2008

Cover design by Mark Sanders

Dedication

To my students. They provided the encouragement for which I am grateful because it gave me the incentive to complete this project.

William L. Traxel, M.D.

Table of Contents

Preface

Dr. William Traxel is a graduate of Northwestern University and Vanderbilt University School of Medicine. He is a graduate of the Naval Aerospace Medical Institute. He has had postgraduate training in internal medicine at Vanderbilt and in ophthalmology at the University of Michigan. He practiced ophthalmology for over twenty-five years. Following his retirement from medical practice, he began teaching Anatomy and Physiology at Three Rivers Community College. *Notes on Anatomy and Physiology* arose from the lecture notes that he compiled to teach the course.

Notes... has been written to fill the gap between lengthy, expensive texts and condensed versions. Although it is not lengthy, *Notes...* is not a condensed text. Teachers and students will find that *Notes...* contains the material that is required learning in any Anatomy and Physiology course.

Notes... is written in a clear, concise style using short sentences and omitting confusing qualifiers. It has been purposely written in a style that is as declarative as possible so as to allow the reader to quickly grasp concepts.

Another goal was for the textbook to be affordable to students. Most of the illustrations are drawings by Dr. Traxel, and the book is done solely in black and white, which holds down the cost, but does not infringe on the book's textual content.

Notes on Anatomy and Physiology has been written for the undergraduate student in nursing, pre-med, and any other related health field. Medical students will find this textbook useful as a "first read" for a particular topic that can instill an initial understanding of a topic before tackling material that is more in-depth.

Teachers, especially instructors of Anatomy and Physiology, may find *Notes...* to be valuable as a quick reference and as the basis for lectures -- for that is what this text is all about; it began as Dr. Traxel's lecture notes for Anatomy and Physiology.

In addition to practicing medicine and teaching Dr. Traxel has found time to be involved in community and church musical events (he plays, tunes and repairs pianos) and to maintain an eight handicap on the golf course. He also has done a stint as host for a health related television program.

Dr. Traxel has published several articles on medical topics. He has also published two full length books, *Footprints of the Welsh Indians*, a work of historical nonfiction, and *The Third Coffin,* a mystery in the historical fiction genre. His previous writing experience gave him the incentive to write this textbook.

Bill and his wife, Mary, live in Poplar Bluff, Missouri. They have two children and five grandchildren.

Chapter One

Principles of Anatomy and Physiology

What are the sciences of **_anatomy and physiology_**? Basically anatomy equals form, and physiology equals function. Anatomy is how your body is put together. It is the shape of things in your body and how they connect. A literal definition of anatomy is **_"to dissect_**," or to cut and separate organs in order to study their relationships. Physiology refers to a **_study of nature_**. Human physiology is the study of how your body works.

I want to congratulate all students who take Anatomy and Physiology. I consider Anatomy and Physiology and any subsequent related courses to be among the most important courses you will ever take because they are the study of your body – how you are made and how your body works.

Anatomy and physiology have been joined in this course to fuse form (anatomy) with function (physiology). This course is a mixture of at least nine different courses, and it necessarily encompasses much material. The individual courses that are encompassed in this single course include: **_General Chemistry_**, which is freshman chemistry; **_Gross Anatomy_**, which refers to the study of the human body without magnification; **_Comparative Anatomy_**, which is the comparative study of vertebrate anatomy; **_Histology_**, which is the microscopic study of tissues; **_Physiology_**, which is the study of how nature works; **_Cellular Physiology_**, which is the study of how nature works on a cellular level; **_Organic Chemistry_**, which is the study of all of the compounds containing the element carbon; **_Biochemistry_**, which is the study of the chemistry of living organisms, and **_Genetics_**, which is the study of inheritance. In addition most medical specialties will be touched on in this course.

It is important that you pay close attention to the **_language_**. Medicine has a whole new and different vocabulary. Learning the subject matter will be much easier if you know the meanings of the **_Latin and Greek_** words and their prefixes and suffixes, because most medical terms have Greek or Latin roots. In 1895 medical nomenclature was simplified to reduce the number of eponyms. A list of terms used in anatomy is included in this chapter.

An **_eponym_** is a name taken from a prominent individual, such as the Kennedy Space Center, Reagan International Airport, Eustachian Tube, or Alzheimer's disease.

An **_acronym_** is a term that has been coined by using the first letters of several words, such as DNA, ATP, PTA or CBC (complete blood count). MRSA is an acronym for methicillin resistant Staphylococcus aureus. Acronyms save time and are intended to promote clarity in speech and writing, but they must be clearly and repetitively defined. Acronyms are detrimental if you do not know the words the acronym represents -- you would be confused, and you would not understand what is being discussed.

A **_mnemonic_** is a poem or other saying to help you remember things such as a word list for bones or nerves.

Two major body cavities develop in the embryo, the dorsal cavity, and the ventral cavity. The **_dorsal cavity_** becomes the cranial cavity and the vertebral canal; the **_ventral cavity_** becomes the **_thoracic cavity, abdominal cavity and pelvic cavity._** The pelvic cavity is below and continuous with the abdominal cavity. In addition two **_pleural cavities_** contain the lungs, and the space between the lungs containing the heart is called the **_mediastinum_**. The areas of the vertebral column are the **_cervical, thoracic, lumbar, sacral and coccygeal._** These areas correspond respectively to the neck, chest, abdomen, pelvis, and tail.

The cavities of the body are lined by thin membranes. Three layers called **_meninges_** line the dorsal cavities. The **_parietal peritoneum_** lines the inner wall of the abdominal cavity; the **_visceral peritoneum_** covers the abdominal organs. The **_parietal pleura_** lines the thoracic cavity, and the **_visceral pleura_** covers the organs of the chest. The heart is surrounded by a three layered membrane called the **_pericardium_**; **_periosteum_** surrounds bones, and **_perichondrium_** surrounds some cartilage.

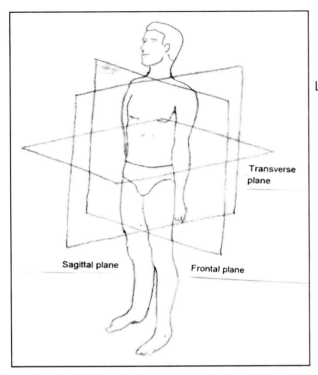

Left: Planes passing through the body need to be understood, especially in radiology and the surgical specialties. The three major planes are frontal or coronal, sagittal and transverse. The ___frontal plane___ is vertical; it passes from side to side (ear to ear). The ___sagittal plane___ is vertical; it passes from front to back. The ___transverse plane___ is horizontal. A sagittal plane may pass through the center of the body, in which case it is called a median or ___midsagittal___ section. Planes that are neither vertical nor horizontal are called ___oblique.___

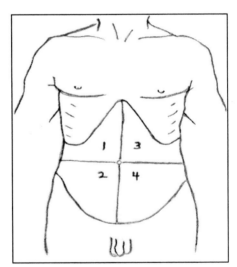

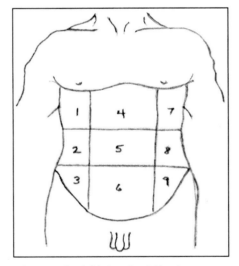

Surgical Abdominal Quadrants
  (1) Right upper
  (2) Right lower
  (3) Left upper
  (4) Left lower

Anatomical Abdominal Regions
  (1) and (7) R and L Hypochondriacal areas
  (2) and (8) R and L Lumbar or Lateral areas
  (3) and (9) R and L Inguinal areas
  (4) Epigastric area
  (5) Umbilical area
  (6) Hypogastric area

Above: The abdomen is divided into four quadrants by ___surgeons:___ the right upper, right lower, left upper and left lower quadrants. ___Anatomists___ divide the abdomen into six areas: right and left hypochondriacal, lumbar or lateral, and inguinal areas. Centrally are the epigastric, umbilical, and the pubic or hypogastric areas. The midclavicular lines separate the three center regions from the lateral regions.

Science is a discipline that follows certain rules. How do scientists evaluate what has been proven and what has not been proven? This does not mean that what has not been proven is not true, merely that it has not been verified scientifically.

The ***Inductive Method of Bacon and Descartes*** is used in the study of anatomy. It amounts to making numerous ***observations*** until you are able to draw generalizations and predictions based on the observations. This is how knowledge of anatomy has developed.

The ***Deductive Method of Experimental Design*** is used in the study of physiology. It requires the formation of a ***hypothesis*** or possible answer to a question, which can be ***tested with experimentation*** to see if the hypothesis holds true or not. Without the possibility of testing it is a theory, not a hypothesis.
Example: a hypothesis may state that epileptic seizures are caused by bursts of abnormal electrical activity in nerve cells of the brain. If the hypothesis is correct, brain waves of patients can be recorded during epileptic seizures, and they should show abnormal bursts of activity.

A ***hypothesis*** differs from a ***fact***. A fact is defined as information that can be independently verified by a trained person. All facts follow the laws of nature, which are the predictable ways that matter and energy behave. Hypotheses can be tested and proved, and a proven hypothesis can be said to have become a fact. Facts can be proven by repeated testing by independent investigators.
A ***theory*** is a statement that may or may not be true. To be credible a theory should be based on facts, laws, confirmed hypotheses or repeated observations. According to scientific philosophy, theories cannot be proven, but they can be disproved. Confidence in a theory builds if it survives scrutiny, but it is not said to be proven without experimentation, in which case it can be said to have become a hypothesis. It can be difficult to determine whether a theory has been disproved or not, and some scientists have become so involved with a theory that they continue to hold to their belief in it, even after new findings apparently have disproved it.

Factors in Experimental design:

The ***sample size*** must be adequate, and a ***control group*** must be included for comparison of result.
Experimental bias is negated by doing ***double blind*** studies where neither the experimenter nor the experimented is aware of which of two substances is being tested - the substance or the control. (The control is usually a ***placebo***, which is a substance that has no effect on the body.)
Others should be able to reproduce your results.
The results need to be statistically significant.

In the nineteenth century ***Robert Koch***, a German microbiologist, outlined a design for proving the cause of an infectious disease. Basically his postulates are: (1) the microorganism must be observed in every case of the disease, (2) the microorganism must be isolated and grown in pure culture, (3) the pure culture must reproduce the disease when inoculated into a susceptible animal, and (4) the microorganism must be observed and recovered from the diseased experimental animal.

In order to produce a meaningful result, an experiment must be properly designed. Consider a misadventure in the life of ***John Hunter***, an eighteenth century Scottish anatomist and physician. Hunter was no amateur at his profession, and his works are credited with laying the foundation for twentieth century developments. One of his students and friends was ***Edward Jenner***, who was the first to employ vaccination for smallpox. Hunter is quoted telling Jenner, "Why think (meaning theorize)? Try the experiment."
Hunter's most infamous experiment came from his belief that two diseases could not exist simultaneously in the same organ, and he considered syphilis and gonorrhea to be different manifestations of the same disease. Hunter designed an experiment to prove his hypothesis, and in 1767 he dipped a lancet into a lesion of a prostitute with gonorrhea. He then used the lancet to puncture the skin of his penis, and lo and behold, he contracted syphilis, which he considered proof of his hypothesis.
Hunter's hypothesis came from inadequate observations because his sample size was too small, he failed to use the double blind technique, he did not use microbiologcal methods, and he had an obvious experimenter bias. Had he followed Koch's postulates he would not have erred, but Hunter lived a century before Koch.

Edward Jenner also formed a hypothesis on the basis of observations (inductive reasoning). Jenner and many others had repeatedly noted that milkmaids who had cowpox scars were immune to smallpox. In 1796 Jenner took material from a cowpox lesion of a dairymaid named Sarah Nelmes and inserted it into the arm of eight year old James Phipps. Phipps came down with cowpox, from which he soon recovered. Six weeks later Jenner introduced scrapings from a patient with smallpox into Phipps' arm. The boy did not contract the deadly infection because of his immunity to cowpox. Both Hunter's and Jenner's hypotheses were based on inductive reasoning or observations. Both of their experiments were flawed (sample size too small, no control group). The difference between them is that Jenner and others had made numerous observations of cowpox affording immunity to smallpox, and his experiment could be duplicated by others. Had Hunter looked further into venereal disease, he would have found patients who had either syphilis or gonorrhea, but not both. Unfortunately for Hunter, the prostitute he chose had both gonorrhea and syphilis, and Hunter, who was forty-one years old at the time and engaged to be married for the first time, had to delay his marriage and take the "cure," which took three years. In those days the cure for syphilis consisted of multiple painful injections of mercury, a toxic heavy metal, over a three year period, and it was not all that effective. Some suspect that Hunter had latent syphilis for the rest of his life.

Characteristics of Living Beings

How do living things differ from nonliving things? What characteristics differentiate you, a tree or a snail from a rock?

Living things exhibit a higher level of _**organization**_ than non-living things, and they expend energy to maintain that order.

Living things are _**composed of cells**_, which are the basis of their organization.

All living things have a _**biochemical unity**_, meaning that they are composed of _**proteins, lipids (fats), carbohydrates and nucleic acids**_.

Living things are constantly undergoing _**metabolism**_, which is the constant change in their molecules resulting in a change in structure, physiology and energy.

Living things are _**responsive**_, which means they have the ability to sense and react to stimuli in their environment.

Living things possess _**homeostasis**_, which is the maintenance of a stable internal environment.

Living things _**develop and change**_ over their lifetime. This includes growth and differentiation.

Living things _**reproduce**_ other organisms similar to themselves.

Life functions on different levels. The smallest level that we will study is the _**chemical level**_ -- the atoms that make up the molecules of the body, which undergo changes through chemical reactions.

Next is the _**cellular level**_. Cells are the basic unit of life, and we will study the anatomy of cells and the functions they perform. Cells are the smallest and most numerous structural units that possess the basic characteristics of living matter. Bacteria, amoebae and paramecia are one-celled organisms. Smaller units that contain some characteristics of life are viruses and prions, but these units are parasitic and require a host cell.

Next is the _**tissue level**_. Cells group themselves into four types of tissues: (_**1) epithelial tissue, (2) connective tissue, (3) muscular tissue, and (4) nervous tissue.**_ Each type of tissue has special properties and functions.

Next is the _**organ level**_. Organs are contiguous bodies that have a specific function. They are composed of several different kinds of tissues, and therefore they are more complex than a single tissue. For instance, the heart is an organ made up of muscle tissue, specialized connective tissue, specialized epithelial tissues, and nervous tissue. Other organs include the brain, kidneys, liver, skin, etc.

Organs are grouped into systems, and the _**organ system level**_ is the next level. An organ system is more complex than an organ, and involves various organs arranged to perform complex functions. Eleven major organ systems are found in the body. They are _**respiratory, urinary, nervous, muscular, reproductive, skeletal, lymphatic-immune, integumentary, digestive, endocrine, and circulatory.**_ A mnemonic for the eleven organ systems is "RUN MRS. LIDEC." The chapters of this textbook are arranged according to organ systems.

The final level is the ***organism level***, which is a study of how the organism functions as a whole.

In spite of our likeness as a species, there are anatomical and physiological differences between all of us, which may include such basic things as the number of muscles, bones and teeth. Our physiology differs according to the proteins that our DNA is coded to synthesize.

For internal constancy (***homeostasis***) to be maintained, the body must have sensors that are able to detect changes from a set point. The ***set point*** is like a thermostat. Your body has set points for temperature, blood glucose concentration and many other things. A ***sensor*** detects a change from a particular set point; the information is transmitted to the nervous system, which then goes about bringing the aberrant parameters back to the set point. This is called ***negative feedback***. Negative feedback involves a loop with three constituents: a ***receptor*** (sensor), a ***control center*** (usually in the nervous system), and an effector (a muscle or organ).

Human thermoregulation is controlled by temperature-sensing nerve cells in the brain. These cells control shivering, sweating and blood flow through the skin by negative feedback. When your body overheats, effectors will cause blood vessels in your skin to dilate and sweating to commence. Dilated skin vessels provide heat loss by radiation, and sweating produces heat loss through evaporation.
When your body is chilled, effectors produce constriction of blood vessels in the skin, which reduces heat radiation. Chilling also leads to shivering, which produces more heat.

Positive feedback loops contrast to negative feedback. Positive feedback is a self-amplifying cycle that leads to a permanent change. Examples of positive feedback include the birth process, blood clotting, and digestion of proteins. ***Negative feedback*** control systems are **inhibitory;** **they oppose a change** by creating a response that is opposite to the initial disturbance; therefore, they are responsible for maintaining a constant internal environment, which is homeostasis. ***Positive feedback*** loops are **stimulatory.** **They result in an even greater** change in the same direction, and they produce a rapid and permanent change.
Control of body temperature involves ***negative feedback loops*** with dilation of blood vessels in the skin, which increases the radiation of heat, and with sweating, which increases evaporative cooling. However, when the body temperature exceeds 108 degrees F, a ***positive feedback loop*** results because the increased metabolic rate produces more heat than can be dissipated. Patients with temperatures over 108 degrees F must be cooled quickly to survive. A temperature of 113 degrees F kills cells and is fatal.

The following is a list of terms that you should know:
Directions:
Anterior (front) and **Posterior** (back)
Ventral (toward the front of the abdomen) and **Dorsal** (toward the back of the abdomen)
Superior (higher) and **Inferior** (lower)
Medial (toward the midline) and **Lateral** (away from the midline)
Proximal (toward the trunk) and **Distal** (toward the end of the extremities)
Supinate (palm facing forward or up) and **Pronate** (palm facing backward or down)
Flex (decreasing the angle of a joint) and **Extend** (increasing the angle of a joint)
Rostral (toward the front of the head) and **Caudal** (toward the back of the head or the base of the brain)

Definitions
a-, an-: prefix meaning "non-" or "un-"
abduct: move away from center
adduct: move toward center
anatomy: the study of structure, literally "to dissect"
andro-: male
anti-: against
ante-: before
anterior: front
-ase: suffix indicating an enzyme

bi-: two
blast-: precursor, producer
brachi-: arm
brady-: slow
calyx: cuplike
carcino-: prefix indicating a cancer of epithelial tissue
cauda: tail
cephalo-: head
cervi-: neck
chondro-: cartilage
cilium, cilia: eyelash(es)
circ-: about or around
cisterna: reservoir, dilated sack
-clast: to break down
contra: opposite
cranium: helmet (the casing for the brain)
crista: crest
cyto-: prefix pertaining to the cell
demi, hemi, semi: half
dendro-: branched like a tree
derm-: skin
desmo-: a band or bond
di-: two
distal: away from the center
dorsal: a directional term meaning toward the back
dur: hard
ecto-: outside of
-ectomy: suffix for a procedure that removes or cuts out something.
encephalo-: prefix pertaining to the brain (literally inside the skull)
endo-: inside of
epi-: upon, above
erythro- or rubro-: red
exo-: out
-form: suffix meaning the shape of
-glia: suffix meaning glue
glosso-: tongue
hallux: big toe
hemo-: blood
histo-: histology, tissues, the study of tissues
holo-: entire, whole
homeo-: constant, unchanging
homo-: same, alike
hydro-: water
hyper-: above, excessive
hypo-: below, deficient
inferior: below
infra-: below
inter-: between
intra-: within, inside of
iso-: the same, equal or normal
itis-: inflammation
juxta-: next to
kali-: potassium
kerato-: horn, skin
labium: lip
lacrimo-: tear, cry

lacto-: milk
lamina: layer
lateral: toward the side
-lemma: husk, covering
leuko-: white
litho: stone
lucid: clear, transparent
lunar: crescent shaped
luteum, lutea: yellow
lyso-: to split apart
macro-: mega-, large
mal-: bad
micro-: small
mammo-, masto-: breast
mano-: hand
medial: toward the midline
melano-: darkly pigmented
meso-: in the middle
meta-: the next in a series
mollé: soft
mono-: uni-, one
morpho-: the shape of
muta-: change
myo-: muscle
natri-: sodium
neuro-: nerve, nervous tissue
oculo-: eye
-oid: like, resembling
oligo-: few, a small number of
-oma: suffix indicating a tumor
orbi-: circle
ortho-: straight
-ose: suffix indicating a sugar, or (2) full, as in adipose
-osis: suffix for a nonspecific abnormality
osteo-: bone
-ostomy: suffix for a permanent opening or fistula
-otic: a general descriptive suffix
-otomy: a suffix meaning to make an incision into
parietal: external covering, wall
pecto-, sterno-: chest
pedi-, pod-: foot
penna-: feather
phago-: to eat
philo-: attracted to or love
phobo-: repelled by, or feared
physiology: the study of natural causes (function)
pilo, tricho, villus: hair
pino-: to drink, imbibe
pollix: thumb
posterior: rear
proximal: toward the center
pterygo-: wing
ptosis-: droopy or sagging
quadri-: four
ramus, rami: a branch
recto-: straight

reticular: a net
retro-: behind
sarco-: muscle
sclero-: hard, tough, fibrous
sepsis: infected
skull: the bones of the head and face
soma, somato-: pertaining to the body
stenosis: a narrowing
stratum, strata: layer(s)
stria: striped
sub-: below
superior: above
supra-: above
sym-, syn-: together
tachy-: fast
telo-: the last of a series
tertiary: third in a series
thrombosis: blood clot
tone, tonicity: force or tension (muscle or solute concentration)
trans-: across
tri-: three
troph-: nourishment
ventral: a directional term alluding to the front of the abdomen or the underside of the brain.
vesicle: bladder or blister
visceral: pertaining to the organs in the chest and belly

Giants in Medical History

Many people have contributed to our knowledge of anatomy and physiology. Some of the most outstanding follow:

1. **Hippocrates** (460-377 B.C.) is regarded as the ***"Father of Modern Medicine."*** He lived in Greece. He applied ***logic, facts and reason*** to medicine in an age full of superstitious thought. He showed that disease had natural causes. He set fractures and reduced dislocations.

2. **Aristotle** (384-322 B.C.) lived in Greece. He argued that ***complex structures are built from smaller components.***

3. **Galen, Claudius** (130-200 A.D.) is known as the ***"Father of Experimental Physiology."*** He was born in Turkey, traveled to Greece and Phoenicia and studied in Alexandria, Egypt. He served as a surgeon to gladiators and eventually went to Rome where he became the foremost physician of his time. ***He wrote over four hundred books, eighty-three of which survive***. He dissected pigs and monkeys (but not humans, which was illegal in Rome), and he described his findings. He discovered that arteries were filled with blood and not air as had been previously taught. His works on Physiology, Anatomy and Surgery were so highly regarded that they were the standard for the world for ***over 1300 years***.

4. **Avicenna, or Ibn Sina** (980-1037) was an Arab physician, philosopher, astronomer and poet who was born in Bukhara in what is now Uzbekistan. He questioned authority when evidence demanded it. He wrote the ***Canon of Medicine***, which was used as a medical text for over six hundred years. Arab medicine was the storehouse of knowledge for the world during the Dark Ages, and for that period of time it was superior to Western medicine due to the efforts of Avicenna and others in the Middle East.

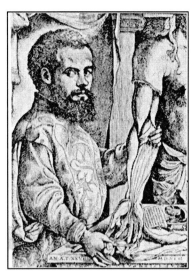 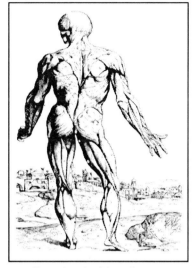

Andreas Vesalius   Drawing by Vesalius

5. Vesalius, Andreas (1514-1564, painting by Jan Stephen van Calcar) is known as the *"Father of Anatomy."* He was born in Brussels and became a professor at the University of Padua, Italy, at the age of 23. Vesalius dissected the bodies of dead criminals, and he published *Concerning the Fabric of the Human Body"* in 1543. Vesalius dared to correct errors in Galen's work, which were based on animal dissection. Followers of Galen bitterly attacked him. He burned most of his writings, left Padua discouraged, and went to Spain where he became physician to King Philip II and King Charles V.

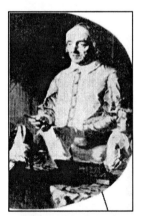

6. William Harvey (1578-1657, painting by Robert Hannah) was an English physician who discovered how blood circulates in the body. He published *An Anatomical Treatise on the Motion of the Heart and Blood in Animals* in 1628. Harvey's treatise is regarded as **the most important** single volume in the history of physiology.

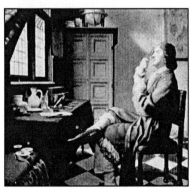

7.   Anton Van Leeuwenhoek (1632-1723, painting by Robert A. Thom) was a Dutch scientist who is known as *"The Father of Microbiology."* He made hundreds of *lenses,* which magnified up to 270x, and he used them to study stagnant water, teeth scrapings, blood cells, muscle fibers, spermatozoa, and silk fibers among other things. He called the tiny organisms that he saw "animalcules" (small animals).

8.   Robert Hooke (1635-1703) was an English scientist with many interests and inventions.   He took Leeuwenhoek's work further and invented the compound telescope. He described plant cells in 1665 and *named them "cells."*

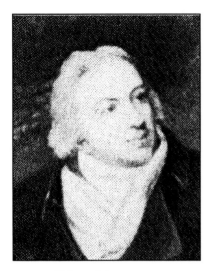

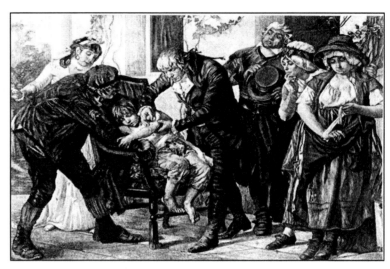

Edward Jenner
from Bettman archive

Jenner, James Phipps and Sarah Nelmes
painting by Ewing Galloway

9. Edward Jenner (1749-1843) was an English physician who observed that milkmaids with scars from a previous cowpox infection were immune to smallpox (an example of inductive reasoning). In 1796 Jenner took material from a cowpox lesion of a dairymaid named Sarah Nelmes and inserted it into cuts he made on the arm of eight year old James Phipps. Phipps came down with cowpox. Six weeks later Jenner introduced smallpox material into Phipps' arm, but the boy did not contract the deadly infection because he was immune. Jenner's success began the practice of immunization for smallpox, which later was done using the less virulent Vaccinia virus (another pox virus which gave an even milder disease than cowpox). Jenner's ***introduction of vaccination*** is an example of the Deductive Method. He published his work in 1798. Smallpox is known to have caused 15% to 90% mortality in the days before vaccination.

10. Karl Zeiss (1816-1888) made further ***improvements to the microscope***. Zeiss microscopes became the most desirable microscopes in the industry, and despite being made in Leipzig, East Germany, they were sought after by the west during the cold war.

11. Matthias Schleiden (1804-1881) and **Theodor Schwann** (1810-1882) concluded that all organisms were composed of cells. From this they put forth the ***"Cell Theory"*** in 1839.

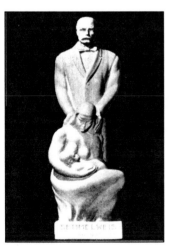

12. Ignatz Semmelweiss (1818-1865, photo from the International College of Surgeons) was a Hungarian physician who practiced in Vienna. He observed (inductive reasoning) that the extraordinarily high rate of female infections at Vienna Lying-In Hospital was associated with the ***failure of physicians to wash their hands*** before examining their patients in labor. His theory was met with hostility in spite of the fact that the infection rate fell drastically with the institution of hand washing.

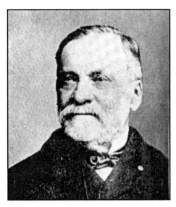

13. Louis Pasteur (1822-1895, UPI photo) was a French physician-scientist who is credited with the finding that **_life comes only from other life,_** and spontaneous regeneration does not occur as had been previously thought. He studied bacteria and infections, and he invented the process of **_pasteurization_** to keep wine from spoiling. He then used pasteurization to keep beer, milk and food from spoiling. He developed the **_first vaccination for rabies_** and used it successfully on a patient who had been bitten by a rabid dog.

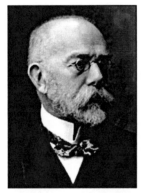

14. Robert Koch (1843-1910) was a German physician who established the science of bacteriology. He suffered from tuberculosis and won the Nobel Prize in 1905 for his work on the microorganisms that cause tuberculosis, cholera and plague. The tubercle bacillus is still known as "Koch's bacillus." In 1878 Koch published his thesis on the cause of infections, and he put forth **_"Koch's Postulates_**," which outline the proper design for an experiment regarding infectious diseases. He won the Nobel Prize for Physiology or Medicine in 1905.

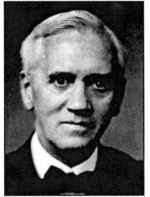

15. Sir Alexander Fleming (1881-1955) was an English bacteriologist who was born in Scotland. He observed that bacteria would not grow on his cultures if they were near a mold colony. His inductive observations were published in 1929. Fleming's **_discovery of penicillin_** ushered in the age of antibiotics, and he won the Nobel Prize for Physiology and Medicine in 1945.

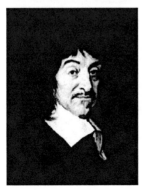

16. Rene Descartes (1596-1650) was a French philosopher, mathematician and scientist who sought to find truth through the use of reason. His observations (inductive reasoning) led him to say his most famous quote: **_"I think, therefore, I am."_**

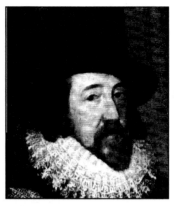

17. Sir Francis Bacon (1561-1626, painting by Paulus van Somer) was an English nobleman of giant intellect, who was also a lawyer, scientist and author. He published a plethora of works in philosophy and science under his own name, and there is evidence that he wrote the plays and sonnets credited to William Shakespeare. It is thought that he did not take credit for Shakespeare's work because Queen Elizabeth considered the works to be seditious. He is ***credited with describing inductive reasoning*** as a means of proving a scientific point, but he also put forth the idea that a ***preliminary hypothesis*** would aid an investigation.

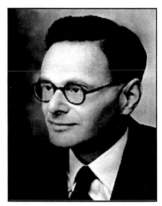

18. Hans Adolph Krebs (1900-1981) was a German biochemist-pharmacologist who discovered the ***urea cycle*** in 1932 and the ***citric acid cycle*** in 1937. The urea cycle rids the body of nitrogenous wastes. The citric acid cycle (Krebs cycle or tricarboxylic cycle) is the aerobic method of extracting energy from carbohydrates, fats and proteins. Krebs did most of his work in England. He won the Nobel Prize for medicine and chemistry in 1953.

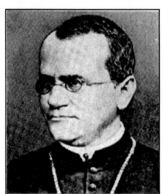

19. Gregor Mendel (1822-1884, Bettman archive) was an Austrian monk and botanist who discovered the principles of heredity through his work on garden peas. He observed that some of his peas had smooth skin and some had wrinkled skin. His experiments showed that heredity was due to dominant and recessive characteristics. He published his findings in 1866, but the importance of his work was not appreciated until 1900. He is now regarded as the ***"Father of Genetics."***

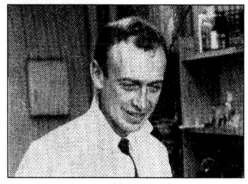
James Watson

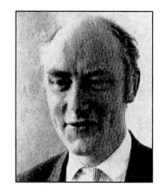
Francis Crick

20. James Watson (1928-) and **Francis Crick** (1916-2004) (UPI photos) were the first to ***discover the structure of DNA,*** describing it as a double helix in a paper they published in 1953. Watson was an American, and Crick was an Englishman. They shared the Nobel Prize in 1962 for their discovery.

Study Guide

1. Review the definitions in this chapter.
2. Review the "Giants in Medical History."
3. Understand body planes (sagittal, transverse and coronal or frontal).
4. Be able to demonstrate the anatomical position.
5. Know the location and contents of the body cavities (dorsal, ventral, cranial, thoracic, abdominal, pelvic).
6. Know where to find the pelvis, thorax, mediastinum, cervical area, lumbar area, sacral area and coccyx.
7. Know the meaning of the terms *acronym, eponym, and mnemonic.*
8. Know the meaning of the directional terms *superior, inferior, posterior, anterior, dorsal, ventral, caudal, rostral, proximal, distal, medial, lateral, superficial and deep.*
9. Know the meaning of terms relating to joint movements (flex, extend, supinate and pronate).
10. Know the meaning of *visceral, parietal, pleura, peritoneum, mesentery, pericardium, periosteum and perichondrium.*
11. Know the difference between a tissue, an organ, and an organ system.
12. Know the four principle tissue types (epithelial, connective, muscle and nervous).
13. Understand the terms *homeostasis, negative feedback, and positive feedback,* and appreciate how they relate.
14. Know what is meant by inductive reasoning and deductive reasoning.
15. Understand the difference between a theory, a hypothesis and a fact.
16. Recognize the four types of compounds that make up all living things (proteins, lipids [fats], carbohydrates and nucleic acids).

Chapter Two

Chemistry

Everything that exists is either in the form of matter or energy. ***Matter*** has mass and takes up space. Energy exists as a capacity to do "work," and is in the forms of heat, light and movement. Matter exists as a solid, liquid or gas. Matter is formed into over one hundred ***elements***, each of which is unique. Chemistry is the study of elements and the reactions they undergo. Each element is identified by its ***atom.*** The atom of each element is unique to that element, and the atom is the simplest form of an element. Atoms are made up of ***protons*** and ***neutrons*** in their core, or nucleus, and ***electrons*** in their shell. The apparent resemblance of the atom to the solar system led English physicist, Ernest Rutherford, in 1911 to describe the atom as like the solar system. In 1913 Danish physicist, Niels Bohr, described electron rings and related the planetary theory to ***quantum mechanics***. Rutherford and Bohr envisioned the nucleus to contain protons and neutrons and be encircled by electrons.

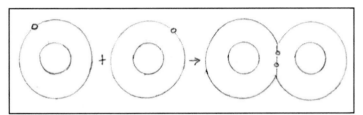

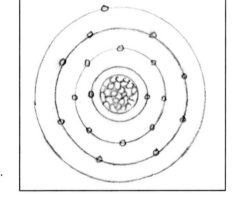

In the illustrations above the nucleus is in the center, surrounded by electron rings.

Right: A potassium atom.

Quantum mechanics is a scientific theory developed by German physicist, Max Planck, in 1900. It describes radiant energy waves as tiny measurable packets or particles called quanta. Light is energy that is in the form of waves. ***Photons*** are quanta of light waves that may be thought of as particles.

Protons have a positive charge; ***electrons have a negative charge***, and ***neutrons have no charge.*** What is meant by a charge? In the wiring of your home, in your automobile battery, and in the cells of your body a charge is the ***movement of electrons*** in one direction or another. ***Oppositely charged particles attrac***t; ***like charged particles repel***.

The ***periodic table*** lists all the elements. Note that each element has an ***atomic number*** written below its symbol, which reflects the number of protons in the nucleus of an atom of that element. The atomic number of each element is ***unique to that element, and it identifies the element.***

All nuclei of an element contain the same number of protons, but ***the number of neutrons may vary***. The ***atomic mass*** is the number of protons plus the number of neutrons in the nucleus of ***the most common form*** of an element. Protons and neutrons have a mass of ***one atomic mass unit (amu).*** The ***atomic weight*** is similar but not identical to the atomic mass. The difference is reflected by the ***number of neutrons in the nucleus*** of different forms of a given element, and these different forms are called ***isotopes.*** The number of protons in the nucleus of the various isotopes of a given element is always the same; otherwise, they would not be isotopes of the same element. However some isotopes contain more or fewer neutrons than the most common form, and the atoms of those isotopes will weigh more or less than the atomic mass. The ***atomic weight*** of an element is the ***average mass*** of the isotopes of the element. The atomic weight is written in the periodic table above the symbol for the element.

The mass of a proton is approximately equal to that of a neutron, but the mass of an electron is only 1/1836 of a proton; the mass of the electrons is disregarded when totaling the total mass or weight of an atom.

Ninety-one elements occur naturally on earth and 27 more have been created artificially in the laboratory. Most of the commonly found elements in the body are relatively small elements with a good deal of stability. 98.5% of your body's weight is composed of the elements hydrogen (H), carbon (C), nitrogen (N), oxygen (O), phosphorus (P) and calcium (Ca). Next in the total are sodium (Na), magnesium (Mg), sulfur (S), chlorine (Cl), potassium (K) and iron (Fe). Also necessary for life but present in small quantities are vanadium (V), chromium (Cr), manganese (Mn), cobalt (Co), copper (Cu), zinc (Zn), silicon (Si), fluorine (F), selenium (Se), molybdenum (Mo), tin (Sn), and iodine (I). These 24 elements are essential to human life. In addition Boron (B) and Germanium (Ge) have recently been added to the list of trace elements that serve a function in the human body. The other elements have no known function in the human body and are sometimes harmful.

hydrogen 1 **H** 1.0079																	helium 2 **He** 4.0026
lithium 3 **Li** 6.941	beryllium 4 **Be** 9.0122											boron 5 **B** 10.811	carbon 6 **C** 12.011	nitrogen 7 **N** 14.007	oxygen 8 **O** 15.999	fluorine 9 **F** 18.998	neon 10 **Ne** 20.180
sodium 11 **Na** 22.990	magnesium 12 **Mg** 24.305											aluminium 13 **Al** 26.982	silicon 14 **Si** 28.086	phosphorus 15 **P** 30.974	sulfur 16 **S** 32.065	chlorine 17 **Cl** 35.453	argon 18 **Ar** 39.948
potassium 19 **K** 39.098	calcium 20 **Ca** 40.078	scandium 21 **Sc** 44.956	titanium 22 **Ti** 47.867	vanadium 23 **V** 50.942	chromium 24 **Cr** 51.996	manganese 25 **Mn** 54.938	iron 26 **Fe** 55.845	cobalt 27 **Co** 58.933	nickel 28 **Ni** 58.693	copper 29 **Cu** 63.546	zinc 30 **Zn** 65.39	gallium 31 **Ga** 69.723	germanium 32 **Ge** 72.61	arsenic 33 **As** 74.922	selenium 34 **Se** 78.96	bromine 35 **Br** 79.904	krypton 36 **Kr** 83.80
rubidium 37 **Rb** 85.468	strontium 38 **Sr** 87.62	yttrium 39 **Y** 88.906	zirconium 40 **Zr** 91.224	niobium 41 **Nb** 92.906	molybdenum 42 **Mo** 95.94	technetium 43 **Tc** [98]	ruthenium 44 **Ru** 101.07	rhodium 45 **Rh** 102.91	palladium 46 **Pd** 106.42	silver 47 **Ag** 107.87	cadmium 48 **Cd** 112.41	indium 49 **In** 114.82	tin 50 **Sn** 118.71	antimony 51 **Sb** 121.76	tellurium 52 **Te** 127.60	iodine 53 **I** 126.90	xenon 54 **Xe** 131.29
caesium 55 **Cs** 132.91	barium 56 **Ba** 137.33	57-70 ✱	lutetium 71 **Lu** 174.97	hafnium 72 **Hf** 178.49	tantalum 73 **Ta** 180.95	tungsten 74 **W** 183.84	rhenium 75 **Re** 186.21	osmium 76 **Os** 190.23	iridium 77 **Ir** 192.22	platinum 78 **Pt** 195.08	gold 79 **Au** 196.97	mercury 80 **Hg** 200.59	thallium 81 **Tl** 204.38	lead 82 **Pb** 207.2	bismuth 83 **Bi** 208.98	polonium 84 **Po** [209]	astatine 85 **At** [210]	radon 86 **Rn** [222]
francium 87 **Fr** [223]	radium 88 **Ra** [226]	89-102 ✱✱	lawrencium 103 **Lr** [262]	rutherfordium 104 **Rf** [261]	dubnium 105 **Db** [262]	seaborgium 106 **Sg** [266]	bohrium 107 **Bh** [264]	hassium 108 **Hs** [269]	meitnerium 109 **Mt** [268]	unnnilium 110 **Uun** [271]	unununium 111 **Uuu** [272]	ununbium 112 **Uub** [277]		ununquadium 114 **Uuq** [289]			

*Lanthanide series	lanthanum 57 **La** 138.91	cerium 58 **Ce** 140.12	praseodymium 59 **Pr** 140.91	neodymium 60 **Nd** 144.24	promethium 61 **Pm** [145]	samarium 62 **Sm** 150.36	europium 63 **Eu** 151.96	gadolinium 64 **Gd** 157.25	terbium 65 **Tb** 158.93	dysprosium 66 **Dy** 162.50	holmium 67 **Ho** 164.93	erbium 68 **Er** 167.26	thulium 69 **Tm** 168.93	ytterbium 70 **Yb** 173.04
**Actinide series	actinium 89 **Ac** [227]	thorium 90 **Th** 232.04	protactinium 91 **Pa** 231.04	uranium 92 **U** 238.03	neptunium 93 **Np** [237]	plutonium 94 **Pu** [244]	americium 95 **Am** [243]	curium 96 **Cm** [247]	berkelium 97 **Bk** [247]	californium 98 **Cf** [251]	einsteinium 99 **Es** [252]	fermium 100 **Fm** [257]	mendelevium 101 **Md** [258]	nobelium 102 **No** [259]

Above: The Periodic Table of the Elements. The atomic number is given above the symbol for each element. The atomic weight is given below the symbol.

Hydrogen is the lightest and smallest element, having only one proton, one electron and no neutrons. Hydrogen has an atomic number of one (one proton), and an atomic mass of one (one proton plus zero neutrons). The atomic weight is the ***average*** of the atomic masses of all the isotopes in a sample of that element.

**Deuterium** is an isotope of hydrogen that contains one proton and one electron _**and one neutron**_. Therefore, it has an atomic number of one and an atomic mass or weight of two. Because hydrogen is a mixture of hydrogen and a small amount of its isotope, deuterium, hydrogen has an atomic mass of one, but an atomic weight of 1.0079.

In this illustration a hydrogen atom is on the left. It has one proton in its nucleus.

On the right is a deuterium atom, an isotope of hydrogen. Deuterium has one proton and one neutron in its nucleus.

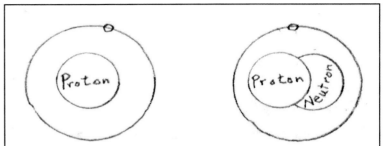

A normal carbon atom has 6 protons and 6 neutrons in its nucleus and an atomic mass of 12. But one isotope of carbon (called C 14) has 6 protons and _8_ neutrons and has an atomic mass of 14 (6+8). Because C 14 exists normally in small quantities among all carbon on earth, the atomic weight of carbon is 12.0112, which represents mostly C 12 but also includes a small amount of C 14.

Whereas the neutrons and protons of an atom exist in the nucleus, the electrons exist in a series of shells around the nucleus. Exposure of the electrons allows them to form bonds with other atoms. The inner shell of electrons is filled with a maximum of only two electrons. The second shell becomes filled when it has eight electrons. In atoms where the third shell has eight electrons, the fourth shell begins to fill. However, once the fourth shell has begun to accept electrons, the third shell can build up to eighteen electrons. _**The outermost shell of any atom never contains more than eight electrons**_, even though the third shell and beyond may contain more than eight when an outer shell has begun to fill. The maximum number of electrons in the third or fourth ring can build to 18 and the fifth ring can build to 32, but not until the ring beyond has begun to fill. Elements with atomic numbers of 84 or higher have six or seven electron rings, and they are unstable. They are naturally radioactive and give off subatomic particles as they decay to lighter elements. Uranium and radon are examples.

The periodic table lists the elements. Similarities exist among the elements in each column. The atomic numbers and atomic masses and weights gradually get larger going toward the bottom of the table. The atoms in each specific column are similar and react similarly because their electrons behave similarly. The elements listed in a single column of the periodic table have the _**same number of electrons in their outer rings.**_ Different elements in a single column simply have a different number of electron rings. The electrons in the outer ring are called _**valence electrons**_, and they are what determine how that element reacts with other elements. _**Reactions involving any element will tend to move electrons so that each reacting atom has a full quota of electrons in its outer ring.**_ For example in the right hand column of the periodic table are listed helium, neon, argon, krypton, and xenon. All of these elements all have the maximum number of electrons in their outer ring - two for helium, eight for the others. Because their outer rings are full, they do not accept electrons from other elements, nor do they give up electrons. In fact they rarely react, and they are called "inert." In the far left column are listed hydrogen, lithium, sodium, potassium and several other larger atoms. The atoms of these elements all have one electron in their outer ring, which they readily give up. In the second column from the right are listed fluorine, chlorine, bromine and iodine. These elements are called _**halogens**_. Each of the halogens has seven electrons (one less that a full quota) in its outer ring, and it readily accepts one electron from other atoms when they are made available.

Elements react depending upon the number of electrons in their outer rings (their valence electrons). Thus does carbon, with 4 electrons it its outer ring, readily accept 4 electrons as well as it will readily give up 4 electrons. Nitrogen has five electrons in its outer ring and its usual valence is -3 because it tends to accept three electrons, which then fill its outer ring. However, nitrogen can also achieve a full quota of electrons in its outer ring by giving up five electrons. This means that nitrogen may react by donating up to five electrons or accepting as many as three electrons. In other words, the valence of nitrogen can vary anywhere between –3 and +5. _**The negativity or positivity of the valence refers to the charge the atom assumes after it has gained or lost electrons.**_ A valence of -3 means that atom will tend to pick up three electrons; a valence of +5 means that it will tend to lose 5 electrons. This property of nitrogen and some other elements makes it possible for multiple compounds to be formed by a few elements. An element that has given up electrons or accepted electrons from another atom is called an *ion.* *Cations* have lost one or more electrons and have a positive charge. *Anions* have gained one or more electrons and have a negative charge.

It is possible to have different numbers of electrons in the outer ring of elements in which the fourth ring has begun to fill. For example the atomic number of iron is 26. Iron has 26 protons in its nucleus, and it has 26 electrons in its unionized state. The first ring has two electrons; the second ring has eight electrons, and the third ring theoretically has between eight and fifteen electrons. The fourth ring theoretically has between one and eight electrons. All of these possibilities do not exist in nature; the two possibilities that commonly exist are iron with a valence of +2, having two electrons in the fourth ring and fourteen electrons in the third ring, and iron with a valence of +3, having three electrons in the fourth ring and thirteen electrons in the third ring. Iron with the *lower valence (+2) is called ferrous*, and iron with the *higher valence (+3) is called ferric*. When ionized, Fe++ has lost two electrons and is the reduced form; Fe+++ has lost three electrons and is the oxidized form. Compounds made by the two different forms of iron reflect this difference in valence. Ferrous chloride is $FeCl_2$, and ferric chloride is $FeCl_3$. The difference is significant in physiology because the ferrous form is better absorbed, and it is the ferrous form that is present in hemoglobin. Cells are able to interchange the two valences of iron, however, so the difference is less important once iron has been absorbed.

A *molecule* is composed of two or more atoms linked by chemical bonds that involve the sharing of a pair of electrons. This sharing of a pair of electrons, one from each of two atoms, defines a *covalent bond,* which is the *strongest* type of chemical bond. The atoms of a molecule may be of the same element. For example, two hydrogen atoms may bond to form a hydrogen molecule (H_2). One pair of electrons is shared with each hydrogen atom donating an electron to the bond; this is called a *single covalent bond*. Or two oxygen atoms may bond and form an oxygen molecule (O_2). Oxygen has six electrons in its outer ring; it readily accepts 2 electrons, and it has a valence of –2. In the molecular form of oxygen (O_2) *two pairs* of electrons are shared; each of the oxygen atoms shares two of its electrons with the other. This amounts to each atom having eight electrons in its outer ring (four unshared, two of its own shared with the other atom, and two of the other atom's electrons which it shares). The resulting bond is a *double covalent bond* because two pairs (four total) of electrons are shared. An oxygen molecule may, therefore, be written O=O. A nitrogen molecule is formed by two nitrogen atoms linked by three pairs (six total) of electrons, which is a triple covalent bond. A molecule may also be composed of different elements such as when sodium bonds with chlorine and produces sodium chloride. Molecules range in size from quite small (an H_2 molecule) to extremely large. A single DNA molecule may be several inches long.

Right: This illustration shows two atoms of hydrogen, oxygen and nitrogen on the left. To the right of the arrows is a molecule of each element. The atoms have been linked by covalent bonds to form a molecule of each element.

Top: Hydrogen

Center: Oxygen

Bottom: Nitrogen

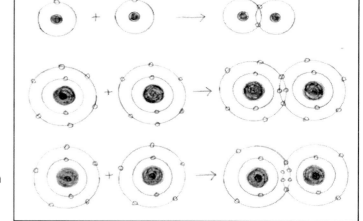

A *compound* is a molecule that is composed of atoms of at least two different elements. Thus sodium chloride and DNA are compounds, but O_2 and H_2 are not.

The *atomic weight* of an element is standard and can be obtained from the periodic table. It represents an average of the number of protons plus neutrons in the nucleus of all the existing atoms of an element, which includes the isotopes of that element. The *molecular weight* of a molecule is simply the sum of the atomic weights of all of the atoms in that molecule. The molecular formula expresses those atoms. For example, the molecular formula for glucose is C6H12O6. That means that there are six atoms of carbon, twelve atoms of hydrogen and six atoms of oxygen in one glucose molecule. We learn from the periodic table that carbon has an atomic weight of about 12; hydrogen has an atomic weight of about one, and oxygen has an atomic weight of about sixteen. The molecular weight of glucose is calculated as follows:

(6x12) + (12x1) + (6x16), or 72 + 12 + 96 = **180.**

A **_mole_** is the molecular weight of a molecule expressed in grams. Thus for glucose, one mole would be 180 grams. A **_one molar solution_** (**_1 M_**) is the molecular weight of a molecule in grams dissolved in one liter of water. Thus 180 grams of glucose would equal a **_one molar solution_** when dissolved in one liter of water, and 90 grams of glucose dissolved in one liter of water would equal a 0.5 Molar (0.5 M) solution.

Because scientific measurements are done according to the metric system, you must learn this system. This means being able to convert ounces and pounds to and from grams and kilograms; inches and feet to and from meters, centimeters and millimeters; liquid ounces and quarts to and from milliliters (cubic centimeters) and liters; and Fahrenheit to and from Centigrade (Celsius). The prefix **_deci-_** means one tenth; **_centi-_** means one hundredth; **_milli-_** means one thousandth; **_micro-_** means one millionth; and **_nano-_** means one billionth. The prefix **_kilo-_** means a thousand times, so one kilogram equals 1000 grams and one kilometer equals 1000 meters. One milligram equals 0.001 gram.

Listed below are useful conversion figures to commit to memory.
1 ounce equals approximately 28.4 grams;
1 fluidounce equals approximately 29.6 ml;
1 pound equals 0.45 kg, and 1 kg equals 2.2 pounds;
1 inch equals 2.54 cm, and 1 cm equals 0.394 in;
1 quart equals 0.946 liter, and 1 liter equals 1.057 qt
(Degrees Fahrenheit -32) x 5/9 = degrees C   (You MUST subtract before multiplying.)
(Degrees Centigrade x 9/5) +32 = degrees F   (You MUST multiply before adding.)

Glucose   Galactose   Fructose

Above: An **_isomer_** is a compound with an identical number of the same kind of atoms as the original, but with a different structure. In other words, the same atoms are put together in a different way. For example, glucose, galactose and fructose are isomers because they share the same molecular formula, C6H12O6. But they are different because those atoms are linked differently to create a different structure. Glucose is the primary sugar that is metabolized by your body. You can easily convert fructose and galactose to glucose. Glucose and fructose are in most foods. Galactose is found only in milk and dairy products.

When the atoms of elements like sodium and chlorine are placed in water, they dissolve.   Sodium (Na) has one electron in its outer ring, which it readily gives up in solution. It becomes **_ionized_** and forms a sodium ion (Na+). Chlorine has seven electrons in its outer ring; it readily accepts any electrons that are in solution and also becomes ionized. The ionized form of sodium lacks an electron; therefore, it lacks the negative charge that was the lost electron. Sodium ions, therefore, bear a positive charge and are **_cations_**. In contrast ions of chlorine have gained an electron, bear a negative charge and are **_anions._**   **_Electrolytes_** are ions such as Na+ and Cl- that are able to conduct an electric current. Salts are derivatives of acids where the acidic hydrogen atom has been replaced by a metallic ion such as sodium. Thus sodium chloride (NaCl) is a derivative of hydrochloric acid (HCl). The names of salts often end in –ate, -ite, or ide. When an acid and a salt of that acid are placed in solution and ionize, the anions are identical. For example:

$$H_2CO_3 \quad \rightarrow \quad H+ \; + \; HCO_3-$$
Carbonic acid   Bicarbonate ion

$$NaHCO_3 \quad \rightarrow \quad Na+ \; + \; HCO_3-$$
Sodium bicarbonate   Bicarbonate ion

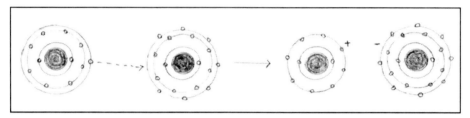

Sodium atom   Chlorine atom   Sodium ion   Chlorine ion

Sodium chloride exists as a molecule when not in solution. When placed in water, sodium chloride dissolves and ionizes. The ions separate; sodium loses an electron and develops a positive charge; chlorine gains an electron and develops a negative charge.

Isotopes of most of the lighter elements are rare or uncommon. Isotopes of the heavier elements are often unstable and are called ***radioactive isotopes*** because they gradually give off neutrons, electrons, protons and/or smaller particles in what is termed radioactive decay. This transforms them either into the common form of the element, another isotope of that element, or (if one or more protons are given off) into another element altogether with a smaller atomic number. The particles given off in radioactive decay include (1) neutrons, (2) protons (hydrogen nuclei), (3) helium nuclei or ***alpha particles*** (two protons and two neutrons), (4) electrons or ***beta particles***, and (5) ***gamma rays*** or x-rays. The larger radioactive particles such as alpha particles cannot penetrate the skin, and beta particles penetrate only a few millimeters. However, gamma rays with short wavelengths are highly energetic and can easily go through your entire body. Such radiation is dangerous because it produces ***free radicals.***

Free radicals are highly reactive charged molecules that have lost or gained one or more electrons due to exposure to such things as radioactivity, ultraviolet light, or some chemicals. Like ions they have an unequal number of electrons and protons. Unlike ions, however, free radicals are harmful. They can cause cancer and are a cause of aging because they trigger reactions in your body that destroy necessary molecules by converting them into free radicals. Free radicals can be controlled by vitamins A, C and E, the element selenium, and other substances that act as ***antioxidants***. Antioxidants are substances that readily accept or give up electrons as the situation dictates, and they are capable of stopping the chain of molecular destruction.

Exposure to radiation is measured in units called ***Sieverts.*** The average American receives about 3.6 millisieverts (mSv) in background radiation per year and about 0.6 mSv from diagnostic health sources and consumer products such as smoke detectors. A dose of five Sieverts (5000 mSv) or more is usually fatal.

Atoms in proximity may form a molecular bond by ***sharing*** one or more pairs of electrons. The result is a strong ***covalent bond.***

When the atoms of sodium chloride and other salts are separated in solution, they become cations and anions. An attraction between them continues to exist when they are in solution because of the attraction between negative and positive charges. This bond between a cation and an anion is a relatively weak ***ionic bond.***

The third type of chemical bond is the ***hydrogen bond.***   Although it is the weakest of the types of bonds, hydrogen bonds are physiologically important because they give structure to proteins and DNA. A ***hydrogen bond*** is the result of a ***polar covalent bond*** where a polar molecule like water (H_2O) has one atom that has a slight negative charge (oxygen), and one atom that has a slight positive charge (hydrogen). This results from a difference in the ability of the nuclei of oxygen and hydrogen to attract electrons. The larger oxygen nucleus exerts more attraction to electrons than does the small nucleus of the hydrogen atom. The result is a small negative charge around the oxygen atom and a small positive charge around the hydrogen atoms. This gives water molecules *polarity*. Water molecules are attracted to each other by this polarity, the oxygen atom of one water molecule being mutually attracted to hydrogen atoms of other water molecules. Polarity gives water molecules adhesive and cohesive properties, which give water its surface tension or "wetness." In contrast a *nonpolar* covalent bond is one in which there is equal affinity for the electrons being shared. The carbon-to-carbon covalent bonds of oils and other lipids are typically nonpolar. The polarity of a substance is a prime determinate of that substance's solubility in water. Polar compounds are generally soluble in water; nonpolar compounds are not.

Most covalent bonds are single, meaning that one pair of electrons is shared between two atoms, but they can be also double, in which two pairs of electrons are shared. This can occur only between atoms having a valence of two or greater. All of the essential fatty acids (arachidonic, linoleic and linolenic acids), have double carbon-to-carbon bonds. A triple covalent bond can also occur between atoms having a valence of three or greater. An example is cyanide, CN-.

Metabolism is all the chemical reactions of the body. If a metabolic reaction involves breaking apart molecules, it is called a *catabolic* reaction. If a metabolic reaction involves building up molecules, it is called an *anabolic* reaction. Catabolic reactions give off energy and are called *exergonic*; anabolic reactions require energy input and are called *endergonic.*

Chemical reactions may be classed into *decomposition reactions*, wherein a molecule is broken apart and energy is released; *synthesis reactions,* wherein a molecule is put together and energy is required; and *exchange reactions,* wherein one part of one molecule, called a *moiety,* is exchanged for a different moiety from another molecule. Decomposition reactions usually involve the addition of water, and they are called *hydrolysis* reactions. Synthesis reactions typically involve the removal of a water molecule, and they are called *dehydration synthesis* reactions.

Reacting molecules must make contact with each other in order for a chemical reaction to take place. This can happen only in a fluid medium such as a liquid or gas. When molecules or atoms are in a liquid or gaseous medium, they are constantly in motion, and therefore, they can collide and react. This is called the *collision theory. This theory does not apply to solids.* The movement of molecules in a liquid can be demonstrated by microscopically visualizing small particles under the high power of a microscope. The molecules are too small to be seen, but the particles exhibit a jiggling movement that is due to the collision of moving molecules with the particles. This movement is called *Brownian movement.*

The *rate* of a chemical reaction depends on several things. (1) The higher the *temperature,* the faster the rate because the molecules move faster and collide more often; (2) the higher the *concentration* of the reactants the faster the rate; and (3) the presence of a *catalyst* will speed up the rate. A catalyst is a nonreacting substance, which has the effect of speeding up a reaction, often by physically bringing the reactants together. The primary catalysts of the body are proteins called *enzymes.*

A *solution* consists of a liquid called the *solvent* and dissolved substances called *solutes*. In living situations the solvent is *water.* A solution is usually transparent and does not separate on standing. The solutes are small particles, less than 1 nanometer (nm) in diameter, and they pass through most membranes of the body.

A *colloid* may exist as a liquid or a gel. It is usually cloudy and will not pass through most membranes, but it does not separate on standing. The particles of a colloid are from 1-100 nm in size. Albumin is the main protein in blood where it exists in a colloid state.

A *suspension* is cloudy to opaque. The particles in a suspension are over 100 nm in size and will not pass through membranes. Suspensions separate on standing.

An *emulsion* is a suspension of tiny droplets of one liquid in another. Examples are many salad dressings, mayonnaise and the fat in homogenized whole milk.

Solutions, colloids, suspensions and emulsions may exist concomitantly. For example, in milk the fat is in emulsion, the protein is in a colloid state, and the calcium is in solution. The homogenization of milk entails the application of heat and pressure to break up fat globules. The small globules of fat then go into emulsion.

The basis of all bodily fluids is **_water,_** which constitutes between 50% and 75% of your weight. Because of the presence of so much water, H2O is the most common molecule in your body; hydrogen is the most common element in your body, and oxygen is the element with the largest amount of weight in your body. The properties of water determine how your body functions. These properties include its **_polarity_**, which in turn determines what substances are soluble in water. Substances that are soluble in water are called **_hydrophilic._** Most substances in the body are hydrophilic including sugars and salts. Substances that do not dissolve in water are called **_hydrophobic_**. Lipids (fats) are hydrophobic because they are not soluble in water or other polar solvents. They are also called **_lipophilic_** because they are soluble in oils and other nonpolar organic solvents.

Right: The upper figure is a non polar bond, as exhibited by a carbon to carbon bond. The nuclei of the atoms have an equal ability to attract protons. The bottom figure is a polar bond, as exhibited by water. The larger oxygen nucleus has a greater ability to attract electrons than the hydrogen nucleus.

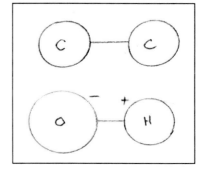

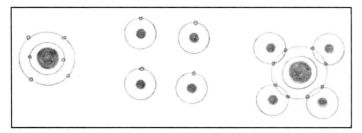

Left: A carbon atom + four hydrogen atoms make up methane. Methane is a non-polar molecule.

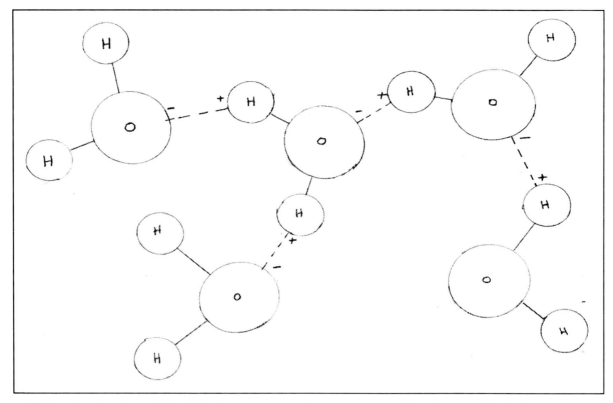

Above: Water showing its polarity. The larger oxygen atoms have a negative charge. The hydrogen atoms have a positive charge.

Water is thermally stable, meaning that it takes an inordinate amount of energy to raise or lower its temperature. This helps to control of your body's temperature at a constant level. The high heat capacity of water helps to retain the body's heat, and it also effectively removes heat when it evaporates from the skin. **It takes one calorie of energy to raise the temperature of one gram of water one degree Centigrade.** A few molecules of water in a sample will fully ionize producing hydrogen (H+) and hydroxyl (OH-) ions, which are then free to react with other substances. One thousand calories equals one Calorie (capitalized), which is a unit of energy in food.

Many of the chemical reactions of the body, especially those involving the production of energy, are **oxidation-reduction or REDOX reactions. When a molecule has lost electrons it has been oxidized.** The oxygen atom is effective in attracting electrons from the atoms of many elements, and oxidation may involve the addition of oxygen, but not necessarily. Oxidation in the body often involves the loss of a hydrogen nucleus in addition to its electron. When one molecule is oxidized in a reaction, another molecule **must necessarily be reduced**. The oxidized molecule **loses electrons, and it loses energy.** The reduced molecule **gains electrons, and it gains energy**. Niels Bohr was the first to hypothesize that it is the movement of electrons that determines the gain or loss of energy by a substance. In redox reactions electrons are transferred from one substance to another. One reactant gives up electrons and is oxidized; the other reactant gains electrons and is reduced. The reactant that loses electrons has been oxidized and is called a **reducing agent.** The reactant that gains electrons has been reduced and is called an **oxidizing agent.**

A solution is judged to be acidic or basic depending on the concentration of hydrogen ions (H+) in the solution. **A hydrogen ion is the same thing as a proton**. An **acid** is any molecule that tends to lose a hydrogen ion when placed in solution. A **base** is any molecule that tends to accept hydrogen ions (protons) and remove them from solution. A strong acid will ionize nearly completely and release a great many hydrogen ions. A weak acid ionizes to a much lesser extent and releases only a few hydrogen ions. A strong base avidly accepts hydrogen ions and pulls them out of solution. A weak base takes up hydrogen ions much less avidly.

The concentration of hydrogen ions in a solution is measured in **pH units**. The pH scale expresses the **concentration of the hydrogen ions in solution in the negative logarithm format.** Thus the lower on the pH scale you go, the more hydrogen ions are in solution and the more acidic the solution is. The higher on the pH scale you go, the fewer hydrogen ions are in solution, and the more basic the solution. In pure water one in 10 million molecules of water is ionized. This results in a concentration of 0.0000001 Molar or 1×10^{-7}. The negative logarithm of 10^{-7} is seven, and seven is neutral on the pH scale. The pH scale extends from 0 to 14; zero being a situation where the entire liquid mass is a strong acid that is fully ionized to hydrogen ions (protons). A pH of fourteen would exist if the concentration of protons were one in one hundred trillion, which is essentially zero. Because the scale is exponential, each integer is ten times more or less acidic than the next.

The **pH** of your blood must stay within a narrow range around 7.4. The body manages strict control over the pH of its fluids by the use of **buffers.** Buffers are weak acids and weak bases. Strong acids such as hydrochloric acid (HCl) and sulfuric acid (H2SO4) ionize almost completely releasing a large number of hydrogen ions into solution. A weak acid ionizes only slightly, which keeps many hydrogen ions tied up and out of solution. Strong bases such as sodium hydroxide (NaOH) or ammonia (NH3) have a strong tendency to bind hydrogen ions and remove them from solution. Weak bases do not exert as strong an affinity for hydrogen ions; consequently their ability to remove hydrogen ions from the solution and raise the pH is limited. An **alkaline** substance is synonymous with a base. When a solution contains buffers (weak acids and weak bases), the result is **stabilization** of the pH around 7, which is neutral.

Organic chemistry is the study of compounds of **carbon**. Carbon is unique in that it has the ability to form chains and ringed compounds that are the chemical backbone of all life as we know it. If extraterrestrial life is ever identified, it will probably be based on carbon. It has been postulated that silicon, which, like carbon, has a valence of four, would be the only possible substitute for carbon in life forms.

Organic compounds are derived from living matter, and they contain hydrogen as well as carbon. Organic molecules in chains are called **aliphatic** compounds. Organic molecules that contain one or more rings are called **aromatic** compounds.

Some organic molecules are extremely large and complicated. A **_polymer_** is a large molecule made up of identical subunits called **_monomers._** Examples are starch and cellulose, both of which are huge polymers that are made up of glucose monomers. The process of making a polymer involves **_dehydration synthesis_**, in which water is removed and monomers are linked to form a polymer.   The opposite of dehydration synthesis is **_hydrolysis,_** which is a decomposition reaction involving the addition of water to a polymer. Hydrolysis refers to the break-up of a polymer into smaller units by the breakage of the covalent bond between two monomers. Digestion consists of hydrolysis reactions.

The major organic molecules in your body and all living things are **_carbohydrates, lipids (fats), proteins, and nucleic acids._** **_Carbohydrates_** are sugars and starches. Sugars have ring structures with either five or six carbon atoms. The names of most sugars end in -ose. The sub words glycol-, glycans, and saccharide refer to carbohydrates. **_Monosaccharides_** are simple sugars.   Some examples are glucose, fructose, ribose, and galactose.   **_Starches are polysaccharides,_** which are polymers of a simple sugar, usually glucose.   A disaccharide has two sugar monomers. Sucrose (glucose + fructose) and lactose (glucose + galactose) are disaccharides. Domino sugar is sucrose; lactose is milk sugar. Glycogen is animal starch, which is a glucose polymer. Pectins and amylopectins are plant starches that form gels in the intestines and are designated as soluble fibers in the diet. Cellulose is a plant polysaccharide that is a polymer of glucose, but cellulose is not digestible by man, and it is designated as insoluble fiber in the diet. Termites and bacteria in the stomachs of cattle and other ruminants are capable of breaking down cellulose into glucose. Cellulose differs from starch by having alternate glucose monomers upside down. Most of the animal kingdom lacks the enzymes necessary to break bonds between the monomers of cellulose.

Carbohydrates can link with proteins to produce **_glycoproteins_** and **_proteoglycans,_** and they can link with lipids to produce **_glycolipids and liposaccharides_**. The **_dominant part of these molecules is given last_**. (In a glycoprotein, the protein moiety is larger than the carbohydrate moiety; in a proteoglycans the carbohydrate moiety is the larger.)

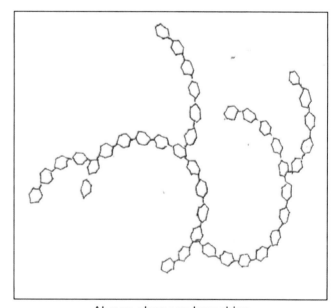

Above: "A" is glycogen; "B" is cellulose.   Above: glycogen branching

Fats and oils are known as **_lipids;_** they include fatty acids, triglycerides and cholesterol. Lipids are lipophilic and hydrophobic, which means they are soluble in nonpolar solvents such as oils, but they are insoluble in polar solvents like water. Three fatty acids are essential for human life and must be in the diet. They are **_arachidonic acid, linoleic acid and linolenic acid._** All three consist of a long chain of 18 or 20 carbon atoms, and each contains double carbon to carbon bonds. A saturated fatty acid contains only single carbon bonds (it is saturated with hydrogen). A fatty acid is "unsaturated" when it contains one or more double carbon-to-carbon bonds. Nearly all fatty acids in nature contain an even number of carbon atoms because fatty acids are synthesized from acetate, which has two carbon atoms. A **_triglyceride_** is a molecule that contains three fatty acids linked to a **_glycerol_** molecule (C3H5(OH)3). Triglycerides are called "neutral fats" because the acidic portion of the fatty acid (the carboxyl group or COOH) has been neutralized in the synthesis to a triglyceride. Lecithins and cephalins are combinations of glycerol, fatty acids and phosphate linked to another moiety. These compounds are called **_phospholipids._** Whereas other fats are hydrophobic, phospholipids are **_amphiphilic,_** meaning that part of the molecule (the fatty acids) is hydrophobic, and part of the molecule (the phosphate moiety) is hydrophilic. Therefore, phospholipids and other amphiphilic compounds are soluble in both water and oils. **_Cholesterol_** is a lipid that is produced by animals but not by plants. However, plants produce sterols, which have the same basic complicated four ring structure as cholesterol.

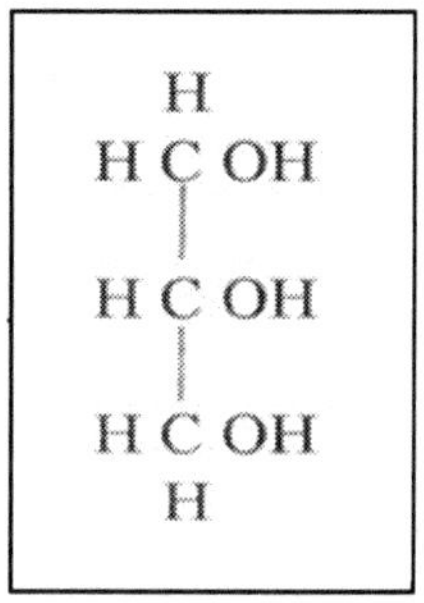

Right: A

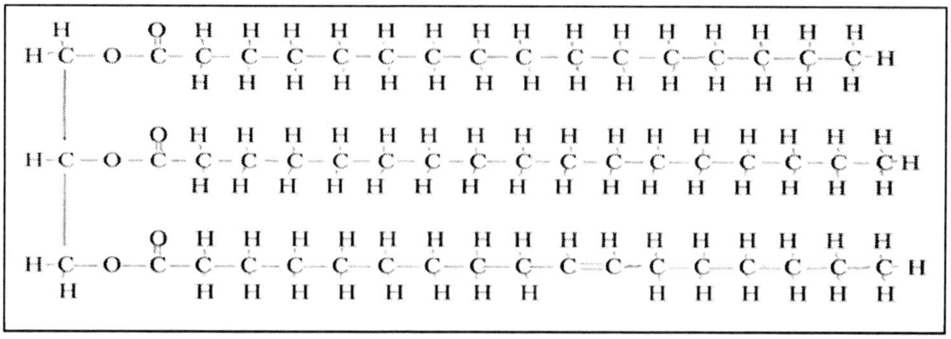

Above: Glycerol

Right: "A" is the structure for cholesterol.
"B" is the structure for testosterone.

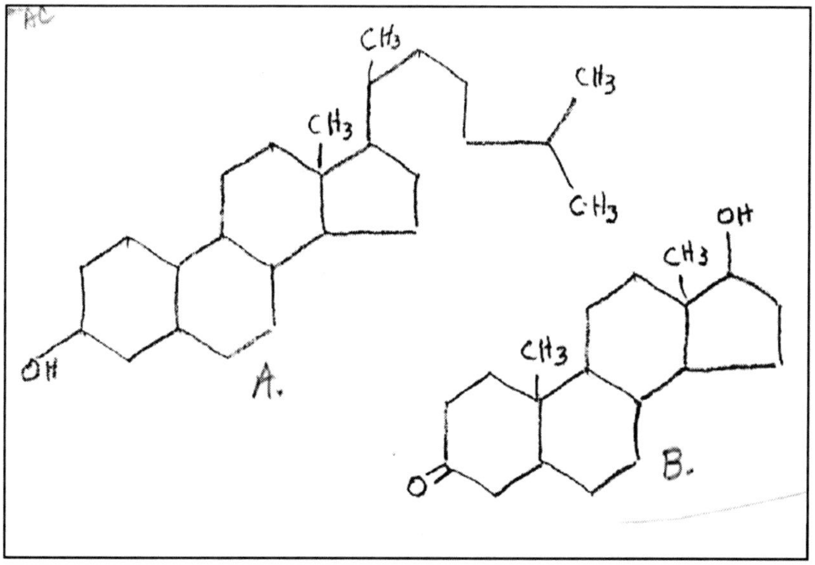

Proteins have many functions including acting as enzymes and hormones. **_Amino acids_** are the building blocks for proteins, and the body uses twenty different amino acids in protein production. All twenty amino acids and consequently all proteins contain **_nitrogen, oxygen, hydrogen and carbon_**. Three amino acids contain **_sulfur._** Eight of the amino acids are called "essential," meaning that they cannot be synthesized and must be present in the diet. The essential amino acids are leucine, valine, isoleucine, methionine, glycine, threonine, phenylalanine, and tryptophan. Your body can synthesize the other twelve amino acids from the eight essential ones. All amino acids contain an **_amino group (-NH2)_** at one end and a **_carboxyl group (-COOH)_** at the other end. Amino acids are linked by a **_peptide bond,_** which links the amino group of one amino acid to the carboxyl group of another in a dehydration synthesis reaction. This forms a **_peptide._** A small peptide containing ten to fifteen amino acids is called an **_oligopeptide._** A peptide becomes a **_polypeptide_** when multiple amino acids have been linked. A polypeptide becomes a protein when it has grown to be a large molecule, and it has been molded into a specific shape. The final shape the protein assumes is determined by several factors including **_(1) the amino acid sequence, (2) disulfide bonds between distant amino acids, and (3) hydrogen bonds._**

25

```
            Carboxyl
             group      Amino                                       Peptide
            (acidic)    group                                        bond
               ↓        (basic)
               O          ↓          O  Dehydration synthesis        O ↓           OH
    H    H   //       H   "R2"  //   ----------------------→   H   H  II ↓   "R2"   /
      N --- C --C  +    N -- C -- C                             N -- C -- C -- N -- C -- C   +   H2O
    H    "R"  \       H    H   \        ←---------------------  H   "R"      H   H   \\
               OH              OH    Hydrolysis                                       O

       Amino acid        Amino acid                                  dipeptide           water
```

Above: Peptides are synthesized by the process of dehydration synthesis. Peptides are broken down by hydrolysis. "R" and "R2" stand for different "radicals," moieties that are different in each amino acid.

Enzymes are proteins that serve as catalysts for chemical reactions. The names of newly discovered enzymes end in **-ase**. In order to catalyze a reaction, enzymes frequently require the presence of a **coenzyme**, which is a nonprotein that often acts to transfer electrons in a redox reaction. Examples of coenzymes include some B vitamins and ions of the metallic elements, iron, magnesium, copper, and zinc.

Nucleotides provide our genetic structure and store energy. **Nucleic Acids** are polymers of nucleotides. A nucleotide consists of a sugar (ribose or deoxyribose), a phosphate moiety, and a nitrogenous (nitrogen containing) base. The nitrogenous bases are either **purines,** which are structures with two rings, or **pyrimidines,** which have only one ring. Nucleotides in **DNA (deoxyribonucleic acid)** provide the basis for our genetic heritage. Nucleotides in **RNA (ribonucleic acid)** are responsible for the amino acid sequence in proteins. **ATP (adenosine triphosphate)** is a nucleotide that is responsible for energy storage. **Adenine and guanine** are the two purines in nucleic acids. Adenine linked to the sugar, ribose, is called **adenosine,** and guanine linked to ribose becomes **guanosine**. The pyrimidines in DNA are **thymine and cytosine**. The pyrimidines in RNA are **uracil and cytosine**. ATP contains three phosphate groups in addition to adenine and ribose.

```
                              HOC-------COH
                                 /    H  \
                                /         \
       C        N------------------------CH
      // \  / \\                  \         \
     N    C    CH                  \         \              O      O      O
     |    ||                        \         \             II  ↓  II  ↓  II
     HC   C                          O---------C-CH2 -O-P-O~~~P-O~~~P-O-
      \\  / \ /                               H        O  ↑ O  ↑ O
       C    N                                          H     H     H
       |                            Ribose
       NH2
                                       Triphosphate
       Adenine           (The arrows designate high energy phosphate bonds.)
```

Above: The structure of ATP, (adenosine triphosphate), a nucleotide. A nucleotide consists of a nitrogenous base that is a purine or a pyrimidine, a sugar and one or more phosphate groups. In ATP adenine is the purine and ribose is the sugar. Adenosine is adenine plus ribose. ATP stores energy in the form of high energy phosphate bonds.

Many organic compounds are named according to the number of carbon atoms they contain. A list of names that correspond to the number of carbon atoms in a compound follows:

Methyl- is used when the compound contains one carbon atom. Examples are methanol and methane. **Form-** is also used for one-carbon compounds. An example is formaldehyde.

Ethyl- and **acetyl-** are used for two carbon compounds. Examples are ethanol and acetic acid.

Propyl- is used for three-carbon compounds. An example is propane.

Butyl- is used for four-carbon compounds.

Penta- is used for five-carbon compounds.

Hexa- is used for six-carbon compounds.

Hepta- is used for seven-carbon compounds.

Octa- is used for eight-carbon compounds. Octane is an example.

The structure of some of the major chemical bonds and substances in our bodies are diagrammed below.

A hydroxyl group:

OH-

An organic acid (a carboxyl group): Carboxyl groups are acidic because the hydrogen atom may be ionized into solution.

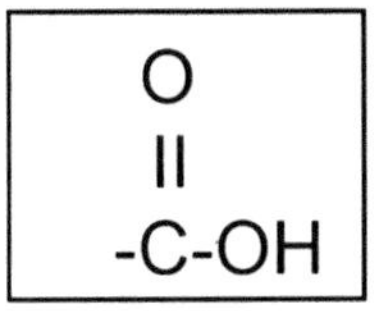

$$O$$
$$\|$$
$$-C-OH$$

An amino group: Amino groups are basic because they attract hydrogen ions.

-NH2

An amino acid:

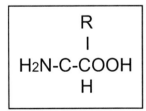

The "R" stands for radical. Each amino acid has a different radical moiety.

A peptide bond:

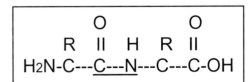

"R" stands for radical, a moiety that is different in each amino acid. Peptide bonds link amino acids. (The underlined portion is the peptide bond.)

A monosaccharide:

Monosaccharides are simple sugars.
They are ring compounds that contain
either five or six carbon atoms. The
names of sugars typically end in –ose.

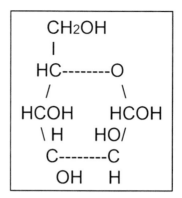

```
        CH₂OH
         |
        HC--------O
        /          \
     HCOH         HCOH
       \ H      HO/
        C--------C
        OH      H
```

An alcohol:

```
    H
   -C-OH
```

The names for alcohols typically end in –ol.

An aldehyde:

```
    H
   -C=O
```

A ketone:

```
     O
     ||
   -C-C-C-
```

The names for ketones often end in –one.

An ester bond:

```
 -C-O-C-
```

A polyester compound consists of moieties linked by ester bonds.

A methyl group:

```
    H
   HC-
    H
```

An ethyl or acetyl group:

```
   H  H
  -C--C-
   H  H
```

Study Guide

1. Organic chemistry is the study of the compounds of which element?
2. Know the definition of *matter, energy, atom, element, molecule and compound,* and know how they exist in nature.
3. Understand atomic structure, protons, electrons, neutrons, electron shells, atomic mass, atomic weight and valence.
4. Be able to define an isotope and an isomer.
5. Be able to calculate the molecular weight of a molecule, and understand the term "mole" (gram molecular weight) and how it relates to the molarity of a solution.
6. Be able to convert measurements of length, weight, volume and temperature between the American system and the metric system.
7. Know what is meant by radioactive isotope and what makes up an alpha, beta and gamma particle.
8. Know the meaning of the terms ion, anion, cation and free radical.
9. Review redox reactions, and understand the terms oxidation, reduction, redox, oxidizing agent, reducing agent, antioxidant, electron donor and electron acceptor.
10. Know what is meant by a Sievert.
11. Know the three types of molecular bonds (covalent, ionic and hydrogen), the relative strength of each, and how each is formed.
12. Be able to discern a polar covalent bond and a nonpolar covalent bond.
13. Know the meanings of the terms *moiety, decomposition reaction, hydrolysis, dehydration synthesis reaction, exchange reaction, metabolism, anabolism and catabolism.*
14. Know the things that can alter the rate of a chemical reaction (concentration, temperature, catalyst).
15. Know how to define a solution, a suspension, a colloid and an emulsion.
16. What is the most abundant molecule in the body according to weight and number of molecules?
17. What is the most abundant atom in the body according to weight?
18. What is the most abundant atom in the body according to the number of molecules?
19. Recognize the elements that have a function in human metabolism and which do not.
20. Understand the terms *hydrophobic, lipophobic, hydrophilic and lipophilic.*
21. Know and understand the following terms: acid, base, buffer and pH.
22. Be able to identify a carbohydrate, a lipid (fat), a protein and a nucleic acid.
23. Understand terms that are related to fats and fatty acids including *triglycerides, glycerol, cholesterol, phospholipids, saturated fatty acids, unsaturated fatty acids and essential fatty acids.*
24. Understand the makeup of a nucleic acid.
25. Know the structure of a peptide bond. Know the four elements that are in all amino acids (C,O,H and N), and know the common structure of all amino acids.
26. Know the difference between a peptide, an oligopeptide, a polypeptide and a protein.
27. Be able to recognize various chemical bonds including those of an ester, alcohol, aldehyde, ketone, carboxyl, hydroxyl, and amino group.
28. Know what makes up a sugar, a disaccharide, a polysaccharide and a starch.
29. Be able to recognize a peptide bond.

Chapter Three

The Cell

Your body is made up of cells. Life began on earth as one-cell creatures. Each organism had to be able to carry out all the essentials of life such as ingestion, digestion, excretion, movement, respiration and reproduction. Cells began to specialize when multicellular organisms came into existence. Bone cells established structure; muscle cells provided movement; sensory cells informed of the environment, and so on.

In 1663 Robert Hooke became the first man to observe cells with a primitive microscope. Two centuries later Theodor Schwann concluded that ___all living organisms were composed of cells.___ Through the work of Louis Pasteur and others it has become apparent that all physiological processes of the body are based on cellular activity. From these observations it can be stated that: 1. All organisms are composed of cells and cellular products. 2. The cell is the simplest structural and functional unit of life. 3. An organism's structure and all of its functions are ultimately due to the activities of its cells. 4. Cells come only from preexisting cells and not from non-living matter. 5. The cells of all species have many fundamental similarities in their chemical composition and metabolic mechanisms, which indicates that cells of all species come from a common ancestry.

The **_fluids_** of the body are all based on water. They may be divided into those fluids **_inside_** the cell, which are **_intracellular fluids_**, and those fluids **_outside_** the cell, which are **_extracellular fluids_**. **_Interstitial fluid_** is that part of the extracellular fluid that is located in the tissues between cells. Extracellular fluid within blood vessels is called **_intravascular fluid_**.

Right: Cell shapes
A. stellate (a neuron)
B. squamous
C. cuboidal
D. columnar
E. fusiform
F. discoid
G. spherical
H. fibrous

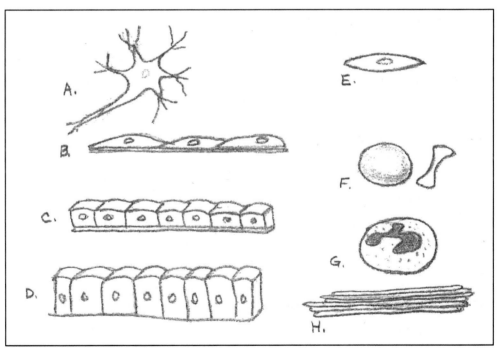

Cells of the body come in all shapes and sizes.
Squamous cells are thin and flat; skin cells are squamous.
Cuboidal cells are square; some cells in the kidneys, testes and intestines are cuboidal.
Polygonal cells have multiple sides; polygonal cells are seen in the lining of the urinary bladder, and they are often located in the middle of a multilayered structure.
Columnar cells are significantly taller than they are wide; some cells in the respiratory tract and the urinary tract are columnar.
Spherical and **_ovoid_** cells have a rounded contour; the ovum (egg cell) is round.
Discoid cells are disc-shaped; red blood cells are discoid.

Fusiform cells are thick in the middle and tapered at the ends; smooth muscle cells are fusiform.
Fibrous cells are threadlike in shape; striated muscle cells are fibrous shaped.
Stellate cells are star-shaped with numerous pointy spikes. Neurons are stellate.

Egg cells (ova) are 100 microns in diameter, and they are visible to the naked eye. (A micron is a micrometer, which is one thousandth of a millimeter.) But most cells are 10-15 microns in diameter. Some nerve cells have an extension (axon) that is over three feet long, stretching from the spinal cord to the feet.

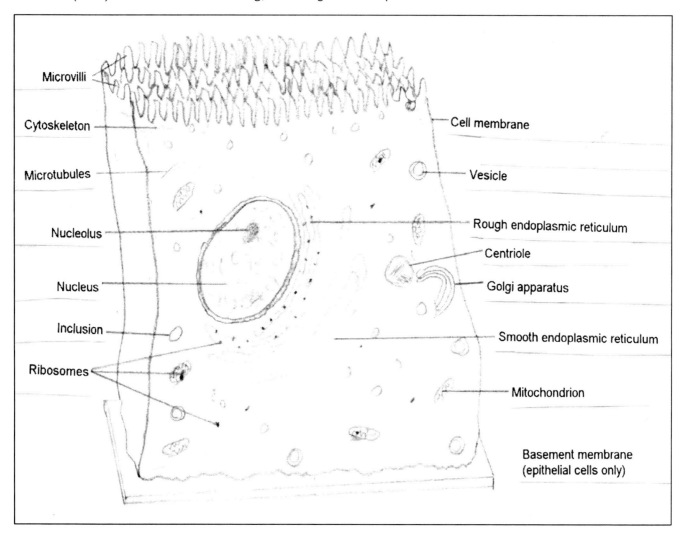

Above: This is a drawing of a cuboidal cell of the intestinal epithelium. The various organelles are identified in the drawing.

Cells are surrounded by a **_plasma membrane_** (or cell membrane), which controls what enters and leaves the cell. The inside of the cell is divided into the **_nucleus_**, which contains the genetic material of the cell, and the **_cytoplasm_**, which contains the fluid and structures of the cell not located in the nucleus.

Genetic material in the nucleus is in the form of **_chromosomes_**, which, except when the cell is dividing, are in the form of **_chromatin_**. Chromatin consists of fine, lacy strands of DNA (deoxyribonucleic acid). The envelope of the nucleus is called the **_nuclear membrane_**, which is a **_two layered_** membrane composed largely of **_phospholipids_**. The nuclear membrane has pores which allow for materials to enter and leave the nucleus. Inside the nucleus is a small, dark body called the **_nucleolus_**, which is the site for the synthesis of ribosomes. Most ribosomes leave the nucleus and enter the cytoplasm where they direct protein synthesis.

The liquid portion of the cytoplasm is the **_cytosol._** The cytosol contains suspended proteins and dissolved amino acids, carbohydrates and other molecules. The cytoplasm contains a high level of potassium (K+) ions and a low level of sodium (Na+) ions. The concentrations of K+ and Na+ are reversed in the extracellular fluid.

Cells may be classified as **_somatic cells or germ cells._** Somatic cells are all of the cells of your body except the eggs and sperm, which are called **_germ cells or gametes._** Somatic cells reproduce by **_mitosis_** and have the full **_diploid_** complement number of 46 (23 pair) chromosomes. Each germ cell has only 23 unpaired chromosomes, which is the **_haploid_** number of chromosomes. Germ cells are produced by a process known as **_meiosis._**

Microvilli are tiny finger-like extensions of the plasma membrane that serve to increase the surface area of the cell. They enhance absorption in the gastro-intestinal (GI) tract and in the tubules of the kidneys. When they are numerous they form a **_brush border_**, which resembles the surface of a brush. Microvilli are also present in the cochlea of the ear and in taste buds. Some microvilli are attached to **_actin_** fibers in the cell. Actin is one of the motor (contractile) proteins, and it can contract and "milk" the microvilli, thereby increasing cellular absorption.

Cilia (singular, cilium) are hair-like processes extending from the cell. Most cilia can move back and forth because they are connected to a contractile protein in the cell named **_dynein_**, which moves them back and forth. In most areas where cilia are present they act together to beat in waves, thereby moving extracellular material on the surface of the cell in one direction. They are present in the respiratory tract and fallopian tubes. Mucus in the respiratory tract is propelled to the mouth by the beating of cilia. The mucus "floats" on a layer of salt water that is secreted by the cell. Without the saline layer the cilia cannot do their job. In the genetic disorder, cystic fibrosis (also known as mucoviscidosis), the secretion of chloride is faulty, and mucus builds up in the respiratory tract causing frequent bouts of pneumonia. In this disease mucus also builds up in glands such as the pancreas, which rely on cilia to propel their secretions. Blockage of the pancreatic duct can result in poor absorption, malnutrition and pancreatitis. Cilia in the eye, ear and olfactory (smelling) apparatus are nonmotile and serve a sensory function.

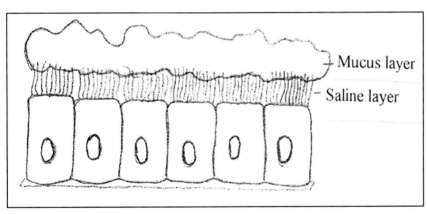

Above: Ciliated epithelium. Cilia are the thread-like
extensions into the saline layer.

Right: A spermatozoon.
The flagellum is the tail.

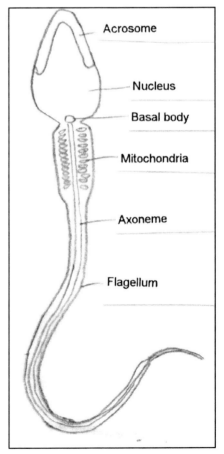

The Cell   Chapter Three

Flagella are long whip-like structures extending from the cell. In the cell they are connected to ***dynein,*** the same motor (contractile) protein that propels cilia. Flagella provide motility. The only flagellum in the human body is the tail of sperm cells.

The various cells of the body are held together by three types of ***intercellular junctions.***
(1) ***Tight junctions*** are zipper-like attachments between cells. They completely surround the cell and hold it tightly to its neighbor; they are functionally leak-proof. They are found in the GI tract, where they restrict the entrance of undigested material into the body. They are also found in the capillaries of the brain, where they restrict the diffusion of materials into the brain. This is called the ***blood-brain barrier.***
(2). ***Gap junctions*** are channels between cells that allow the passage of material directly from one cell to another without having to go through the plasma membranes. ***Intercalated discs*** are gap junctions in cardiac muscle that allow for quick passage of electrical impulses. Pores called ***canaliculi*** are gap junctions in compact bone that allow the diffusion of nutrients and wastes between bone cells.
(3). ***Desmosomes*** are like a rivet or a spot-weld that holds cells together. The structure of a desmosome is a like a tiny piece of Velcro. A desmosome is a connection between two cells. A connection between a cell and an underlying membrane is called a ***hemidesmosome.*** Desmosomes are present in the epidermis of the skin, cardiac muscle and cervix of the uterus. Hemidesmosomes serve to hold the outer layer of the cornea of the eye (the epithelial layer) to the underlying membrane (Bowman's membrane). A corneal abrasion rips hemidesmosomes apart and tears away the epithelium. Although the epithelial cells quickly spread out to cover the defect, the hemidesmosomes are slow to recover, and the eye may remain sensitive and subject to repeated abrasions for months or years.

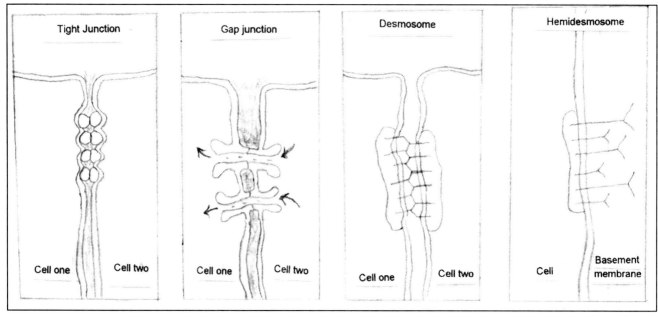

Above: This illustrates four types of cellular junctions: Tight junctions cement cells together so tightly that materials cannot pass between the cells. Gap junctions are an open conduit between cells that allow materials to pass from one cell to another without passing through the plasma membranes. Desmosomes and hemidesmosomes give adherence between two cells or between a cell and a basement membrane.

Cytoplasm is not simply an amorphous gel. It contains several specific structures called ***organelles.*** These are:
1. The ***endoplasmic reticulum ER)*** is a double membranous structure that folds over and winds throughout an area of the cytoplasm. The ER consists of sheets of parallel membranes continuous with the nuclear membrane. It is made up primarily of phospholipids. Endoplasmic means "within the cytoplasm of the cell," and reticulum means "a network." The endoplasmic reticulum is divided into the ***rough endoplasmic reticulum (RER) and the smooth endoplasmic reticulum (SER).*** Attached to the RER are tiny granules of protein and genetic material that give the RER its rough appearance. These granules are ***ribosomes***, and they are the sites of polypeptide production. Polypeptides are later turned into proteins.   Not all ribosomes are attached to the RER;

some are free in the cytosol, some are in the nucleus, and a few are in the mitochondria. The **_SER_** is continuous with the RER, but the SER lacks ribosomes. The SER produces steroid hormones and other lipids. The SER in hepatic cells of the liver is the site for detoxification of alcohol and drugs; the SER is well developed in liver and kidney cells of alcoholics and drug addicts. Sack-like areas in the SER called **_cisternae_** store and release **_calcium ions_**, which are used to initiate a contraction in muscle cells.

2. The **_Golgi complex (Golgi apparatus or Golgi body)_** was first described by Italian histologist Camillo Golgi (1843-1926). It is a system of membranes and cisternae (areas of dilatation) that is continuous with the plasma membrane. It functions to synthesize carbohydrates, and it adds carbohydrate moieties to proteins, thereby creating glycoproteins. The Golgi body inserts glycoproteins into **_secretory vesicles_**, which are surrounded by a membrane and can be excreted from the cell.

3. **_Other vesicles_** made by the cell include **_lysosomes_** and **_peroxisomes_**, both of which contain enzymes. The contents of vesicles may be excreted, or the enzymes may be used inside the cell. Some enzymes break down polysaccharides and peptides into simple sugars and amino acids and make them available to the cell. Enzymes also break down worn out organelles and cellular compounds no longer of use to the cell. **_Autophagy_** is the process of digestion of worn out organelles. **_Autolysis_** is the programmed digestion of products of dead cells.
Peroxisomes are similar to lysosomes. They contain the enzyme **_catalase_**, which breaks down hydrogen peroxide (H_2O_2) into water and oxygen. Cells create peroxide because it is useful in the destruction of bacteria and in drug and alcohol detoxification. But hydrogen peroxide can produce free radicals through oxidation, so it must be broken down as well as created.
Although vesicles are enclosed by a unit membrane, cellular inclusions are not; therefore, inclusions are not classified as organelles. Such things as glycogen granules, fat droplets, melanin pigment, bacteria, viruses and foreign bodies are inclusions.

4. **_Mitochondria_** are prominent organelles in the cytoplasm that, like the nucleus, are surrounded by a double membrane. The inner membrane of a mitochondrion has folds called **_cristae,_** which are the sites where energy that has been extracted from carbohydrates, proteins and fats is converted into **_ATP_**. ATP is adenosine triphosphate, the energy storage nucleotide of the body. The inner membrane of mitochondria contains enzymes for ATP synthesis. The **_matrix_** of the mitochondria is the central area inside the inner membrane. The matrix contains ribosomes and a small circular bit of DNA. **_The nucleus and the mitochondria are the only places where DNA can be found in animal cells._** The presence of DNA in the mitochondria is fascinating. It suggests that mitochondria originated as bacteria that were inculcated into larger organisms early in evolution. Mitochondrial DNA is more durable than nuclear DNA; both have been used in anthropological studies and criminal investigations.

Right: A mitochondrion. The parts of a mitochondrion are designated by the pointers. They are
(1) the outer membrane,
(2) the intermembranous space,
(3) the inner membrane,
(4) the matrix cavity,
(5) a crista on the inner membrane.

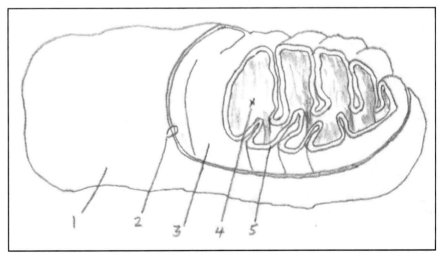

Mitochondria are the energy factories of the cell. The simple sugar, **_glucose_**, is the primary source of energy on a day to day basis. Energy is stored in ATP as high energy phosphate bonds. Glucose is broken down to two molecules of **_pyruvate_** in the cytoplasm. These steps are called **_glycolysis_**; glycolysis is **_anaerobic_** (does not require oxygen). Pyruvate is further broken down to carbon dioxide and water through chemical reactions in the mitochondria. These steps include the Krebs cycle and the electron transport chain; they are aerobic (require oxygen), and they are called **_aerobic respiration_**. Glycolysis provides only two molecules of ATP for each molecule of glucose. Aerobic respiration is far more efficient; it provides a theoretical maximum of 36 molecules of ATP for each molecule of glucose.

5. **_Microtubules_** are small cylindrical structures made up of the protein **_tubulin._** Microtubules form "railroads tracks" through the cytoplasm that guide organelles and molecules to their destinations. **_Basal bodies and axonemes_** are microtubular structures that anchor cilia and flagella to the inside of the cell. **_Centrioles_** are groups of microtubules that produce the **_mitotic spindle_**, which plays an essential role in guiding chromosomes during cell division. The **_cytoskeleton_** consists of bundles of microtubules that hold organelles in place and provide for cellular shape and rigidity. Microtubules are being continuously assembled and disassembled, and they are short lived, except for the axonemes and basal bodies that anchor cilia and flagella.

6. The **_nucleus_** is an organelle. It has a double membrane of phospholipids that is continuous with the RER. DNA in the nucleus is usually in the form of **_chromatin,_** which consists of long, lacy strands of DNA. Chromatin condenses into chromosomes during cellular division. The **_nucleolus_** is a dark staining area in the nucleus; it is the site where ribosomes are assembled.

The Plasma Membrane (Unit Membrane)

The plasma membrane is a **_single layered structure_** that surrounds the cell. Seventy-five percent of the molecules that make up the plasma membrane are **_phospholipids, which are in a double layer_**. Phospholipids are made up of glycerol (CH_2OH-$CHOH$-CH_2OH) with attached fatty acids, phosphates and other moieties. Lecithin is an example. Phospholipids are **_amphiphilic_**, meaning that they are both hydrophilic (water soluble) and lipophilic (fat soluble). Double solubility is accomplished by the coexistence of fatty acid moieties, which are fat soluble, and phosphate moieties, which are water soluble. The amphiphilic nature of phospholipids leads to a constant spinning of the molecules and a constant movement of material through the membrane.

Twenty percent of the molecules in the plasma membrane are **_cholesterol_**. Cholesterol provides rigidity to the plasma membrane; however, when cholesterol is present in high concentrations, the plasma membrane becomes more fluid because the phospholipid molecules become more separated.

Right: The plasma membrane includes phospholipids, cholesterol and protein molecules.
The proteins are large molecules that include channel proteins and receptors.
The glycocalyx is a polysaccharide moiety of a glycoprotein that allows the immune system to identify the cell. The cytoskeleton is made up of microtubules.

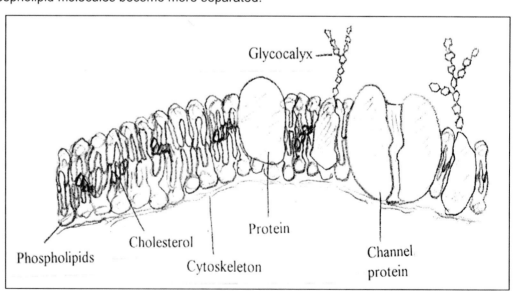

Less than 10% of the molecules of the plasma membrane are **_proteins,_** but proteins are such large molecules that they constitute 50% of the weight. Proteins that extend across the width of the plasma membrane are called **_integral proteins_**. **_Peripheral proteins_** are those that are adherent to the inner surface of the membrane and serve to anchor integral proteins to the cytoskeleton.

Proteins in the plasma membrane serve several functions:

1 **_Receptors_** are proteins that bind to such things as neurotransmitters and hormones on the surface of the cell. Receptors are typically specific for one hormone or neurotransmitter. Once bound, a receptor subsequently causes a change inside the cell. An intracellular chemical that acts as an intermediary in this change is termed a **_second messenger._** One second messenger is 3'5'cyclic AMP (adenosine monophosphate), a breakdown product of ATP.

2 **_Enzymes_** are located in the plasma membrane including those that breakdown neurotransmitters and hormones and those that function in the GI tract for digestion. Lactase, which breaks down the disaccharide, lactose, into glucose and galactose is an example of an enzyme in the plasma membrane of the digestive tract.

3 **_Channel proteins_** create pores in the plasma membrane for the ingress and egress of specific substances. The ions of sodium and potassium travel through specific pores, and these pores have the capacity to be open or closed. A **_ligand-gated channel_** is one that is opened when a specific chemical binds to a receptor that also functions as a channel protein. A **_voltage-gated channel_** is one that is opened by an electrical impulse.

4 A **_Carrier_** is a type of channel protein that binds to dissolved molecules and transports them across the plasma membrane (discussed below).

5 The **_motor molecules, dynein, actin and myosin_** are contractile proteins that arise in the cytoplasm and attach to the plasma membrane. They are capable of causing movement of the cell, movement of organelles within the cell, or the movement of cilia and flagella.

6 **_Cellular adhesion proteins_** are plasma membrane proteins that cause cells to adhere to each other and to extracellular material. Cells do not usually grow or survive unless they are mechanically linked. The **_glycocalyx_** is made up of glycoproteins with polysaccharide moieties that extend from the plasma membrane of a cell forming a surface coating. The glycocalyx is unique in everyone except identical twins; the glycocalyx is instrumental in allowing the body to determine its cellular identity. The glycocalyx of red blood cells establishes the blood type of an individual.

Movement across Membranes

The plasma membrane is selectively permeable due to the amphiphilic nature of the phospholipids and the ability of the proteins to act as carriers. The plasma membrane allows certain molecules to pass through, and it excludes the passage of others. Molecules move about in liquids and gases in several ways. Those include the following:

Simple diffusion results from the constant, random motion of molecules in a fluid. In diffusion molecules move from an area of higher concentration to an area of lower concentration; this is called down gradient. The **_rate_** of diffusion depends upon several factors including: (1) **_temperature_** (the higher the temperature the more energetically the particles move, and the faster the diffusion rate), (2) **_molecular size_** (smaller molecules are more mobile), (3) **_the steepness of the concentration gradient_**, (the greater the difference between the concentrations of a substance across a membrane, the faster the diffusion rate), (4) **_the surface area of a membrane_** (the larger the surface area, the faster the diffusion rate, and (5) **_the permeability of a membrane_** (a more porous membrane allows for faster diffusion).

Osmosis is the **_diffusion of water_** across a **_selectively permeable membrane_**. Water can travel across these membranes, but larger molecules cannot. The direction of water flow is from the more dilute concentration with fewer dissolved substances, to the solution with more dissolved particles. (The concentration of water is less in the solution with more solutes). The **_osmotic pressure_** is the hydrostatic pressure that is required to stop osmosis. Osmotic pressure has the ability to raise a column of fluid a certain amount, which can be measured in mm of Hg (mercury) or mm of water. **_Osmolarity_** refers to **_the total concentration of all the solutes_** in a solution and is expressed by the number of moles per liter of solution. One **_mole_** of a substance is that substance's molecular weight in grams. Because salts such as sodium chloride ionize when placed in solution, one mole of sodium chloride dissolved in water produces two particles, and the resulting osmolarity would be double that of one mole of an unionized substance such as glucose. From the periodic table we can see that the atomic weight of carbon is 12, hydrogen is 1, and oxygen is 16. The molecular weight of **glucose** (C6H12O6) can then be determined to be 180. [(12x6) + (1x12) + (16x6) = 180]. Therefore, 180 grams of glucose equals one mole of glucose, and 180 grams of glucose dissolved in one liter of water constitutes a one molar solution of glucose. The osmolarity of ninety grams of glucose in one liter of water, therefore, would constitute a 0.5 molar or 500 millimolar solution. However, when **sodium chloride** is placed in solution, each molecule is completely ionized producing two particles, one Na+ ion and one Cl- ion. Therefore, when one mole of sodium chloride is dissolved in one liter of water, the resulting solution has an **osmolarity of two.**

Osmolarity is based on the volume of a solution (dissolved particles in one liter of water). **Osmolality** is based on the weight of the solvent (dissolved particles in one kilogram of water). Osmolarity and osmolality are similar, but they are the same only when water is at the temperature at which it is densest (immediately above freezing), because the volume of one kilogram of water varies with the temperature.

Tonicity depends on the osmolarity of a solution; it describes the ability of an extracellular solution to affect the fluid volume and osmotic pressure inside a cell. Tonicity depends on the concentration and permeability of the solutes. An **isotonic** solution is an extracellular solution that is in balance with the solution inside the cell. A **hypotonic** solution contains too few solute particles, which would cause water to move across the plasma membrane into the cell. Cells placed in a hypotonic solution would swell and possibly burst. That is why pure water cannot be given intravenously. A **hypertonic** solution contains too many solute particles (the osmolarity is too high), and water would move out of a cell placed in a hypertonic solution. The cell would lose water and shrivel (become wrinkled or crenated).

Carriers are proteins that bind to dissolved substances and transport them across the plasma membrane. **Sodium and potassium ions** are transported in and out of the cell by carriers. Some carriers use ATP (require energy to function) and are called **pumps.** The process of utilizing energy (ATP) to pump a substance across the cell membrane is called **active transport.** Active transport is required to move molecules **up a concentration gradient** (the movement of the molecule is from an area of lower concentration to an area of higher concentration). When all carriers are saturated with the substance they are transporting, the rate of transport is at maximum and cannot be raised any higher.

If passage of a molecule across the plasma membrane involves a carrier but is **down gradient** and consequently does not require ATP, it is called **facilitated diffusion, or passive transport.** In facilitated diffusion the solute binds to a carrier that carries material across to the other side where the material is released. The carrier protein does not move its position in the plasma membrane while it is transporting; rather the carrier changes shape to usher the material in or out of the cell.

Some molecules are transported across the membrane by facilitated diffusion, but depend on the active transport system for some other substance. An example is the entrance of glucose from the kidney tubules into the kidney cells. A carrier pumps sodium through the plasma membrane and out of the cell. When the carrier returns to the inner surface of the membrane, glucose tags along and enters the cell. This system whereby glucose enters the cell is called **secondary active transport;** it keeps glucose from being excreted in the urine.

The **sodium-potassium pump** **involves active transport** and is **the most energy consuming activity in the body**. In this system three sodium ions bind to a carrier and are transported out of the cell. Once out of the cell, the sodium ions enter the extracellular fluid, and two potassium ions are picked up by the carrier. The potassium ions are transported to the cytoplasm. The Na-K pump is a system of **cotransport,** meaning that one substance (sodium) is pumped out of the cell, and another (potassium) is pumped into the cell by the same carrier. The Na-K pump regulates cell volume, ion concentration, and osmolarity. It maintains an electrical potential across the plasma membrane (the inside of the cell is kept negatively charged relative to the outside). Because it utilizes so much energy, the Na-K pump produces a significant amount of heat. The pump is amazingly effective, for it keeps the sodium concentration at 144 mEq/L outside and 10 mEq/L inside the cell, and it keeps the potassium concentration at 4.5 mEq/L outside and 141 mEq/L inside. (A mEq is a milliequivalent, which is the molarity times the valence of an ion.)

Larger substances are taken into the cell and removed from the cell by a different method. ***Endocytosis*** is the process by which large particles or droplets are engulfed by outfoldings of the plasma membrane and taken into the cell. ***Phagocytosis*** is a type of endocytosis whereby cells engulf bacteria and small foreign particles. ***Pinocytosis*** is the taking in of small droplets by surrounding them in a dimple in the plasma membrane; the dimple is pinched off, bringing the droplet into the cell. ***Exocytosis*** is the process by which vesicular material leaves the cell. In exocytosis the membrane of a vesicle unites with the plasma membrane. The plasma membrane then develops a pore for the extrusion of the contents of the vesicle. Sweat glands of the skin and mammary glands produce their secretions by exocytosis.

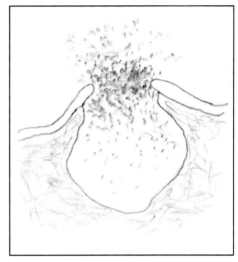

Above: Exocytosis

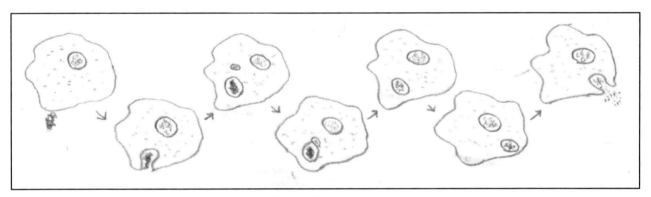

Above: Phagocytosis.

Endocytosis and exocytosis may involve ***receptors***. ***Clathrins*** are receptors in the plasma membrane where endocytosis and exocytosis occur. Insulin is transported across the endothelial cells that line capillaries in this way, as are the polio virus, HIV virus and hepatitis virus. Low density lipoproteins (LDLs) are taken up by endothelial cells in the blood vessels by a receptor mediated technique. Individuals with familial hypercholesterolemia are subject to cardiovascular disease at a young age because they lack these receptors. LDLs build up to high levels in the blood of these patients, and they develop fatty deposits in their arteries.

Study Guide
1. Appreciate the anatomic and physiologic importance of the cell.
2. Know the terms intracellular, extracellular, interstitial and intravascular as they relate to bodily fluids.
3. Know the terms used to describe the shapes of cells (cuboidal, columnar, squamous, fusiform, spherical, ovoid, discoid, fibrous, and polygonal.)
4. Know the cellular physiology and microscopic anatomy of the following cellular structures: plasma membrane, nucleus, nucleolus, cytoplasm, cytosol, Golgi body, rough and smooth endoplasmic reticulum, ribosomes, mitochondria, vesicles (lysosomes and peroxisomes) inclusions, cytoskeleton, microtubules, centrioles, microvilli, cilia and flagella.
5. Be able to name the three motor molecules of the cell (actin, myosin and dynein).
6. Know the term "glycocalyx" and what it signifies.
7. Know the three types of cellular junctions (tight, gap and desmosomes).
8. Understand how the term "amphiphilic" relates to phospholipids in the plasma membrane.

9. Know the various compounds that can be found in the plasma membrane, their prevalence and function.
10. Know the meanings of a "ligand-gated channel" and a "voltage-gated channel."
11. Understand the terms diffusion, osmosis, osmotic pressure, osmolarity, down gradient, tonicity, hypotonic, isotonic and hypertonic.
12. Understand active transport, cotransport, secondary active transport and passive transport (facilitated diffusion).
13. Understand how the sodium-potassium pump works, and appreciate that it requires more energy (ATP) than any other metabolic function of the body.
14. Define exocytosis, endocytosis and pinocytosis.

Chapter Four

Protein Synthesis and Cellular Division

Protein Synthesis

After fertilization a human **zygote** consists of one cell with the **diploid** number of 46 chromosomes (twenty-three pairs). At maturity an individual is made up of about 100 trillion cells. **Mitosis** is the process by which the **somatic** cells in the body divide. All the cells of the body are **somatic cells** except the **germ cells** (eggs and sperm). Cell division is necessary for growth and for the replacement of cells. One cell becomes two; two become four and so forth. Cells begin to specialize in the third week of gestation, and by the eighth week they have developed into distinct types such as bone cells, skin cells and nerve cells. Undifferentiated cells are immature **stem cells** that can later differentiate into many types. Cells live for a predetermined length of time. **Apoptosis** is the natural death of cells. **Necrosis** is cellular death that is premature and pathologic (abnormal).

The nucleus of the cell contains the genetic material of the cell, which is **DNA** (deoxyribonucleic acid). The DNA molecule contains a code for the synthesis of proteins -- nothing else. Many of the proteins coded by DNA are enzymes that direct the synthesis and breakdown of proteins, fats, carbohydrates, nucleic acids and other compounds. DNA in the nucleus directs cell division, but not all cells have a single nucleus; some, such as striated muscle cells, have multiple nuclei, and mature red blood cells have no nucleus at all; consequently, they cannot divide. DNA in the nucleus is contained in chromosomes. Each chromosome is actually one incredibly long DNA molecule. Except when undergoing mitosis, the chromosomes are in the form of **chromatin,** which is a lacy tangle of DNA in the nucleus. The nucleus is surrounded by a double unit membrane called the **nuclear envelope,** which is selectively porous. The **nucleolus** is a small dark area within the nucleus where **ribosomes** are assembled.

The Nucleic Acids, DNA and RNA

The structure of DNA was described by **James Watson and Francis Crick** in their monumental paper, which was published in 1953. They found DNA to be in the form of a double helix. A double helix is a structure that can be described as two spiral staircases wound around each other. The two strands, or backbones, of DNA in the double helix are composed of alternating moieties of the sugar, **deoxyribose, and phosphate**. Attached to each sugar moiety (deoxyribose) is a nitrogen containing alkaline compound called a **nitrogenous base**. The combination of a sugar, a phosphate moiety and a nitrogenous base makes up a **nucleotide**. The nitrogenous bases are either **purines** or **pyrimidines.** The chemical structure of a purine contains two rings, one with five atoms and one with six. Purines are larger molecules than pyrimidines, which contain only one ring with six atoms. A purine and a pyrimidine connect to each other by **hydrogen bonds**, which hold the two strands of the helix together. A purine of one strand **always** connects to a specific pyrimidine of the other strand. This is called the **law of complementary base pairing**. The purines in DNA are **adenine** and **guanine**. Adenine and guanine are similar but different compounds. The pyrimidines of DNA are **thymine and cytosine**, which are similar but different compounds. **Adenine is always connected to thymine, and guanine is always connected to cytosine**. Adenine and thymine are linked by two hydrogen bonds; guanine and cytosine are linked by three hydrogen bonds.

The DNA molecule of a chromosome is incredibly long and wispy. An average chromosome contains 300 million nucleotides. If the length of a single nucleotide were one foot, one DNA molecule could circle the globe more than twice. DNA is supported by proteins called **histones,** which are grouped into granules called **nucleosomes.** The DNA molecule is wrapped around nucleosomes in a supercoil.

Right: The molecular structure of DNA is shown in this drawing. The sugar-phosphate backbones are the columns on the right and left. "A" represents adenine; "G" represents guanine; "T" represents thymine, "C" represents cytosine, "P" represents phosphate, and "D" represents the sugar, deoxyribose. The dotted lines are hydrogen bonds linking the nitrogenous bases. Note that the purines, adenine and guanine, have two rings and are larger molecules than the pyrimidines, thymine and cytosine.

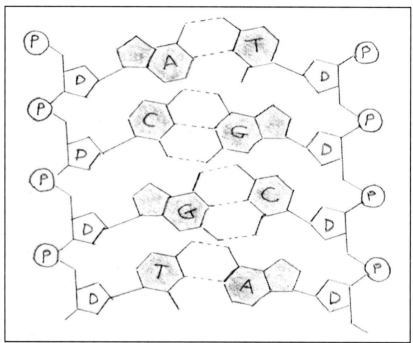

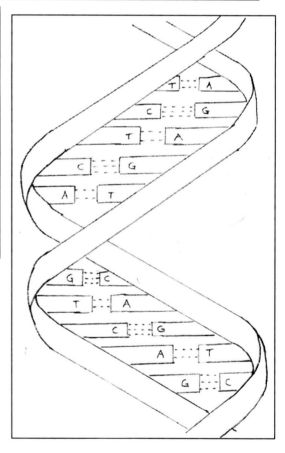

Above: The chemical formulae for complementary base pairing in DNA. The arrows point to hydrogen bonds. The upper drawing shows two hydrogen bonds between thymine (T) and adenine (A). The lower drawing shows three hydrogen bonds between cytosine (C) and guanine (G).

Right: The double helix structure of DNA. "A, T, G and C" are the nitrogenous bases. The dotted lines are hydrogen bonds. The ribbons are the deoxyribose-phosphate backbones.

The various proteins produced under the direction of genes perform many tasks, including functioning as enzymes. DNA codes for the production of proteins, but it does **_NOT_** code for the synthesis of fats, carbohydrates or anything except proteins. Enzymes produced under the direction of DNA accomplish the synthesis and metabolism of the other compounds.   A sequence of three DNA nucleotides (three base pairs plus the deoxyribose-phosphate backbone) is called a ***base triplet***. Each mathematical possibility for base pairing in a triplet (there are 64 [4x4x4] possibilities) is a code for one of the 20 amino acids used in human protein production. A ***codon*** is the RNA equivalent of the DNA base triplet. It is the sequence of codons that determines the amino acid sequence in a protein molecule.

Right: These drawings show one way an enzyme works. The figure on the left represents an enzyme. The reactants are being linked to form a new compound.

The middle figure shows how the enzyme has brought the reactants into a position where they will react.   The figures on the right represent the enzyme and the newly synthesized molecule.

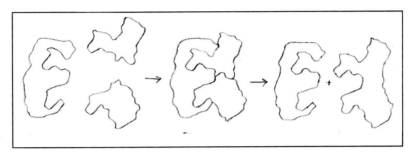

Enzyme   Reactants   Catalytic process   New molecule

   RNA serves to interpret the code in DNA and direct the synthesis of proteins. RNA works mainly in the cytoplasm while DNA remains in the nucleus. RNA is a much smaller molecule than DNA. RNA has only one strand, and it is not in a helical form.   RNA contains the sugar, ***ribose***, instead of deoxyribose, and RNA lacks the pyrimidine, thymine, substituting the pyrimidine, ***uracil***, in its place.

   There are three types of RNA. ***Messenger RNA (mRNA)*** is a strand of RNA that is copied from a section of DNA in the nucleus through the action of enzymes. Messenger RNA leaves the nucleus and connects with a ribosome in the RER or in the cytosol. Ribosomes are made up of ***ribosomal RNA (rRNA)*** and enzymes. Messenger RNA links with rRNA in the ribosome, and mRNA is gradually pulled through the ribosome as its code is being read. ***Transfer RNA (tRNA)*** molecules are relatively small. Each tRNA molecule binds to a specific amino acid in the cytosol and delivers that amino acid to the ribosome. The base sequence of the mRNA directs the sequence of amino acid placement into a peptide. Because there are 64 possible codons, and only 20 amino acids are used in protein production, most of the amino acids are represented by more than one codon. One specific codon serves as a "start" codon, which tells the ribosome where to begin the peptide; another codon is read as the "stop" codon. The start codon is always the sequence AUG (adenine-uracil-guanine). The stop codons are UAG, UGA and UAA. Because the A-U-G sequence codes for the amino acid, methionine, all peptides initially begin with methionine, although methionine may be removed later.   All three types of RNA are synthesized in the nucleus. Ribosomes are assembled in the nucleolus. Ribosomes, mRNA and tRNA are released from the nucleus into the cytoplasm after their synthesis. ***Transcription*** is the process of synthesizing mRNA from DNA in the nucleus. ***Translation*** is the process of putting together a polypeptide in the ribosome from the mRNA code.

   Chaperones are proteins that serve to guide newly synthesized proteins to their destinations in the cell, such as to the Golgi apparatus where carbohydrate moieties are added. Chaperones also help to model a polypeptide into its functional structure as a protein.

   The ***twenty amino acids*** that are used by the body to manufacture proteins include eight that are required to be in the diet and are called ***"essential."*** The other twelve can be synthesized from the essential amino acids. The eight essential amino acids are leucine, isoleucine, valine, lysine, threonine, methionine, phenylalanine, and tryptophan.   The nonessential amino acids are alanine, arginine, asparagine, aspartic acid, cysteine, glutamic acid, glutamine, glycine, histidine, proline, serine and tyrosine.
   The basic structure of an amino acid is diagrammed below.

R
|
NH2—CH—COOH

The "R" stands for radical, which represents a moiety of the compound that is unique to each amino acid. The R may be as simple as a hydrogen atom, in which case the amino acid is ***glycine***, or it may be a complicated moiety. The R moiety in *__tryptophan__* contains a six atom ring and a five atom ring.

Linkage of amino acids to form peptides and proteins is done by the *__peptide bond__*, which links the carboxyl group of one amino acid to the amino group of another. Water is lost in this reaction.

```
             R    O                  R
             |    ||                 |
         NH2—CH—C—------------NH—CH--COOH
                  Peptide bond
```

All the amino acids contain at least one carboxyl group, which is acidic, and one amino group, which is basic. *__Arginine and lysine__* contain two amino groups and are basic; *__aspartic acid and glutamic__* acid contain two carboxyl groups and are acidic. *__Methionine and cysteine__* contain a *__sulfur__* atom. Disulfide bonds are bonds between sulfur atoms of methionine or cysteine. Disulfide bonds provide structure to proteins.

Valine   Leucine   Isoleucine   Tryptophan

Threonine   Lysine   Phenylalanine   Methionine

Above: The structures of the eight essential amino acids.

The speed at which metabolic processes occur in the cell is phenomenal. A single cell may continuously synthesize as many as 2000 different proteins, and the human body makes over 2 million different proteins. A single cell may have 300,000 identical mRNA strands being produced simultaneously, and it may produce over 150,000 proteins per second. Ribosomes constitute twenty-five percent of the dry weight of the liver.

Genetics

You have 23 pairs of chromosomes -- 46 chromosomes total. Forty-four of those chromosomes are autosomes; two are sex chromosomes. The autosomes are paired; they are numbered 1-22, and each pair shares a distinctive appearance. Two chromosomes that are a pair are called *__homologous chromosomes;__* they share the same gene loci, but not the same genes. The largest chromosomes are assigned the small numbers; the chromosomes get smaller as their number gets higher. Each numbered chromosome pair includes one chromosome inherited from the mother and one chromosome inherited from the father. The twenty-third pair of chromosomes are the sex chromosomes -- X and Y, which are not homologous; they differ considerably. Females have two homologous X chromosomes. Males have one X chromosome and one Y chromosome.

A *__gene__* is a nucleotide sequence in DNA that codes for one polypeptide, which eventually is turned into a protein. *__Alleles__* are the different forms that a gene can take. Each gene is located on a specific section of a chromosome called its *__locus.__* Humans have approximately 35,000 genes. All the genes of one person constitute that individual's *__genome.__* An individual's *__genotype__* represents the particular alleles of his genes. An individual's *__phenotype__* represents those genes that are "expressed" (functional or visible). *__Karyotype__* is an individual's chromosomal make up. **_Pleiotropy_** refers to the production of multiple phenotypic effects by one gene. **_Polygenic inheritance_** means that more than one gene contributes to a phenotypic trait. **_Penetrance_** refers to the ability of a gene to be expressed. For example 80% penetrance of a particular gene means that the gene is expressed in only 80% of the individuals who possess the gene. Penetrance of a homozygous recessive gene may depend upon polygenic inheritance. The inheritance of a trait can be predicted by outlining an individual's genotype on a **_Punnett square._**

Genes vary **_according to their base sequence_**. The **_homozygous_** state is one in which both alleles of a gene are identical on a pair of homologous chromosomes. If the alleles are not identical, the state is called **_heterozygous_**. An allele is termed to be **_dominant_** if it functions while being present on only one of a pair of chromosomes. It is called **_recessive_** if it is expressed only when it appears on both chromosomes of a pair. **_Co-dominance_** is a heterozygous state in which both alleles are expressed. An example of co-dominance is the A-B-O blood type system. A **_carrier_** is an individual who is heterozygous for a trait, but does not express that trait phenotypically.

A dominant gene usually codes for the production of a normal enzyme and a **_recessive gene for the production of a faulty enzyme._** Faulty recessive genes can be passed on from generation to generation because carriers are not symptomatic. Sometimes a dominant gene is faulty and harmful. Any dominant gene that leads to destruction of a necessary physiologic process could not continue to be present in the population unless it was not expressed until after puberty. An example of a disorder carried by a destructive dominant gene is Huntington's disease (Huntington's chorea), a fatal neurological disease that often does not become manifest until middle age.

A faulty recessive gene is not expressed unless the individual is homozygous for the recessive gene. When that is the case, both of the individual's parents are phenotypically normal, but both would be heterozygous carriers of the defective recessive gene. Phenylketonuria (PKU) is caused by the homozygous state of a defective recessive gene; it is fatal if not detected early. In PKU the amino acid, phenylalanine, cannot be converted to tyrosine, and phenylalanine builds up to toxic levels in the cells. Another example of a disorder carried by a defective recessive gene is galactosemia. In galactosemia the sugar, galactose, cannot be metabolized, and it builds up in the cells leading to cellular destruction, liver failure, kidney failure and cataracts. In the heterozygous state of PKU and galactosemia the production of the normal enzyme is lower than normal but sufficient to prevent disease. Most states have laws that require screening for PKU and galactosemia at birth. It has been estimated that before infant testing for PKU became available, 35% of all long term patients in Missouri state mental hospitals had PKU. Treatment for PKU and galactosemia is simple but difficult. Dairy products must be withheld from the diet of patients with galactosemia. In PKU only a small measured amount of phenylalanine can be present in the diet. Some phenylalanine is necessary for protein synthesis.

Chromosomes are classified as **_22 pairs of autosomes_** and one **_pair of sex (XY) chromosomes_**. Females have a pair of similar X chromosomes (XX karyotype). Males have one X chromosome and one Y chromosome (XY karyotype). Children of both sexes inherit an X chromosome from their mothers. Females inherit an X chromosome from their fathers; males inherit the much smaller Y chromosome from their fathers. Y chromosomes carry few genes, and those genes are limited to sexual development. **_Recessive sex-linked traits are carried on the X chromosome_**. These traits are much more commonly expressed in males than females because a female must be homozygous for the trait to be expressed. Examples of disorders carried by sex-linked recessive genes on the X chromosome are hemophilia, some forms of muscular dystrophy and red-green color blindness. The defective gene that produces hemophilia is present in about one of every five thousand X chromosomes. Males have one X chromosome, and therefore, males have a one in five thousand chance of inheriting the disease. A female has a two in five thousand chance of inheriting an X chromosome with the defective gene, but she has only a one in 25 million chance (5000 x 5000) of inheriting hemophilia because that would require that she inherit two faulty X chromosomes. Females with hemophilia have a mother who is a carrier and a father who has hemophilia.

Right: The probability of an infant inheriting a genetic disorder can be predicted if the genotypes of the parents and the mode of inheritance are known. A Punnett square is a simple diagram that shows the pattern of inheritance. In this illustration consider that the disorder is caused by the homozygous state of a defective recessive gene.   "P" is the normal dominant gene, and "p" is the defective recessive gene, which is carried on an autosomal chromosome. Each child of the two parents has a 25% chance of being homozygous for the defective gene (pp) and displaying that defect phenotypically.

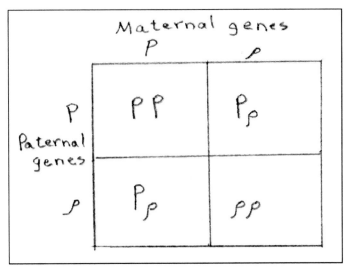

A Punnett square can also be drawn for genetic disorders that are _**carried**_ by the mother on one of her X chromosomes (_**sex-linked recessive inheritance**_). In such cases the maternal genes would be X (normal) and x (defective). The paternal genes would be X and Y (or X and 0 because the Y chromosome does not contain the gene). Daughters of this mother would have a 50% chance of inheriting the mother's defective gene and being a carrier like their mother. But the daughters would inherit a normal gene (X) from their fathers, and they would not have the disorder. Sons of a mother who is a carrier would also have a 50% chance of inheriting her defective gene (x), but sons with the defective gene would have the disorder because they only have one X chromosome.

Right: A Punnett square showing the inheritance pattern of a sex linked recessive disorder. Hemophilia is an example. In this illustration H represents the normal gene; h represents the defective gene; xx are female offspring and xy are male offspring. The Y chromosome does not have a locus for sex linked recessive genes, so males have only one gene for these traits. It can be seen that if the mother is a carrier, her sons will have a 50% chance of inheriting the disease, and her daughters will have a 50% chance of being a carrier.

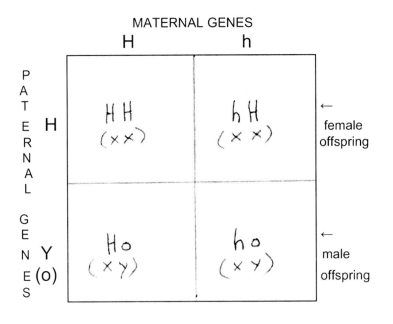

Our ancient ancestors can be traced through their DNA. Two clever ways to do this are by testing mitochondrial DNA, which males and females inherit only from their mothers, and by testing Y chromosomes, which only males inherit from their fathers.

Mitosis

Mitosis is cell division by somatic cells. It produces two cells that are genetically exactly like the parent cell. Cellular division can occur only when several criteria are met. *(1)* The cell must become large enough, *(2)* DNA must have been replicated, *(3)* there must be an adequate supply of nutrients, *(4)* the cell must be stimulated by growth factors, and *(5)* there must be space enough in the tissue. Contact inhibition of cellular division occurs when cells are packed too closely together. Cancer cells have lost that inhibition.

The sequential phases of a cell's life span in relation to mitosis follow:

*1. **The first gap or G-1 phase.*** This phase follows cell division. Somatic cells contain 46 chromosomes, and they are, therefore, diploid. During the G-1 phase the cell undergoes its normal functions; plus it ***synthesizes and stores materials necessary for mitosis***. The first gap phase lasts about 12 hours in cultured fibroblasts, which are connective tissue cells that divide about every 18-24 hours. Some cells (neurons, for example) do not undergo mitosis and do not proceed through the phases of mitosis.

*2. **The synthesis or S phase***. For cellular division to occur the chromatin (DNA) must first double. During the S phase the lacy ***chromatin material is replicated***, producing an exact duplicate of each DNA molecule. In this process an enzyme temporarily separates the strands of DNA by breaking the hydrogen bonds between base pairs. Each strand is then copied according to its base sequence. The S phase lasts about 6-8 hours in cultured fibroblasts. At the end of the S phase each cell contains double the normal amount of DNA. The number of chromosomes has not changed because the new strands of DNA remain connected to the parent strands; the cells remain diploid in spite of the DNA content having doubled.

*3. **The second gap or G-2 phase*** follows the S phase. In this stage the cell prepares itself for division. The ***centriole is replicated*** and enzymes necessary for mitosis are produced. This stage typically lasts 4-6 hours in cultured fibroblasts.

*4. **The Mitotic or M phase*** is the phase in which cell division actually occurs. The M phase begins with ***prophase***. In prophase the chromatin coils itself into the short, dense rods that we recognize as ***chromosomes***. Each chromosome consists of two genetically identical bodies called ***chromatids***, which are joined together at a spot called the ***centromere.*** During prophase there are 46 chromosomes; each of the 46 chromosomes consists of two identical chromatids, with one molecule of DNA in each chromatid. The ***nuclear envelope begins to disintegrate*** and release the chromosomes into the cytoplasm. The ***centrioles*** begin to sprout elongated microtubules; they separate and migrate to opposite poles of the cell.

After prophase comes ***metaphase***. In metaphase the chromosomes ***line up along the midline*** of the cell, and microtubules sprout from the centrioles toward the chromosomes. The ***microtubules*** attach to the centromeres of the chromosomes to form a ***mitotic spindle***. Other microtubules radiate from the centrioles to the plasma membrane to form a star-shaped array called an ***aster.*** Asters serve to anchor the centrioles and mitotic spindles to the cytoskeleton.

After metaphase comes ***anaphase***. In anaphase the ***centromeres*** split and the chromatids separate into ***92 chromosomes***. The two ***daughter chromosomes*** of each original chromosome migrate to opposite ends of the cell, led by their centromeres with their arms trailing behind. They are guided by the mitotic spindles of the centrioles. Within the centromeres is ***dynein***, a motor protein, which propels the chromosome. The daughter chromosomes are exactly alike, and therefore, the daughter cells of mitosis are genetically identical clones, and each contains 46 chromosomes.

The next phase is ***telophase,*** during which the chromosomes cluster at each end of the cell. The rough endoplasmic reticulum forms a ***new nuclear envelope*** around each cluster of chromosomes, and the chromosomes begin to uncoil to form thinly dispersed chromatin. The mitotic spindle breaks up and disappears. Each new nucleus forms a nucleolus, and RNA synthesis and protein production resume.

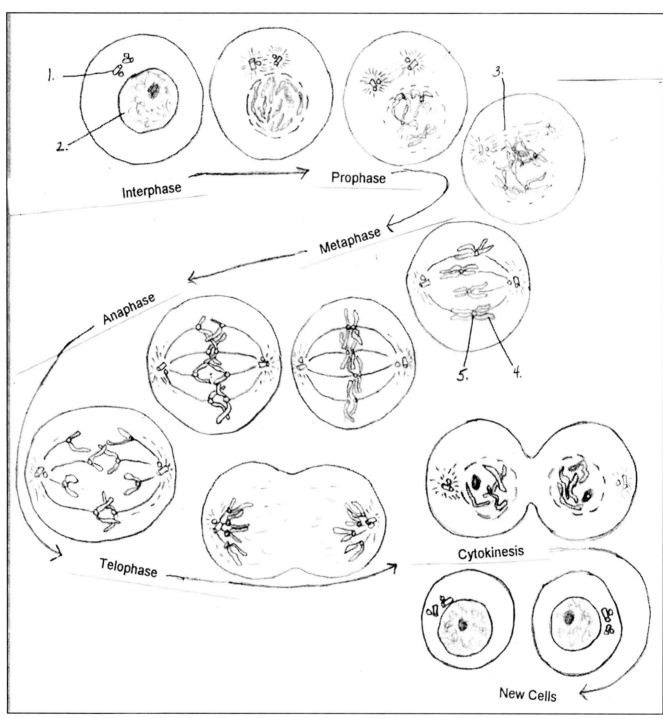

Above: The mitotic phase of mitosis consists of prophase, metaphase, anaphase, and telophase. Interphase is the period between mitotic phases, and cytokinesis is division of the cell membranes following telophase. The structures designated by the numbered pointers are (1) centriole, (2) nucleus, (3) mitotic spindle, (4) chromosome, and (5) centromere.

Telophase overlaps with **_cytokinesis_**, which is division of the cytoplasm of the cell. Cytokinesis is achieved by the motor protein **_myosin_** pulling on small filaments of the motor protein **_actin_** in the cytoskeleton. This creates a **_cleavage furrow_** around the equator of the cell, which pinches it in two.

Meiosis

Meiosis is cell division that results in the production of **_gametes_** -- the sperm and egg cells -- which are **_haploid_**. (They have 23 unpaired chromosomes).

The production of **_sperm_** cells begins with **_spermatogonia_** cells in the testes. Spermatogonia are diploid (they have 46 chromosomes); they divide by **_mitosis_**, and they reproduce themselves. Some spermatogonia cells (called "Type B") develop into **_primary spermatocytes_**, which divide by **_meiosis_**. "Type A" spermatogonia remain as residual spermatogonia.

Meiosis differs from mitosis in four important ways. **(1)** Meiosis occurs only in the primary sperm and egg cells. **(2)** Whereas mitosis results in cells with a **_diploid_** number of chromosomes, meiosis results in a cells with a **_haploid_** number of chromosomes. **(3)** Mitosis results in new cells that have the exact genetic make-up as the parent cell. In meiosis the DNA within each chromosome pair is mixed. Mixing is done by a process known as **_crossing over_**, and it creates a chromosome that is not a copy of an original chromosome; rather the new chromosome contains a new combination of DNA with material from both a maternal chromosome and a paternal chromosome. **(4)** In **_mitosis_** the parent cell produces **_two cloned diploid_** cells. In **_meiosis four haploid daughter cells_**, each with a different genetic content, are produced from one parent cell.

DNA is replicated in the synthesis phase of meiosis as it is in mitosis. This step creates twice the amount of DNA in the nucleus, with each chromosome consisting of two chromatids joined by a centromere. Each chromatid has an amount of DNA equal to that of the chromosome before DNA replication. The cell is still diploid, and it has 46 chromosomes, but each chromosome has twice as much DNA as it had before. The phases of prophase, metaphase and anaphase are similar in meiosis and mitosis, except that in meiosis **_the maternal and the paternal homologous chromosomal pair line up side by side, creating a tetrad_**. Each tetrad consists of a pair of chromosomes, with each chromosome having two chromatids. Therefore, each tetrad consists of four chromatids. **_Crossing over_** is the mixing of genetic material within a tetrad, and it occurs in **_prophase_**. After prophase the **_tetrads separate_** into **_two separate chromosomes_**. The centromere of each new chromosome remains intact, and the chromatids do not separate as the cell undergoes metaphase, anaphase and telophase and becomes two daughter cells. This division is called **_meiosis I._** The daughter cells of meiosis I contain only 23 chromosomes and are haploid; however, each of the 23 chromosomes of these cells contains two chromatids that are linked by a centromere, so the nuclei of these cells contain an amount of DNA equal to that of the parent cell before DNA replication. The products of meiosis I are called **_secondary spermatocytes_** in the male and **_secondary oocytes_** in the female. The centrioles of meiosis I remain intact and function in Meiosis II.

In **_meiosis II_** the chromatids break apart and the centromeres lead single chromatids to opposite sides of the cell. Each daughter cell receives one chromatid from each chromosome of the parent cell. The daughter cells remain haploid, and now they have only half the DNA material of a diploid cell before DNA replication. Sperm and egg cells (ova) are the final product of meiosis; each sperm and each ovum has 23 single chromatid chromosomes when meiosis II is complete. Four sperm cells are formed from the meiotic division of one primary spermatocyte. Potentially four egg cells would be formed from the meiotic division of one primary oocyte, but this does not happen. The first meiotic division in the female results in the formation of a **_secondary oocyte_** and the **_first polar body_**. The first polar body degenerates, and the **_secondary oocyte remains suspended in metaphase of meiosis II until fertilization occurs._** After fertilization, the **_secondary oocyte_** finishes meiosis II by dividing into the **_egg cell_** (ovum) and the **_second polar body_**. The egg cell unites with the sperm, and the second polar body degenerates.

Each **_ovum_** contains 22 **_autosomes_** and one X **_(sex) chromosome_**. Each **_sperm_** cell contains 22 autosomes and **_either one X chromosome or one Y chromosome_**. Thus it is the sperm cell that determines whether the child will have an **_XX karyotype_** (chromosomal make up) and be female, or have an **_XY karyotype_** and be male.

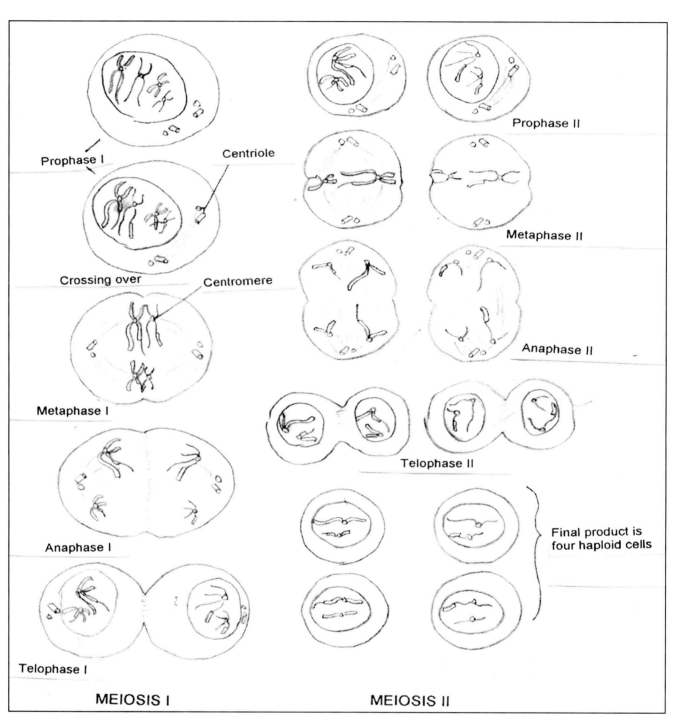

Prophase I

Centriole

Crossing over   Centromere

Metaphase I

Anaphase I

Telophase I

MEIOSIS I

Prophase II

Metaphase II

Anaphase II

Telophase II

Final product is four haploid cells

MEIOSIS II

Above: The first and second meiotic phases are shown in this series of drawings. Tetrad formation and crossing over occurs in prophase of meiosis I. The products of meiosis I are two cells that are haploid, but they contain the same amount of DNA as somatic cells. Each of the daughter cells of meiosis I divide in meiosis II. The products of meiosis II are cells with a haploid number of chromosomes. The daughter cells of meiosis II contain half the amount of DNA as somatic cells.

Division of the secondary oocytes and secondary spermatocytes in meiosis II involves dissolution of the centromeres and separation of the chromatids. If dissolution of a centromere does not occur, one of the daughter cells ends up with 24 chromosomes, and the other daughter cell ends up with 22 chromosomes. Several syndromes result from such an abnormal splitting. ***Down's syndrome is trisomy 21,*** meaning that the 21st chromosome of these people is in triplicate rather than being paired. There are mild and severe cases of Down's syndrome. The more severe cases involve an individual with three #21 chromosomes and 47 chromosomes total. Milder forms have the normal 46 chromosomes, but they have extra genetic material on one of their # 21 chromosomes. Evidently crossing over was faulty and unbalanced in these people. Syndromes involving an abnormal number of autosomes other than #21 occur, but those fetuses rarely survive to be born. They have multiple birth defects, which are uniformly fatal within a few days or weeks of life.

Sex chromosomes are subject to faulty centromere dissolution as well, and some of these people survive. Examples include individuals with the ***XO karyotype***, which is ***Turner's syndrome***. These people are outwardly female; they are of short stature, and they have physical and mental defects.

Another example is the ***XXY karyotype***, which results in ***Klinefelter's syndrome***. These people are male, but their sex organs are underdeveloped. They tend to be tall with long limbs and mental retardation.

Men with the ***XYY karyotype*** were first discovered in prisons in France, and they were originally thought to have a violent nature. But for the most part men with this karyotype appear to be normal, and most live peacefully in society. Their intelligence level is usually at the low end of normal.

Fertility is generally lacking in individuals with an abnormal number of chromosomes with the exception of the XYY males, some of whom have sired children.

DNA testing became possible in 1991. Since that time a few individuals have been discovered who have two types of DNA, but they are normal in all other respects. They are called ***chimera.*** Theories have arisen as to how chimera could come to exist. One theory is that two sperm may rarely fertilize an egg at exactly the same moment while the secondary oocyte is suspended in metaphase. One sperm fertilizes the chromatids that were destined to be the egg, and the other fertilizes the chromatids that would have become the second polar body. In this theory simultaneous fertilization of the ovum by two sperm allows two secondary oocytes to mature into ova, and a second polar body does not develop. The two ova are fertilized by two different sperm. Two nuclei form within the zygote, which divides into two cells with different genetic contents. As the zygote grows and differentiation occurs, one of the fertilized eggs becomes the endoderm (the lungs and future lining of GI tract), and the other becomes the ectoderm (nervous system and epidermis) and mesoderm (muscle and connective tissue), or some other system of differentiation occurs. In this example the two types of DNA of a chimera are related as normal brothers or sisters, but they are not identical twins, who would have the same DNA. It is suspected that simultaneous fertilization of one egg by two sperm occurs more often than is appreciated, but most chimera do not survive. Survivability would be further reduced if one sperm contained an X chromosome and was destined to produce a female offspring, and the other sperm contained a Y chromosome and was destined to produce a male offspring.

Studies on human DNA have found that only three percent of our DNA is coded for protein production. The other 97% serves no known purpose and is called "junk DNA."

Consider the following. Half of a cell's DNA is eliminated in meiosis; crossing over changes the genetic content of individual chromosomes, and only three percent of our DNA is known to be functional. I suggest that it is reasonable to reach these conclusions from the above considerations: (1) After crossing over the four chromatids of the tetrad are all different from one another. (2) After crossing over, none of the four chromatids of a tetrad is like a chromosome of either parent. (3) The inheritance of genetic traits carried by a chromosome can have a decidedly unequal contribution from the two parents and from the four grandparents. These three factors are paramount in accounting for evolutionary change.

Not all genes and genetic traits are shared with parents. A mutation is a change in the base sequence of a gene in a spermatocyte or oocyte. That allele would be lacking in the somatic cells of the parent, but it would be present in some of their gametes. Mutations occur as a result of exposure to radiation and toxic chemicals, and they occur naturally. Most mutations and are innocuous; some are harmful, and rarely a mutation is beneficial. Alleles that produce beneficial mutations are more likely to be passed on to future generations if they help the mutant survive and procreate.

A constant mutation rate and the presence of so much "junk" or unused DNA lead me to conclude that the human species has a great deal of evolutionary possibilities in its future.

The earth's environment can be unforgiving as evidenced by the fact that over 99% of all species that ever existed are now extinct. Biodiversity is a shield against hard times because it allows for more genetic traits to be present in a population, and some of those traits may allow the species to continue in a harsh environment. Therefore, genetic variability became necessary for a species to survive in a changing world. Bacteria increase their chances for survival by mutating rapidly and multiplying with alacrity. Also they are able to share genetic material with their neighbors, even neighboring bacteria of different species. Larger organisms cannot share genetic material, so they need another way to increase their biodiversity. Sex and its associated meiotic cellular division developed as means by which larger organisms could accomplish genetic variability. If multicellular organisms reproduced by mitosis, they would all be clones of a parent. Evolution would slow to a crawl, and the advantages of natural selection would be effectively eliminated. Sharks have been shown to have the ability to reproduce without mating, and sharks have changed little over millions of years. Their skeleton is composed only of cartilage, and their primitive brains do not require sleep.

Genetics Definitions

Mendel, Gregor (1822-1884) was an Austrian monk who discovered the principles of heredity by working with garden peas. The importance of his work was not noted until 1900.

Miescher, Johann (1844-1895) was a Swiss biochemist who discovered the material now known to be nucleic acid, which he considered to be the basis of heredity.

James Watson and Francis Crick worked together in London. They were the first to describe the double helix configuration of DNA. Their paper was published in 1953.

Gene: a segment of DNA that codes for a polypeptide.

Genome: all of the genes possessed by one individual.

Gene pool: all of the alleles present in a population.

Homologous chromosomes: two physically identical chromosomes with the same gene loci but not necessarily the same alleles; one is of maternal origin and the other of paternal origin.

Sex chromosomes: two chromosomes (X and Y) that determine a person's sex.

Autosomes: all chromosomes except the sex chromosomes. Autosomes occur in 22 homologous pairs.

Locus: the site on a chromosome where a particular gene is located.

Allele: any of the alternative forms that a particular gene can take.

Genotype: the alleles that a person possesses for a particular trait.

Phenotype: a detectable trait, such as eye color or blood type.

Karyotype: the chromosomal make up of an individual.

Recessive allele: an allele that is not phenotypically expressed in the presence of a dominant allele and is represented with a lower case letter.

Dominant allele: an allele that is phenotypically expressed even in the presence of another allele and is represented with a capital letter.

Homozygous: having two identical alleles for a given gene.

Heterozygous: having two different alleles for a given gene.

Carrier: a person who carries a recessive allele but does not phenotypically express it.

Co-dominance: a condition in which two alleles are both fully expressed when present in the same individual.

Incomplete dominance: a condition in which two different alleles are both expressed when present in the same individual. Incomplete dominance results in a phenotype that is intermediate between those that each allele would produce alone.

Polygenic inheritance: a condition in which a single phenotype results from the combined action of genes at two or more different loci.

Pleiotropy: a condition in which a single gene produces multiple phenotypic effects.

Sex linkage: inheritance of a gene on the X (or rarely the Y) chromosome, so that the associated phenotype is expressed more in one sex than in the other.

Penetrance: the percentage of individuals with a given genotype who exhibit the phenotype predicted from the allele of that gene.

<u>Study Guide</u>

1. Understand the terms haploid, diploid, mitosis, meiosis, gametes, germ cells and somatic cells.
2. Know how many chromosomes are in human somatic cells and human germ cells.
3. Know the difference between chromosomes and chromatin.
4. Understand the structure of a DNA molecule as determined by James Watson and Francis Crick.
5. Know the moieties that make up DNA and how they are linked.
6. Understand how DNA codes for RNA and subsequently for amino acids.
7. Understand how a protein is synthesized through the processes of transcription and translation.
8. Understand the roles played by the three types of RNA (messenger, ribosomal and transfer RNA), and the roles played by the nucleolus and the ribosomes.
9. Know what a base triplet and a codon are.
10. Appreciate the size of a DNA molecule and the speed of protein synthesis.
11. Know the meanings of the genetic terms listed in this chapter.
12. Know the phases of mitosis.
13. Understand the process of meiosis and how it differs from mitosis.
14. Name one process by which animals and plants increase their genetic variability.

Chapter Five

Histology

The complexity of life took a dramatic leap forward when multicellular organisms began to appear, for then cellular specialization became possible. Cells grouped themselves into organs with specific tasks, and each organ is composed of two or more tissues. ***Histology is the study of tissues; it can also be defined as the study of microscopic anatomy.***

In the first few days of existence of a human being, after a sperm has fertilized an egg to form a ***zygote***, and the haploid (23) number of chromosomes of both the sperm and egg has doubled to the diploid (46) number of an individual human, the cell begins to multiply by mitosis. The first cell division results in a two-celled organism. Later it multiplies to four, then eight, then sixteen and so on. An adult human has about 100 trillion cells, which are divided into about 200 cell types and ***four tissue classes***.

After the first few days of its existence, the early embryo has formed two distinct primary cell layers, the ***ectoderm*** and the ***endoderm.*** The ectoderm layer folds inward; specialized ectodermal cells grow into the fold and become a third distinct primary cell layer called ***mesoderm.*** The ***ectodermal layer*** becomes the nervous system, the epidermis of the skin, mouth, nose, anal canal, the salivary glands and several other glands, and parts of the eye and ear. The ***mesodermal layer*** forms the muscles, gonads, adrenal glands, most of the kidneys and genitourinary tract, and the connective tissues including bone, cartilage and blood. ***Endoderm*** forms most of the mucosal epithelium of the digestive and respiratory tracts, the lungs, the liver and other digestive glands, the thyroid, parathyroid and thymus glands, and the mucosal epithelium of the bladder and urethra.

When one views tissue through the microscope, he sees a two dimensional scene. The microscopic appearance of a thin section of a tubular structure depends upon how the section has been cut. If a tubule has been cut as a transverse section, the tubule appears as a circle. If the tubule has been cut longitudinally, it appears as an elongated passageway. If the tubule has been cut obliquely (on a diagonal), it appears as an oval.

The four tissue types are ***(1) epithelial, (2) connective, (3) muscle, and (4) nervous***. Muscle tissue and nervous tissue are fully discussed in later chapters. This chapter will concentrate on epithelial tissue and connective tissue.

1. Epithelial tissue.

Epithelial tissue is a thin layer of cells that is ***a lining or covering*** over underlying tissues. It also includes the ***cells that make up the tubules*** of the liver, kidneys and glands. Epithelium is derived from either ectoderm or endoderm. (The lining of mesodermal tissues is called mesothelium. Mesothelium is not an epithelial tissue.) All epithelial linings are underlain by a ***basement membrane***. Mesothelium lacks a basement membrane.

Epithelial tissues include the ***epidermis*** (the outer layer of your skin), the inner linings of your respiratory, digestive and urinary tracts, and the cuboidal cells lining tubules in organs and glands are epithelial tissues. The epidermis of your skin contains hair, nails, oil and sweat glands, all of which are epithelial tissues and serve a protective purpose. ***Goblet cells*** are specialized epithelial cells in your respiratory tract and GI tract. Goblet cells secrete mucus, which serves to lubricate and help the body cleanse itself by trapping unwanted debris. The inner surface of blood vessels (***endothelium***) is epithelial tissue.

Epithelial cells are packed closely together, even to the exclusion of blood vessels, and there is little room for any intercellular material. Epithelial cells are held together by ***tight junctions***, which are zipper-like welds between cells, and ***desmosomes***, which are Velcro-like connections between cells. Epithelial cells may be in several layers; the bottom layer ***always*** rests on a ***basement membrane*** of protein, GAGs (glycosaminoglycans) and glycoprotein, which separates the epithelium from underlying connective tissue. Most epithelial cells divide rapidly and have a relatively short life span of only a few days or weeks. Because they divide rapidly, they are subject to cancerous change. A ***carcinoma*** is a malignancy of epithelial tissue. Carcinomas of the lung, colon and breast are epithelial cancers.

Epithelial tissue is described by its histologic appearance. If it has only ***one layer*** of cells, it is called ***simple.*** If it has more than one layer, it is called ***stratified.*** If the cells are square, the epithelium is called ***cuboidal;*** if elongated, ***columnar;*** if flattened, ***squamous.*** Thus epithelium can be identified as "stratified squamous," "simple columnar," and so on. ***Simple columnar*** epithelium lines the trachea, bronchioles, GI tract, uterus and fallopian tubes. ***Simple cuboidal*** epithelium lines the tubules of the liver, kidneys and most glands. ***Simple squamous*** epithelium lines the inner layer of blood vessels (endothelium) and the alveoli of the lungs.

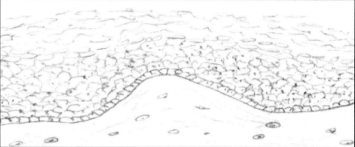

Above: Simple squamous epithelium

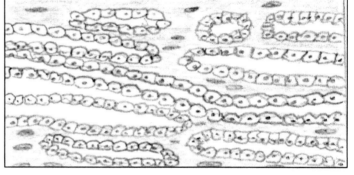

Stratified squamous epithelium

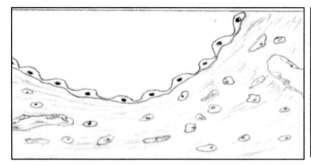

Simple columnar epithelium

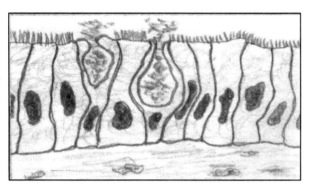

Simple cuboidal epithelium

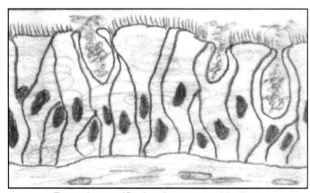

Pseudostratified columnar epithelium

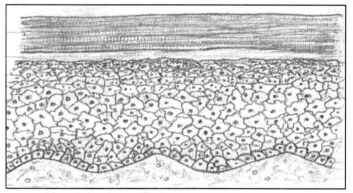

Keratinized stratified squamous epithelium

Stratified cuboidal epithelium is found in sweat glands, ovarian follicles and the seminiferous tubules of the testes. ***Stratified squamous*** epithelium lines the skin (epidermis), oral mucosa, esophagus and adult vagina. The ***epidermis*** is the outer layer of skin; it is an epithelial tissue. The deeper layer of skin is the ***dermis***, which is connective tissue. Stratified squamous epithelium is divided into ***keratinized***, where the outer layer consists of products of a layer of dead cells (keratin), or it may be ***nonkeratinized***. The epidermis is keratinized stratified squamous epithelium. The inside of the mouth, throat, esophagus and adult vagina are nonkeratinized stratified squamous epithelium.

Other descriptive types of epithelial tissue include **_pseudostratified_**, where the epithelium looks to be stratified but is not because all the cells touch the basement membrane; and **_transitional_**, which is a stretchable stratified epithelium of polygonal cells. Transitional epithelium covers the inside of the urinary bladder. Pseudostratified epithelium exists in the respiratory tract and the urinary tract at the junction of stratified squamous and simple columnar epithelia.

2. Connective tissue.

Connective tissue is derived from mesoderm. It is the most abundant and versatile tissue class. It has various functions including physical support, connection of bodily parts, internal communication, immunological protection, and energy storage.   Types of connective tissue include **_adipose tissue (fat), bone, cartilage, tendons, ligaments, blood, marrow_**, and unspecialized **_dense and loose connective tissue_** between the organs of the body. Cells in connective tissue are more dispersed than they are in epithelial tissue, which gives room for blood vessels and fibers. Located between the cells of connective tissue is the **_matrix,_** which varies considerably among the various types of connective tissues. For example the matrix of bone is composed of **_calcium salts_** and **_collagen_** fibers. The matrix of blood is **_plasma_**, and in the dense connective tissue of tendons and ligaments the matrix consists of fibrous bands of **_collagen_**.

Collagen is one of three types of connective tissue fibers. The other two types are **_reticular fibers_** and **_elastic fibers._** **_Collagen_** is a tough, flexible, stretch resistant protein fiber that makes up 25% of the body's protein. Collagen is white in color. It is the primary component of ligaments, tendons, the sclera of the eye and the dermis. Collagen is the basis for gelatin, leather and glue.

Reticular fibers are thin collagen fibers that are coated with a glycoprotein. Reticular fibers form a sponge-like framework for reticular tissue, which includes the spleen, lymph nodes and bone marrow. (Reticulum means "net".)

Elastic fibers are thin, yellow, branching fibers made up of the protein **_elastin_**. They are capable of stretching and recoiling, and they give the skin, arteries and lungs the ability to stretch and recoil.

The primary cell of unspecialized connective tissue is the **_fibroblast._** Fibroblasts produce collagen, the primary fiber of connective tissue. Collagen provides much of the **_matrix_** of connective tissues. (The matrix is the noncellular portion of a connective tissue.) The **_ground substance_** of a connective tissue is that part of the matrix that is nonfibrous. Ground substance may be in the form of a liquid, a chemical polymer or metallic salts. **_Serum_** is plasma minus its clotting factors; it is the ground substance of blood. The ground substance of bone is **_calcium salts_**; the ground substance of cartilage is **_chondroitin sulfate_**, and the ground substance of unspecified connective tissue is made up of **_glycosaminoglycans (GAGS), proteoglycans and glycoproteins._**

GAGS are huge complex molecules of carbohydrate and protein whose chief ingredients are polar disaccharides, which have the ability to attract sodium and potassium ions. Sodium and potassium ions attract water because of their polarity, which gives the GAG molecule the ability to hold water in a **_colloid_** state. Examples of GAGS as ground substance include **_chondroitin sulfate_** in cartilage, and **_hyaluronic acid_**, which is found in joint cavities and the vitreous of the eye.

Proteoglycans are also huge molecules. They are carbohydrate polymers with a protein moiety.   In tissues they are connected to GAGS to form a thin **_colloid_**, like a glue or gravy, which slows progression of an infection. Other proteoglycans are embedded in plasma membranes and bond cells together.

Glycoproteins found in connective tissue are adhesive molecules that bind cells and mark pathways for cellular migration. Hide glues are composed of proteoglycans and glycoproteins.

Other cells in connective tissue include **_macrophages_**, which are derived from monocytes of the blood. Macrophages are relatively large cells with mobility; they are propelled by the motor molecules, actin and myosin. They move through connective tissues and engulf unwanted particles like bacteria and foreign bodies by **_phagocytosis._** They are part of the immune system.

Adipose tissue is fat tissue, where fat is stored by the body. The primary cells of adipose tissue are **_adipocytes_**, large empty-looking connective tissue cells that are filled with fat, primarily as triglycerides. Fat serves to store energy, insulate, fill spaces and establish body contours. Adult fat is white fat, but infants and hibernating animals possess sizeable stores of **_brown fat_**. Unlike white fat, the catabolism of brown fat produces a lot of heat, but little or no ATP. An unusual incident that may involve brown fat has been reported. It involved a fishing vessel that capsized in frigid waters several miles off the coast of Iceland. The men who were on board died in the icy waters, but one successfully swam to shore. He was examined, hospitalized and found have only minimal hypothermia.   He was discharged the next day.   I consider it possible that he had stores of brown fat that were used to maintain his body heat while he was in the water.

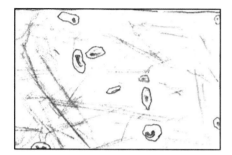

Loose (areolar) connective tissue

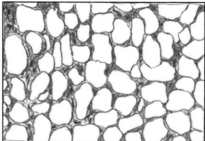

Adipose tissue

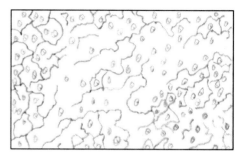

Reticular tissue

Unspecified connective tissue is classified as ***areolar (loose)*** or ***dense***.
Areolar tissue has a loose arrangement of collagen and elastic fibers. The ground substance (proteoglycans and glycoproteins) is abundant and cells are scanty. Areolar tissue is located between muscles, blood vessels and tendons, and it underlies epithelial tissue. Connective tissue under the skin (the ***hypodermis***) is areolar connective tissue, as is ***fascia,*** the connective tissue between muscles and organs.

The collagen fibers in ***dense connective tissue*** are densely packed with scanty ground substance and compressed fibroblasts. When collagen fibers are parallel, as they are in tendons and ligaments, it is called ***dense regular connective tissue***. When the fibers run in several directions or at random as they do in the dermis, periosteum, perichondrium, fibrous part of the pericardium, and the sclera of the eye, it is called ***dense irregular connective tissue.***

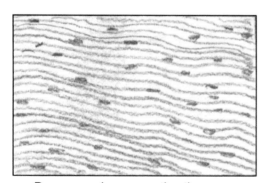

Dense regular connective tissue

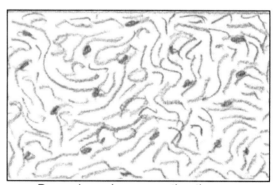

Dense irregular connective tissue

Cartilage helps give the body support. Cartilage consists of a rubbery matrix that is rich in chondroitin sulfate. Most cartilage is surrounded by a fibrous sheath called ***perichondrium***. ***Cartilage has no blood vessels***, so nutrients have to be obtained from blood vessels outside cartilaginous tissue. As a result injured cartilage heals very slowly. Unlike other tissues, some cartilage continues to grow slowly throughout life. Sharks lack bone; their skeleton is purely cartilaginous.

The matrix of cartilage is chondroitin sulfate plus fibers. ***Chondroblasts*** deposit the matrix of cartilage. When a chondroblast becomes embedded in the matrix, it becomes known as a ***chondrocyte***. Spaces in tissue sections of cartilage called ***lacunae*** (lakes) are areas where chondrocytes were located in life. The cells were removed from the lacunae by cutting and fixing the tissue.
A reserve population of chondroblasts exists between cartilage and the perichondrium. These cells contribute to the slow, continuous growth that is detectable in the nose and external ears. It has been reported that one of the signs of pernicious anemia is large ears, but pernicious anemia is a disease of the elderly, who naturally have large ears, and the link is now considered spurious.

There are three types of cartilage, ***hyaline, elastic and fibrous***, depending on the fibers in the matrix. ***Hyaline cartilage*** has a clear glassy matrix with only sparse fine collagen fibers. It is present in the larynx, trachea, bronchi, over the ends of bones at movable joints, and at the sternal ends of ribs. It makes up the fetal skeleton, which is later replaced by bone. Most hyaline cartilage is covered by a layer of perichondrium.

Elastic cartilage contains a web-like mesh of elastic fibers in the matrix. It is flexible, and it is covered by perichondrium. The external ear and epiglottis are examples of elastic cartilage.

Fibrocartilage contains a large amount of collagen fibers, which make it especially strong. It is much more capable of resisting compression and absorbing shock than other types of cartilage. Fibrocartilage lacks a perichondrium; consequently, it does not grow during adulthood. Fibrocartilage fills the menisci of the knee and the intervertebral discs.

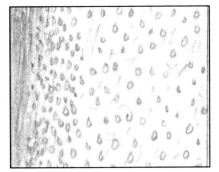
Hyaline cartilage

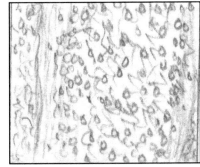
Elastic cartilage

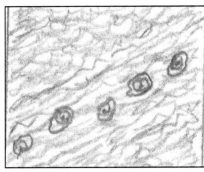
Fibrocartilage

Bone is a type of connective tissue that is specialized for (1) physical support, (2) leverage for muscles and (3) mineral storage for calcium and phosphorus.   The ground substance accounts for two-thirds of the weight of bone. ***Hydroxyapatite*** [$Ca_{10}(PO_4)_6(OH)_2$] makes up ***85% of the ground substance***; calcium carbonate ($CaCO_3$) makes up 10%, and other calcium and magnesium salts make up 5%. The matrix of bone includes collagen fibers in addition to these salts. The hardness of bone is due to the ground substance. Collagen fibers prevent bone from becoming too brittle and breakable. Bone has a supportive function, and the marrow of bone is the area of the body where blood cells are made.

Compact bone occupies the cylindrical areas of long bones and the outer shell of all bones. It is composed of concentric layers of bone called ***lamellae*** with embedded ***lacunae***. ***Osteoblasts*** lay down the bony matrix. An osteoblast that has become surrounded by ground substance becomes embedded in a lacuna, and it becomes known as an ***osteocyte***. An ***osteon*** is the structural unit of bone; it has a ***Haversian or central canal*** in its center. The Haversian canal contains blood vessels, and it is surrounded by lamellae. Osteocytes in the lamellae receive their blood supply from vessels in the Haversian canals. Tiny processes called ***canaliculi*** connect the osteocytes. Canaliculi are ***gap junctions***, which are direct cell to cell connections. Nutrients, oxygen and other materials are passed from one cell to another through canaliculi. ***Osteoclasts*** are large multinucleated cells that reabsorb and shape bone.

Spongy bone fills the heads of long bones and some of the cavities of other bones. It has fingers or spicules of bone called ***trabeculae,*** which appear delicate, but are surprisingly strong in helping bone fill its supportive role. Spongy bone is never on the surface of a bone; it is always covered by a layer of compact bone.

Bone is surrounded by a fibrous sheath called ***periosteum.***   Both the periosteum of bone and the perichondrium of cartilage are derived from mesoderm; they lack a basement membrane, and they are connective tissues.

Right: The units of compact bone are cylinders called osteons. The dark circles are Haversian canals; the concentric circles making up an osteon are lamellae; the small dark ellipsoidal areas are lacunae; the radial lines are canaliculi. Haversian canals contain blood vessels; lacunae contain osteocytes; canaliculi are gap junctions between osteocytes.

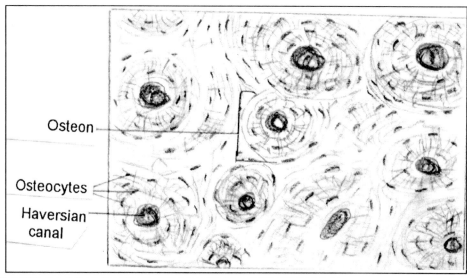

Osteon

Osteocytes

Haversian canal

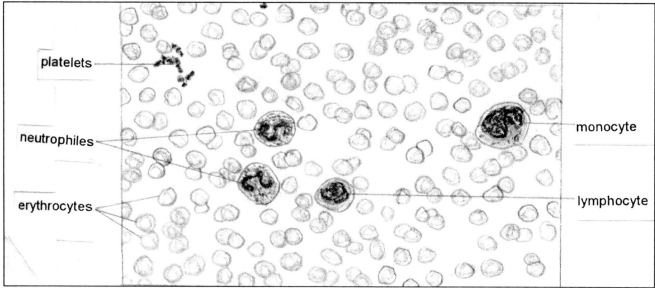

platelets

neutrophiles

erythrocytes

monocyte

lymphocyte

Above: A blood smear. Numerous erythrocytes are visible in this illustration. Thrombocytes (platelets) can be seen in the upper left corner. The white blood cells in this illustration are two polymorphonuclear leukocytes (neutrophiles, or "polys"), one lymphocyte, and one monocyte.

Blood is a liquid connective tissue. The mass of blood is normally 38-50% cells and 50-62% liquid. Men have a higher cellular content in their blood than women. The liquid portion is **plasma**, which is the matrix of blood. Cells of the blood are produced in the bone marrow; they circulate through the heart and blood vessels. The two primary types of blood cells are **erythrocytes** (red blood cells, RBCs, or red corpuscles), and **leukocytes** (white blood cells or WBCs). The red cells are unusual in that they lose their nucleus in the process of maturing. RBCs are essentially tight little packages of **hemoglobin**, a protein-iron complex that transports oxygen to the tissues. White cells serve various immunologic, chemical and scavenger roles. White cells are divided into **granulocytes (neutrophiles, eosinophiles and basophiles)** and **agranulocytes (monocytes and lymphocytes.)** Other marrow cells are normally absent from the blood. **Macrophages** are tissue cells that are derived from monocytes. **Neutrophiles** (polymorphonuclear leukocytes or "polys") are smaller than macrophages, but, like macrophages, they serve to engulf and destroy bacteria by phagocytosis. **Eosinophiles** produce allergic globulins (globulins are proteins in the blood). **Basophiles** contain **histamine** (a vasodilator) and **heparin** (a GAG molecule that is an anticoagulant). **Mast cells** are tissue basophiles, but they are not derived from basophiles in the blood. **Plasma**

cells are derived from a type of lymphocyte ("B" lymphocytes). They are normally absent from the blood. Plasma cells and B lymphocytes synthesize antibodies, which are large proteins that inactivate invasive microorganisms. *Lymphocytes* are produced in the marrow, thymus gland and lymph nodes.   There are two varieties of lymphocytes, type B (from bone) and type T (from the thymus gland). Lymphocytes control antibody production.

A malignancy arising in connective tissue or muscle tissue is called a *sarcoma.* Sarcomas are classified according to the connective tissue in which they arise. Sarcomas include osteosarcomas, chondrosarcomas, lymphosarcomas, fibrosarcomas and liposarcomas.

Several inherited diseases are associated with defective connective tissue fibers. *Marfan's syndrome* is a disorder of *elastin*, the glycoprotein that makes up elastic fibers. Individuals with Marfan's syndrome tend to be tall and lean with long limbs and fingers. They are prone to spinal curvatures, weak heart valves, weak arterial walls, hernias, dislocation of the lenses of the eyes (ectopia lentis), and a pigeon chest deformity (pectus carinatum). Heart failure and rupture of the aorta are complications of Marfan's syndrome.

Ehlers-Danlos syndrome is a hereditary *defect of collagen synthesis* manifest by an amazing looseness and ability of the skin and joints to stretch. Weakness in the arterial walls of these people may lead to rupture of a large artery. People with Ehlers-Danlos syndrome are sometimes on display in circuses because of the laxness of their skin and joints.

Osteogenesis imperfecta, or "brittle bone disease," is a disorder manifest by *defective collagen* throughout the body. Patients with this disease suffer multiple fractures because the collagen fibers in their bones does not provide adequate flexible support. Multiple fractures often lead to deformities in these patients. The sclera of the eyes of individuals with osteogenesis imperfecta is blue; the defective collagen allows the brown pigment (melanin) inside the eye to show through the sclera as a blue color. They also typically suffer from deafness due to otosclerosis, which is fibrosis (scarring) around the tiny bones of the middle ear.

Rickets is a debilitating and deforming disease of childhood that is due to insufficient ground substance (calcium salts) in bones. The adult counterpart to rickets is *osteomalacia.* Rickets and osteomalacia can result from a dietary insufficiency of calcium or from inadequate absorption of calcium. A lack of vitamin D is the most common cause for poor calcium absorption.

Scurvy is a disease caused by the lack of vitamin C (ascorbic acid). This vitamin is needed for the synthesis of the amino acids, tyrosine and proline, which are necessary for *collagen synthesis*. Poor wound healing and subcutaneous hemorrhages are symptoms of a lack of vitamin C.

3. Muscular tissue.
The body has three types of muscular tissue: skeletal, smooth and cardiac.

A muscle cell is a muscle fiber, and *skeletal* muscles have long cylindrical threadlike fibers.   The cells are multinucleated. Skeletal muscles are *voluntary*, meaning that the conscious brain tells them when to contract. They are the strong muscles in your extremities and trunk, and they are the muscles of facial expression and eye movement.   Skeletal muscles are called *striated* muscles because the cells have visible striations when viewed under a microscope

Cardiac muscle cells are also striated, but the striations are not as pronounced as they are in skeletal muscle fibers. They differ from skeletal muscle in other ways: (1) Cardiac muscle cells are shorter, and they are branched. (2) Most cardiac myocytes (muscle cells) contain only one nucleus. (3) There are prominent dividers between cardiac muscle cells called *intercalated discs*; these are *gap junctions* that speed nerve conduction.

Smooth muscle fibers are relatively short, and they are *fusiform* in shape. They lack striations; they are *involuntary* (they contract without the conscious brain telling them to), and they contain only one nucleus. Smooth muscle controls the autonomic functions of the body, including those of the GI tract, blood vessels, uterus, bronchi, and the constrictor and dilator of the pupil.

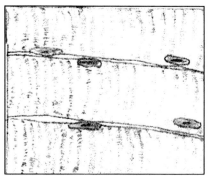
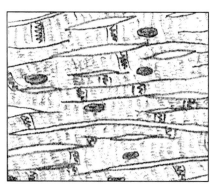
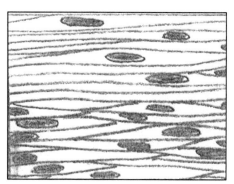

| Skeletal muscle | Cardiac muscle | Smooth muscle |

4. Nervous tissue.

Nervous tissue consists of the brain, spinal cord and peripheral nerves. The basic cell of nerve tissue is the **neuron**, which is a large stellate cell with long cell processes called **dendrites** and **axons** that are used to communicate with other cells. Neurons are found in the brain, spinal cord and peripheral ganglia. Neurons in the central nervous system and the ganglia are surrounded by abundant cells called **glial cells**. Glial cells come in three types, **astrocytes, oligodendrocytes and microglia.** Each type has a special function. Astrocytes serve a protective and nutritive role to neurons. Oligodendrocytes surround nerve tracts and serve to hasten the nerve impulse. Microglial cells are scavengers that remove unwanted debris and fight infection.

Right: Tissue of the central nervous system. The large cell is a neuron. The processes extending from the cell body of the neuron are numerous dendrites and one axon (lower right). The small dark cells are glial cells.

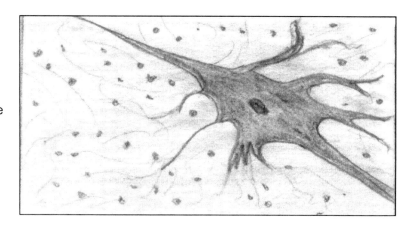

An **organ** is a structure in the body that contains two or more tissue types. Organs serve a special function and have boundaries.

A **gland** is an organ that **secretes** a particular substance that has a function for the body.

Exocrine glands release their secretions into a duct or tube that leads to a surface, such as the skin or the inside of the GI tract.

Endocrine glands are "ductless" and secrete their products directly into the blood stream.

Hormones are the chemical secretions of endocrine glands that exert an effect elsewhere in the body.

Paracrine glands secrete hormone-like chemicals into local tissues, and they have only localized effects.

Some organs have both exocrine and endocrine secretions. For example the **liver** is an exocrine gland that secretes bile into the GI tract through the bile duct. The liver is an endocrine gland that secretes albumin and other proteins into the blood. The **pancreas** secretes enzymes into the GI tract through the pancreatic duct (an exocrine function); it also secretes the hormones, insulin and glucagon, directly into the blood (an endocrine function).

The **parenchyma** of a gland is made up of epithelial cells that produce secretions.

The **stroma** of a gland is the connective tissue framework that includes a capsule with extensions called septae, which divide the gland into regions called lobes and lobules.

A **simple** exocrine gland is a small gland with only one unbranched duct. A **compound** exocrine gland has a duct that is branched.

A *serous* gland produces a thin watery secretion.

A *mucous* gland produces the glycoprotein, *mucin*, which becomes a thick, sticky secretion called *mucus* after it is hydrated. (Mucus is the noun; mucous is the adjective form). A *goblet cell* is a one-cell gland in the epithelium of the respiratory tract and the GI tract that secretes mucin.

A *mixed* gland produces both a serous and a mucous secretion.

Salivary glands are all three types. The *parotid* glands are serous, the *sublingual* glands are mucous, and the *submandibular* glands are mixed.

Cytogenic glands are exocrine glands that release whole cells. The only examples of cytogenic glands in humans are the testes, which secrete sperm cells, and the ovaries, which secrete ova.

Holocrine glands secrete breakdown products of dead cells. Sebaceous glands in the skin and meibomian glands in the eyelids are holocrine glands.

Merocrine glands produce their secretions by *exocytosis.* Sudoriferous (sweat) glands in the skin and ceruminous glands in the external ear canals are merocrine glands.

Apocrine glands are specialized merocrine glands; the mammary glands and sweat glands in the axilla (arm pit) and the groin are apocrine glands.

Membranes are epithelial or connective tissue linings of organs or cavities. The *epidermis of the skin* is the cutaneous membrane of the body. It is a relatively dry *epithelial* tissue of ectodermal origin that consists of several layers. The outer layer is the *keratin layer*, which is derived from dead cellular remains. The *dermis* lies beneath the epidermis, and it supports the epidermis. The dermis is *connective tissue* of mesodermal origin. Membranes that are connective tissue include the peritoneum, pleura, periosteum, perichondrium, the synovial lining around joints, the outer layer of pericardium surrounding the heart, and the dura mater surrounding the brain and spinal cord. Epithelial tissue membranes contain a basement membrane; connective tissue membranes lack a basement membrane.

A *serous* membrane, or *serosa*, is a thin connective tissue membrane that covers organs and cavities in the body. A serous membrane is *kept wet* by the constant secretion of a serous (watery) fluid by cells of the membrane. The peritoneum and pleura are serosal membranes derived from mesoderm. Serosal membranes of connective tissue are called *mesothelia,* (singular, mesothelium).

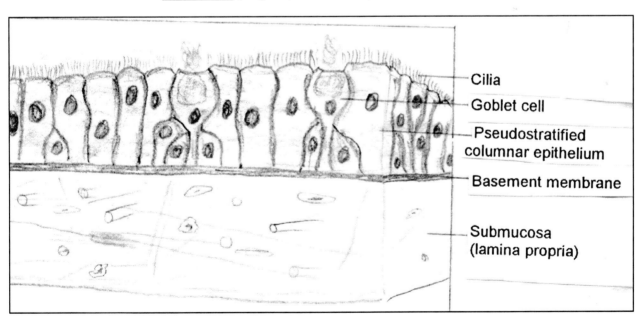

Above: A mucous membrane of the respiratory tract.   Cilia can be seen as projections from the cell membrane above. Two goblet cells can be seen secreting mucin. The epithelium is pseudostratified columnar. The submucosa (lamina propria) with its blood vessels is seen below. The basement membrane separates the epithelial tissue above from the submucosa, which is connective tissue.

A **_mucous_** **_membrane_**, or **_mucosa_**, is lubricated and kept wet by serous and mucus secretions of its cells and glands. Mucus serves to lubricate and trap foreign particles and bacteria. Mucous membranes consist of **(1)** an **_epithelial layer_**, **(2)** a deeper layer called the **_lamina propria_** or **_submucosa_** that is connective tissue and contains blood vessels, and **(3)** a basal layer containing smooth muscle called the **_muscularis mucosae_**. Mucous membranes are found in the digestive, respiratory, urinary and reproductive tracts.

Epithelial cells of mucous membranes may contain appendages. **_Microvilli_** are extensions of the plasma membrane of epithelial cells that serve to greatly increase the surface area of the plasma membrane, which increases the absorptive powers of a cell. **_Cilia_** are hair-like projections from the cell that propel mucus and debris. Cilia allow removal of unwanted inspired material from the respiratory tract.

Tissues sometimes change from one type to another. This change may be simply due to maturity, such as the change from mesenchyme to muscle tissue or the change from simple cuboidal to nonkeratinized stratified squamous in the adolescent vagina. The change of a tissue from one type to another is called **_metaplasia_**. Metaplasia is not always innocuous. An actinic keratosis is a precancerous skin lesion that has undergone a metaplastic change as a result of excessive sun exposure.

Hyperplasia is tissue or organ growth through cell multiplication.

Hypertrophy is enlargement of an organ by the enlargement of preexisting cells.

Neoplasia is a malignant (cancerous) tumor.

Atrophy is shrinkage of an organ from loss of cellular size or number.

Necrosis is the pathological (abnormal) death of an organism, a tissue or a cell.

Apoptosis is the programmed death of a cell. Billions of cells in your body die every hour and are replaced. Cells in the GI tract live an average of 3-6 days. The products of the dead cells are rarely seen because they are quickly engulfed by macrophages.

Damaged tissue can be repaired by **_regeneration_**, in which dead cells are replaced by the same type of cells, or by **_fibrosis_**, where the dead tissue is replaced by collagen fibers producing scar tissue. A scar will hold tissue together, but it does not restore function. Skin and liver have the ability to regenerate to an extent, but most organs do not have that ability and heal by fibrosis.

When skin is lacerated, healing occurs in several stages. First, damaged mast cells leak histamine, which dilates the blood vessels, increases capillary permeability and increases blood flow. Plasma seeps into the wound accompanied by antibodies, clotting factors and leukocytes. A clot then forms with an **_eschar_** (scab) on the surface. Macrophages and neutrophiles get to work cleaning up debris and fighting bacteria. Next, new capillaries grow into the wound creating **_granulation tissue,_** a loose, friable tissue that bleeds easily. Fibroblasts grow into the wound, and after 3-4 days they have begun to deposit new collagen. Surface epithelial cells multiply and spread beneath the eschar. The eschar falls off when the epithelium has **_regenerated,_** spread over the entire wound and thickened.

Keloids are elevated, firm, rubbery, benign tumors that develop within skin scars at sites of healing. They result from excessive fibrosis secondary to an excessive production of fibrocyte growth factors. They occur most commonly in Negroes.

Study Guide

1. Define histology.
2. Know the three primary germ cell layers of the embryo (ectoderm, mesoderm and endoderm), and what tissues are derived from each.
3. Know the four tissue types (epithelial, connective, muscle and nervous) and the characteristics of their histology.
4. Know that the presence of a basement membrane defines a tissue as epithelial.
5. Recognize the various types of epithelia and know where they are found (simple squamous, stratified squamous, simple columnar, pseudostratified columnar, transitional, cuboidal, keratinized and nonkeratinized.
6. Know the various types of tissues that are classified as connective tissue (blood, adipose tissue, cartilage, bone, areolar connective tissue, and dense connective tissue).
7. Understand the meaning of the terms matrix and ground substance.

8. Know the three types of fibers in connective tissue (collagen, elastic and reticular). Appreciate the tremendous importance and prevalence of collagen fibers and fibroblasts in your body.
9. Recognize the following compounds: hydroxyapatite, calcium carbonate, glycosaminoglycans (GAGS), chondroitin sulfate, hyaluronic acid, proteoglycans and glycoproteins. Know their characteristics and where they may be found.
10. Know the terms leukocyte, erythrocyte, neutrophile, lymphocyte, monocyte, eosinophile, basophile, mast cell, plasma cell, and macrophage as they relate to cells found in tissues and blood.
11. Know the functions and characteristics of adipose tissue (fat).
12. Know the differences between yellow fat and brown fat.
13. Know the differences between the three types of cartilage (hyaline, elastic and fibrous) and where each can be found.
14. Define perichondrium and periosteum. Are they connective tissues or epithelial tissues?
15. Know the cell types of bone and their function (osteoblasts, osteocytes and osteoclasts).
16. Understand the structure of compact bone, spongy bone, and bone marrow.
17. Appreciate the structure of an osteon and its parts including canaliculi, lamellae, osteocytes, lacunae, and the central (Haversian) canal.
18. Recognize the following disorders: rickets, osteomalacia, Marfan's syndrome, Ehlers Danlos syndrome, osteogenesis imperfecta and scurvy.
19. Know the three types of muscle tissue (skeletal, smooth and cardiac) and their identifiable histological characteristics.
20. Be able to identify the following terms relating to glands: endocrine, exocrine, paracrine, stroma, parenchyma, mucous, serous, cytogenic, holocrine, sebaceous, merocrine, and apocrine.
21. Know the following terms in relation to mucous membranes: goblet cells, mucin, mucus, epithelial layer, lamina propria, submucosa, and muscularis mucosa.
22. Know the meaning of these terms: necrosis, apoptosis, metaplasia, neoplasia, hyperplasia, hypertrophy and atrophy.

Chapter Six

The Integument

The integument is the skin with its associated glands, hair and nails.

Functions of the skin

Skin can correctly be termed an organ of the body because it is a contiguous structure with uniform functions, and it contains more than one type of tissue. As such it is the largest organ in the body, constituting around 15% of the body's weight. Skin functions as a ***protective barrier***. Skin secretions have a pH of about 5.5, due to the presence of fatty acids and lactic acid. This gives skin an ***acid mantle*** that is fungicidal and bactericidal. Oils in the secretions of skin glands and glycolipids in the epidermis provide water resistance. Vitamin D undergoes activation in the skin when it is exposed to ultraviolet (uv) light. A small amount of oxygen is absorbed through the skin, and the skin gives off small amounts of carbon dioxide and volatile chemicals. The fat-soluble vitamins (A, D, E, and K) can be absorbed through the skin. The skin is sensitive to touch, heat, cold, pressure and pain, through which it alerts the body to the environment. Blood vessels in the skin can dilate or contract, and sweat glands in the skin can increase or decrease their activity.   Both of these functions help to control the body's temperature.

Skin consists of an outer layer, the ***epidermis,*** and an inner layer, the ***dermis.*** The ***hypodermis*** is a layer consisting mostly of adipose tissue that is located beneath the dermis, but the hypodermis is not regarded as part of the integument. The hypodermis is connective tissue; it is otherwise known as the ***superficial fascia***. The word ***cutaneous*** refers to the skin and its associated hair, nails and glands.

The thickest skin covers the palms and soles. The thinnest skin is in the eyelids.

Epidermis

The epidermis is a ***keratinized stratified squamous epithelial*** layer that is derived from ectoderm; it has closely packed cells and very little intercellular material. Hair, nails, and the glands of the skin are epidermal in origin. The epidermis lacks blood vessels and must receive nutrients from the underlying dermis. The epidermis is composed of up to five layers. The deepest layer is the ***stratum basalis***, or basal layer. This layer sits on a ***basement membrane***, which separates the epidermis from the dermis and is present in all epithelial tissues. The ***basement membrane*** is a thin, tough layer of glycoproteins, GAGS and collagen that acts as a barrier to large molecules and pathogens (germs).   The stratum basalis is anchored to the basement membrane by hemidesmosomes.

Cells of the stratum basalis are cuboidal to low columnar in shape. A majority of the cells in the stratum basalis are keratinocytes, which undergo frequent mitosis. Pigment producing cells called ***melanocytes*** are also present in this layer. Melanocytes produce several related pigments that are collectively called melanin. Melanin granules are picked up by neighboring keratinocytes. The darker form of melanin (eumelanin) is highly effective as a barrier to ultraviolet light, and it is effective in preventing skin cancer.

 If skin darkened by melanin is protective, why have some races of people evolved to have pale skin? The answer may be that melanin blocks ultraviolet rays that activate vitamin D in the skin. Days are brief in higher latitudes during the winter, and the Sun never rises very high above the horizon. People in cold climes are accustomed to covering nearly all of their bodies in order to keep warm. As a result little sunlight reaches their skin and little vitamin D is activated. A lack of vitamin D leads to rickets and osteomalacia, which are crippling, deforming diseases.

Deeper layers of the epidermis contain sensory nerve endings, specifically ***Merkel discs*** and ***bare nerve endings***.

External to the stratum basalis is the ***stratum spinosum***, or spiny cell layer. The stratum spinosum contains several layers of keratinocytes, which have been pushed outward by the constantly dividing cells of the stratum basalis. Keratinocytes in the stratum spinosum pick up melanin granules produced by the melanocytes in the stratum basalis. Some of the deeper cells in the stratum spinosum undergo mitosis. Keratinocytes in the stratum spinosum are rich in RNA, and they produce precursors of ***keratin,*** the protective protein that comprises the outermost layer of skin. ***Macrophages*** called Langerhans cells or dendritic cells migrate to the spiny cell layer from the dermis and serve to phagocytize bacteria and debris. The stratum spinosum gets its name from the appearance of the keratinocytes in this layer following fixation, which causes cells to shrink and have spiny processes that they do not have in life.

Above the spiny cell layer is the granulosa cell layer or ***stratum granulosum***. This stratum consists of several layers of keratinocytes whose prekeratin molecules have begun to coalesce into granules. Also present in the stratum granulosum are ***glycolipids*** that help to waterproof the skin. Cells in the outer part of the stratum granulosum are removed from their blood supply in the dermis, and they are at the edge of survivability. Cells in the outer portion of the stratum granulosum are beginning to die.

The ***stratum lucidum*** is external to the stratum granulosum. The stratum lucidum is only present in areas where skin is thickest, such as the palms and soles. This layer contains dead or nearly dead keratinocytes that have indistinct boundaries and have lost their nuclei and organelles. They are packed with ***eleidin***, a translucent precursor to keratin. Eleidin is present in the skin of the lips, where it makes the skin more translucent and, therefore, redder, although the lips do not contain a stratum lucidum layer.

The outermost layer of epidermis is the ***stratum corneum***, which consists of keratin from the remains of dead cells. Layers of the stratum corneum exfoliate (flake off) and are constantly being replaced. When subjected to pressure over a period of time, the stratum corneum responds by increasing in thickness, which results in calluses or "corns." The word corneum means "horn."

The lifetime of a skin cell averages about 30-40 days, but the replacement time for these cells can be reduced to 1-3 days following an injury.

Dermis

The dermis is ***connective tissue***, and it is derived from mesoderm. The thickness of the dermis varies from 0.2mm in the eyelids to 4mm in the palms and soles. The dermis contains blood vessels, nerve endings, hair follicles and skin glands.   Hair and the glands of skin are epithelial (epidermal) in origin, but these structures extend from the epidermis into the dermis. The dermis contains ***papillae***, which are ridge-like extensions of the dermis toward the epidermis.

The outer layer of the dermis is called the ***papillary layer***. It is an ***areolar connective tissue*** that contains ***papillae***, which are responsible for the ridges that make fingerprints, palm prints and footprints.   When doing a finger stick for a drop of blood, you will have more success if you puncture perpendicular to the ridges of a fingerprint because that technique will puncture capillaries in several dermal papillae. ***Meissner corpuscles*** (also known as ***tactile corpuscles***) are present in the papillary layer. They are nerve endings that respond to light touch.   Meissner corpuscles are more concentrated in sensitive areas such as the fingertips, eye lids, lips and genitalia.

The ***reticular layer*** of the dermis is deep to the papillary layer. The reticular layer contains a greater amount of collagen fibers, which run in all directions, and it is classified as ***dense irregular connective tissue***. ***Piloerector (arrector pili)*** muscles are smooth muscle cells that are attached to hair follicles in the reticular layer. Piloerector muscles elevate hair when they contract. ***Pacinian corpuscles*** are ***lamellated*** nerve endings sensitive to pressure that are located deep in the reticular layer. Collagen fibers in the reticular layer can be pulled apart due to stretching during pregnancy and in patients with Cushing's syndrome   Cushing's syndrome involves an overproduction of glucocorticoid hormones by the adrenal glands, which may produce ***striae*** or "stretch marks."

Hypodermis

The hypodermis is not part of the skin. It is a layer of ***subcutaneous fascia,*** which is loose ***areolar connective tissue***. The hypodermis is rich in ***adipose*** tissue, and it is highly vascular. It serves to insulate the body from cold temperatures, and it helps to protect deeper structures against trauma.

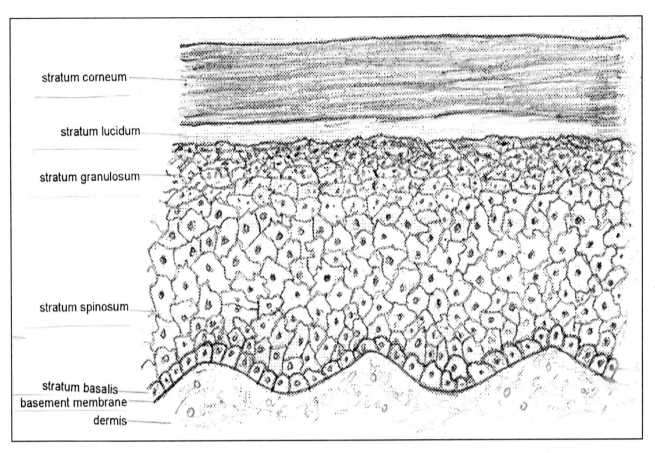

Above: The layers of the epidermis. The outer layer is at the top in this drawing.

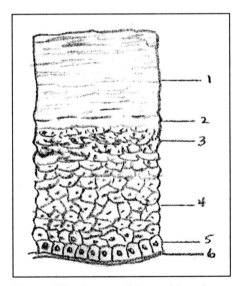

Above: The layers of the epidermis are numbered. (1) the stratum corneum, (2) the stratum lucidum, (3) the stratum granulosum, (4) the stratum spinosum, (5) the stratum basalis, (6) the basement membrane. (The stratum lucidum is only present where skin is thickest.)

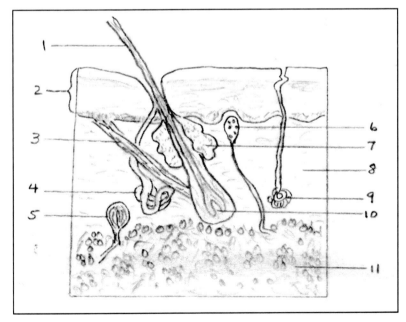

Above: An illustration of skin. (1) hair shaft, (2) epidermis, (3) piloerector muscle, (4) apocrine gland, (5) pacinian corpuscle, (6) Meissner corpuscle, (7) sebaceous gland, (8) dermis, (9) sweat gland, (10) hair bulb, (11) hypodermis.

Hair

Hair is an appendage of the epidermis that extends into the dermis. Whereas the stratum corneum is composed of soft, pliable keratin, the keratin of hair and nails is of the ___hard___ type. Keratin is hardened by the formation of ___disulfide (S-S) bridges___ between sulfur-containing amino acids. Hair is found throughout most of the skin of the body exclusive of only a few areas. Areas lacking hair include the lips, palms and soles. ___Lanugo___ hair is fine, unpigmented hair that is found only in the fetus. ___Vellus___ hair is fine, unpigmented hair of children, and it makes up two-thirds of the hair of women. ___Terminal___ hair is pigmented and coarse. It makes up the hair of the scalp. Ninety percent of all hair in men is terminal hair.

A hair is a filament of dead keratinized cells. The ___shaft___ is that part of the hair that is above the surface of the skin. The ___root___ is that part below the skin surface. The root is surrounded by an invagination of the epidermis called the hair ___follicle___. The follicle is situated obliquely in the skin, and the ___piloerector muscle___ is attached to the follicle.

In cross section the shaft of a hair can be seen to consist of an inner ___medulla___ that is surrounded by a central ___cortex___, which contains ___melanin___. The ___cuticle___ is the outer portion that surrounds the cortex. Hair grows at the ___bulb___, a swollen area at the base of the root where cellular division takes place. A tuft of dermal capillaries is present at the base of the bulb, which nourishes the growing hair.

___Determinate___ hair grows to a specific length and then stops. ___Indeterminate___ hair continues to grow. Scalp hair is indeterminate. If the shaft of a hair is ___round,___ that hair will be straight. If the shaft is ___flattened,___ the hair will be kinky. If the shaft is ___oval,___ the hair will be wavy

___Melanin___ is a variety of yellow, red, brown and black pigments produced by polymers of the amino acid, tyrosine. ___Eumelanin___ is quite dark; it is highly effective as a barrier to ultraviolet light and in the prevention of skin cancer. The choroid of the eye in all races of humans is full of eumelanin. ___Pheomelanin___ is a form of melanin that contains iron and sulfur. Pheomelanin and eumelanin are found in the hair and skin of blondes in varying amounts. Pheomelanin offers considerably less protection against uv radiation; fair skinned redheads are the most vulnerable group for the development of skin cancer. White hair contains no melanin.

Hair grows at an average speed of one mm every three days. After two to four years, an indeterminate hair becomes dormant and stops growing. When the bulb resumes activity, the old hair falls out and a new hair begins to grow.

___Alopecia___ is the medical term for baldness. Baldness may be genetic, or it may have a pathologic etiology (be caused by a disease). ___Hirsutism___ is a term that means "hairiness." The eyelashes are called ___cilia___, and hairs in the nostrils and ear canals are called ___vibrissae___. The eyebrows should not be shaved because they sometimes fail to regrow, especially in elderly women and those with a thyroid deficiency. Normally the hair follicles of eyebrows and eyelashes are actively growing for periods of only 3-4 months.

Nails

The suffix ___-nychium___ refers to nails. Nails are composed of dead cells of the stratum corneum that have produced layers of clear, hard keratin. Nails grow from a specialized area of the epidermis (the ___nail bed___) that is covered by skin (the ___cuticle or eponychium___). The flat, exposed part of the nail is called the ___nail plate___.

Thickened, disfigured nails are often the result of a fungus infection (___onychomycosis___). Psoriasis is a generalized skin disorder that can produce similar nail changes. White spots in the nail plate are due to anomalous keratinization; they may be caused by trauma, and they have been linked to a magnesium deficiency.

Fingernails grow approximately one millimeter per week. Toenail growth is much slower. Six weeks of medical treatment is recommended for onychomycosis of the fingernails; six months is recommended for toenail infections.

___"Clubbing"___ of the fingers is the enlargement of the distal phalanx and nail. It results from chronic cyanosis (chronic cardio-pulmonary dysfunction).

___Beau's lines___ are transverse depressions in the nails that reflect a temporary lack of nail growth. Any severe generalized disorder may produce Beau's lines. ___Mee's lines___ are transverse white lines in the nails that occur in arsenic poisoning.

Cutaneous glands

Sweat glands are called *sudoriferous* glands.   They are *merocrine* glands, all of which produce their secretions by *exocytosis*. The ducts of sudoriferous glands open through the skin to the outside.

Apocrine glands are specialized merocrine glands in the axillae and the groin that open into a hair follicle. The *mammary glands* are specialized apocrine glands. Mammary glands are active only during late pregnancy and lactation. Following delivery, the first secretion of *mammary glands* is a thin, protein rich, antibody rich liquid called *colostrum*. Breast milk, which has a high fat content, does not begin to be secreted until a few days after birth.

Sebaceous glands are *holocrine* glands, which produce secretions by *cellular apoptosis* (the normal death of glandular cells). Sebaceous glands have a short duct that opens into a hair follicle. The secretion of sebaceous glands is known as *sebum*. Sebum is oily, and it helps to protect and waterproof the skin. Lanolin is the name for sheep sebum that is sold commercially.

Ceruminous glands are merocrine glands in the ear canal. Ceruminous glands and sebaceous glands produce *cerumen*, or earwax, which is waterproof, acidic, bactericidal and fungicidal. Its bitterness repels mites and other insects.

Meibomian glands are modified sebaceous glands in the eyelids. An infected meibomian gland is called a *hordeolum* or sty.

Right: A sebaceous gland. Sebaceous glands are holocrine glands, which produce their secretions from the remains of dead cells.

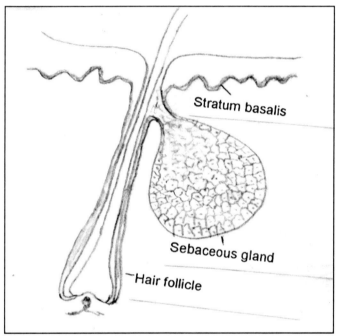

Disorders

Lightly pigmented skin is not totally opaque, and the body takes on different shades of color in some disease states. *Cyanosis* is a blueness of the skin that is due to the presence of more carbaminohemoglobin (hemoglobin with carbon dioxide) and less oxygenated hemoglobin. Cyanosis occurs primarily in heart and lung disorders. Oxygenated hemoglobin is red; carbaminohemoglobin is much darker. (Look at the color of your superficial veins and note that they are blue or nearly blue. This is because venous blood carries less oxygenated hemoglobin and more carbaminohemoglobin).

Polycythemia is the condition of having an excessive number of red cells in the blood. People with polycythemia are called "plethoric." They have a plethora of red blood cells, which gives them a distinctive dusky, cyanotic appearance because their lungs are unable to oxygenate all of their hemoglobin.

In *carbon monoxide poisoning* the patient has good color in spite of a lack of oxygen because the combination of carbon monoxide and hemoglobin produces a cherry red compound called carboxyhemoglobin.

Groups of related individuals in eastern Kentucky and other parts of the world have been found to have blue skin. Studies have shown that they have an unusually large amount of *methemoglobin*, an oxidized form of hemoglobin that is blue in color.

Erythema is an unusual redness of the skin due to dilated blood vessels, such as occurs during a fever or after exercise. Localized erythema is produced by local trauma or disease.

Jaundice is a yellow discoloration of the skin due to an excess of *bilirubin* in the blood. Bilirubin is a breakdown product of hemoglobin that is excreted into the bile by the liver, and jaundice is often associated with liver disease. Jaundice can be detected in the sclera (the whites of the eyes) as well as the skin.

Carotenemia is a yellowing of the skin produced by the excessive consumption of carotene, a form of vitamin A that is found in yellow, orange and red vegetables and in egg yolks. It is not associated with disease, although the liver of polar bears has been said to be toxic due to the large amount of vitamin A it contains.

Addison's disease is an adrenal gland disorder that results in a lack of steroid hormone production. To compensate the pituitary gland produces a large amount of ACTH (adrenocorticotropic hormone), which stimulates the adrenals. The excessive production of ACTH is accompanied by an excessive production of MSH (melanocyte stimulating hormone), which darkens the skin. *Sunlight* also stimulates melanocytes and darkens the skin.

Albinism is a genetic inability to synthesize melanin, and it is present in all races. Besides having pale skin, albinos have poor vision due to the lack of melanin pigment in their eyes.

Anemia produces pallor due to a low level of hemoglobin in the blood. A hemolytic anemia is caused by an excessive and premature breakdown of erythrocytes. Chloasma is a term that was formerly used for the anemia of young women whose pallor had a greenish tint, which was possibly due the presence of *biliverdin*, a precursor of bilirubin in the breakdown of hemoglobin.

Hemorrhage (bleeding) into or under the skin can take several forms. A *hematoma* is an elevated area filled with blood. *Petechiae* are small "splinter" hemorrhages. An *ecchymosis* is an extensive area of hemorrhage. *Purpura* are multiple dark localized hemorrhagic areas in the skin that are frequently raised. A *bruise* is a hemorrhage into or under the skin. A bruise may exhibit several different colors, depending upon its age. A bruise may be bright red from oxygenated blood; dark red or purple from carbaminohemoglobin; green from biliverdin, or yellow from bilirubin.

A *hemangioma* is a benign tumor of blood vessels. Hemangiomas are often present at birth, and many spontaneously disappear as the infant grows. Other types of hemangiomas do not disappear. Hemangiomas composed of capillaries are called *capillary hemangiomas*. If a hemangioma contains larger, thin walled vessels, it is known as a *cavernous hemangioma*.

A *hemangiosarcoma* is a malignant tumor of blood vessels. *Kaposi's sarcoma* is a type of hemangiosarcoma that is most common in older men and in immune disorders such as AIDS (acquired immuno-deficiency syndrome).

A *freckle or lentigo* is a flat hyperpigmented area resulting from an aggregation of melanocytes.

A *mole or nevus* is a benign tumor of melanocytes.

A *melanoma* is a malignant tumor of melanocytes. The individuals who are most likely to develop malignant melanomas are lightly pigmented individuals who have suffered sunburns, especially sunburns in childhood.

Skin develops creases as a result of muscle and joint actions. Creases can reveal underlying abnormalities. For example in *Down's syndrome (trisomy 21)* one of the horizontal creases of the palm of the hand is lacking. Detecting the lack of a palmer crease can lead to the diagnosis of Down's syndrome in a newborn.

Due to its exposure, skin is especially vulnerable to injury and disease. Ultraviolet light is a type of ionizing radiation that can produce free radicals, which are responsible for most skin cancers. Those cancers include (1) *basal cell carcinomas*, the most common type. Basal cell carcinomas grow locally but do not metastasize (establish new tumors at distant sites); (2) *squamous cell carcinomas*, which are more difficult to excise completely and can metastasize to local lymph nodes; and (3) *malignant melanomas*, which can metastasize rapidly and be deadly. A carcinoma can also arise from a sebaceous gland.

Burns to the skin are painful and can be life threatening. A first degree burn involves only the epidermis. A mild sunburn is an example of a first degree burn. Antioxidants such as vitamin E can reduce the number of free radicals in burned epidermal tissue and lead to more rapid healing of a first degree burn. A second degree burn involves a portion of the dermis. In second degree burns, the epidermis must regenerate from cells in the hair follicles and sweat glands, both of which are epidermal structures that extend into the dermis. A third degree burn destroys the epidermis and the dermis. Skin has lost its ability to protect deeper tissues in second and third degree burns; the dermis and deeper tissues have become exposed, which increases the vulnerability to infection.

If a large area of skin has suffered a third degree burn, debridement to clean away dead tissue and skin grafting to cover the defect will be necessary. Otherwise fluid loss and protein loss from the burned area could be fatal. Third degree burns destroy connective tissue in the dermis and lead to scarring and disfigurement. Some drugs, including some antibiotics (tetracyclines) and tranquilizers (phenothiazines), increase the sensitivity of the skin to ultraviolet light and can lead to a severe sunburn in a short period of exposure.

Study Guide

1. Define the integument.
2. Is the skin an organ? Explain.
3. Review the composition and the origin of the acid mantle.
4. Know the layers of the skin, the layers of the epidermis and the layers of the dermis.
5. Know where each layer of the skin is thickest, thinnest and missing.
6. What is the hypodermis, and how does it relate to the skin?
7. Review the basement membrane.
8. Review the types, function and location of melanin.
9. Know the types of nerve endings in the dermis and the epidermis.
10. Review the piloerector muscles.
11. Review the structure and characteristics of hair and nails. Know the terms alopecia, hirsutism, vibrissae and cilia as they relate to hair.
12. Know the names for various types of cutaneous glands including sudoriferous, sweat, apocrine, merocrine, mammary, sebaceous, meibomian, ceruminous and holocrine.
13. Know what sebum is and how it is produced.
14. Know the meaning of the following terms as they relate to skin: erythema, jaundice, carotinemia, Addison's disease, albinism, pallor, anemia, polycythemia, plethora, hemorrhage, ecchymosis, purpura, petechia, hemangioma, mole, nevus, melanoma, lentigo and freckle.
15. Know what keratin and eleidin are and where they are found.
16. What is onychomycosis?
17. What are Beau's lines?

Chapter Seven

Bone Tissue

Bone, or osseous tissue, is a type of connective tissue, and it is, therefore, derived from mesoderm. ***Bone, cartilage and ligaments*** make up the ***skeletal system***. Functions of the skeletal system include **(1)** support, **(2)** protection, **(3)** movement, **(4)** blood formation (hematopoiesis), **(5)** mineral storage (calcium, magnesium and phosphorus), **(6)** pH balance (phosphoric acids), and **(7)** isolation of toxic heavy metals such as lead and arsenic. Isolation limits their toxicity.

Bones are ***ossified***, meaning they contain salt crystals of several calcium and magnesium phosphates. Most bones are closely associated with ***cartilage*** in the body. Cartilage is an avascular (lacks blood vessels) tissue with a matrix of fibers and chondroitin sulfate. The ***perichondrium*** is a connective tissue membrane that surrounds some cartilage.

Bones are classified according to their shape and process of development. ***Long bones*** are cylindrical and longer than they are wide. The cylinder, which encloses the ***medullary cavity***, is composed of dense ***compact bone***. ***Spongy bone*** consists of ***trabeculae,*** which are spicules of bone at the ends of long bones and within the medullary cavity. Spongy bone is always encased in compact bone. Spongy bone weighs less than compact bone, and although it is not solid bone, it contributes appreciably to the strength of a bone because the trabeculae develop along lines of stress. ***Marrow*** is inside the medullary cavity. Marrow contains both adipose tissue and ***hematopoietic*** (blood forming) tissue. The cells and platelets of the blood are formed in hematopoietic tissue. The ***periosteum*** is a fibrous dense connective tissue membrane around bone. Compact bone is perforated by ***nutrient foramina*** (openings) which admit blood vessels to bone and the medullary cavity.

Examples of ***long bones*** include bones of the hands, feet, legs and arms. The wrist and ankle bones are classified as ***short bones***. The vertebrae, ethmoid and sphenoid bones are classified as ***irregular bones.*** The ribs, sternum, scapulae, pelvis and most cranial bones are classified as ***flat bones***. Cranial bones are constructed as a sandwich of compact bone with a layer of spongy bone in the center. They are called ***diploë***, or ***cancellous bones***. ***Sesamoid bones*** are bones that develop within a tendon, and ***wormian bones*** are small bones within a suture joint of the skull.

Long bones and short bones develop from a ***template of hyaline cartilage***. A ***primary ossification center*** develops in the center of the cartilaginous template, and the primary ossification center expands toward each end of the bone. A collar of ossification forms from the perichondrium. This collar becomes compact bone; it is the beginning of the area known as the ***diaphysis.*** The primary ossification center develops a cavity which becomes the ***medullary cavity***. ***A secondary ossification center*** develops at each end of the larger long bones. Bones of the fingers and toes are long bones, but they develop only one secondary ossification center. The ends of long bones become an area of spongy bone called the ***epiphysis***.

The cartilaginous area between the primary and secondary ossification centers is known as the ***metaphysis.*** The metaphysis contains five histological zones of transformation from cartilage to bone.

The epiphysis at each end of a long bone is larger in diameter than the diaphysis, but the diaphysis has greater length. The larger diameter of the epiphysis provides more area for tendons and ligaments to insert, and it strengthens joints. As the bone matures, an ***epiphyseal plate,*** or growth plate, forms in the metaphysis between the diaphysis and the epiphysis. Long bones increase in length at their ***epiphyseal plates***. Bone is laid down at both the epiphyseal end of the plate and the diaphyseal end. In this process ***chondrocytes*** of the epiphyseal plates undergo mitosis and hypertrophy, thereby lengthening the area of cartilage. Then the cartilage begins to ossify, and chondrocytes give way to ***osteoblasts***, which transform calcified cartilage into bone. The longitudinal growth of a long bone stops when chondrocytes cease multiplying, the cartilage in the epiphyseal plates becomes completely transformed into bone, and the diaphysis and epiphysis fuse. This "closes" the epiphyseal plate and turns it into the ***epiphyseal line,*** which is visible on an x-ray. The whole process of ossification in long bones is called ***endochondral ossification***.   Short bones and irregular bones also develop through the process of endochondral ossification, but they lack epiphyseal plates.

The ***articular cartilage*** is a thin covering of hyaline cartilage around the ends of a bone. The articular cartilage provides a smooth surface over bone at a joint. Periosteum does not cover articular cartilage.

The flat bones of the skull and most of the clavicle form by the process of ***intramembranous ossification***. In this process mesenchyme condenses into a sheet of fibrous connective tissue. The cells of this sheet become ***osteogenic cells,*** which differentiate into ***osteoblasts***. The osteoblasts lay down bone. Trabeculae form and calcify into spongy bone in this process.   The peripheral surfaces calcify into compact bone, which become covered with periosteum. Periosteum contains sensory nerves with pain receptors; it is the most sensitive part of bone.

All bones grow at their surfaces; this is called ***appositional growth***. Appositional growth adds diameter to long bones, and it increases the size of irregular and short bones, which lack epiphyseal plates.

Long bones have epiphyseal plates and grow lengthwise, a feature that is lacking in bones without epiphyseal plates. Fracture of an epiphyseal plate in childhood leads to a lack of growth or an irregular growth of that bone, which produces a deformity.

Right: The process of endochondral ossification.
(A.) The long bones of a fetus are cartilaginous. (B) Osteoblasts form in the perichondrium. (C) A marrow cavity with a primary ossification center forms. (D) Secondary ossification centers form at both ends of the larger long bones.
(E) Epiphyseal plates can be seen in the metaphyseal areas.

The numbered pointers indicate
(1) Cartilage.
(2) Diaphysis.
(3) Primary ossification center (medullary space or marrow cavity).
(4) Epiphysis.
(5) Metaphysis (epiphyseal plate).
(6) Calcified cartilage.
(7) Secondary ossification center.

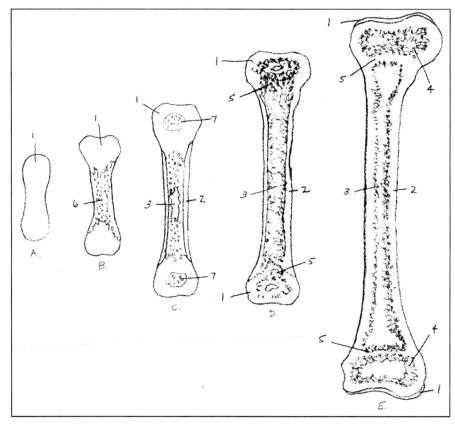

The embryonic cells of osseous tissue (bone) are stem cells called ***osteogenic cells***. After birth residual osteogenic cells reside in the ***periosteum*** and the ***endosteum***. The periosteum is a tough, fibrous connective tissue membrane surrounding the bone. The endosteum is not a membrane; it is the area at the junction of the medullary cavity and the cylinder of compact bone. ***Osteoblasts*** are bone forming cells that create the organic matter of the matrix (chiefly collagen fibers) and cause crystallization of the mineral salts that make up the ground substance.   When an osteoblast has created enough osseous tissue to have become surrounded by bone, it is called an ***osteocyte***. In living tissue osteocytes fill the small holes in bone called ***lacunae.*** Osteocytes are living cells that connect to each other and to blood vessels in the ***central canals*** by means of ***canaliculi,*** which are long tubular ***gap junctions*** between osteocytes.

Osteoclasts are large multinucleated cells that are capable of reabsorbing bone. They increase the calcium level in the blood, and they serve to shape bone as it is forming or being repaired. Osteoclasts are located in pits called **_reabsorption bays_** in the endosteum (the inner surface of compact bone). Osteoclasts develop from **_monocyte precursors_** in the marrow, and not from osteogenic cells.

One-third of the dry weight of bone is organic matter, consisting primarily of **_collagen fibers_**, glycosaminoglycans (GAGs), proteoglycans and glycoproteins. Two-thirds of the dry weight is inorganic matter, consisting of crystallized bone salts that have been laid down by osteoblasts. Eighty-five percent of all bone salt is a large complex compound of calcium and phosphorus called **_hydroxyapatite_** [$Ca_{10}(PO_4)_6(OH)_2$]. Ten percent is calcium carbonate (limestone, or $CaCO_3$), and five percent is other calcium and magnesium salts. Osteoblasts cause these bone salts to crystallize and become the ground substance of bone. The collagen and other organic molecules provide flexibility and tension resistance to bone, and they help to prevent fractures. Hydroxyapatite and the other bone salts provide hardness and rigidity. A calcium deficiency leads to deficient mineralization of bone, which may result in rickets or osteomalacia. In these disorders bones lose their rigidity; they become soft and flexible, and crippling physical deformities can result. The salts of calcium and magnesium make up the **_ground substance_** of bone. These salts plus collagen fibers, GAG compounds, glycoproteins and proteoglycans make up the **_matrix_** of bone.

The histological unit of compact bone is the **_osteon._** An osteon consists of a **_central canal (Haversian canal)_** and several surrounding layers of bone called **_lamellae._** The lamellae are filled with bone matrix that has been laid down by osteoblasts. In cross section the lamellae resemble layers of an onion. In the lamellae are **_lacunae_** (lakes) where the osteocytes (former osteoblasts) reside. Most lacunae are empty in tissue sections because their osteocytes are lost in the fixation process. **_Canaliculi_** are tiny tubes that radiate from the central canals and osteocytes.

Spongy bone contains lamellae like compact bone, but it has few true osteons, and it lacks Haversian canals. Haversian canals are not required in spongy bone because the osteocytes are near a surface of the bony matrix where nutrients are available.

Right: Osteons consist of Haversian canals in their center, surrounded by layers of crystallized bone salts called lamellae.
Osteocytes are located between lamellae; osteocytes connect with each other through tiny gap junctions called canaliculi.

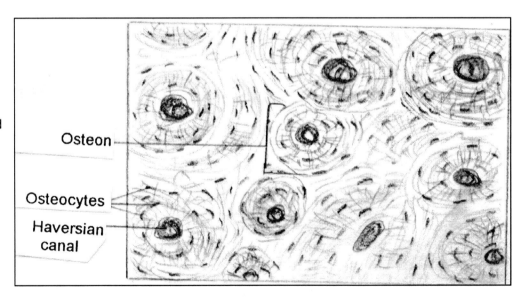

The crystallization of bone salts (mineralization) begins with the appearance of crystals on collagen fibers. Osteoblasts neutralize inhibitors that prevent this calcification. One crystal serves as a seed for others in a process of **_positive feedback_**.

Bone marrow occupies the area within the medullary cavities of long bone and between trabeculae of spongy bone. The structural framework of marrow is formed by reticular fibers. There are three types of marrow. **(1) _Red_** marrow contains hematopoietic tissue (blood cell forming). It is present in many bones of children. But in adults red marrow is found only in the sternum, pelvis, ribs, vertebrae, head of the humerus and head of the femur. **(2)** **_Yellow_** marrow consists of fat, and it fills the medullary cavities of most adult long bones. **(3)** **_Gelatinous_** marrow is yellow marrow that has deteriorated in older individuals.

Bone is a reservoir for calcium and phosphorus. **_Phosphorus_**, in the form of phosphate, serves as a buffer, and it is an ingredient in ATP, DNA, RNA and phospholipids. 85-90% of all the phosphorus in the body is in the bones. The compounds mono-hydrogen phosphate (HPO_4=) and di-hydrogen phosphate (H_2PO_4-) are important buffers in the blood. The normal level of phosphorus in plasma is 3.5-4.0 mg% (mg per 100 cc).

Calcium is needed for the conduction of nerve impulses, muscle contraction, blood clotting and exocytosis. It also serves as a second messenger and a coenzyme. Ninety-nine percent of the body's calcium is located in the bones. Of that reservoir, only 1% is easily exchanged with the blood. The other 98% can be mobilized gradually. The skeleton exchanges 18% of its calcium per year. The normal level of blood calcium is between 9.2 and 10.4 mg/deciliter (mg%, or mg/100cc) in plasma. (Plasma is the acellular portion of unclotted blood; serum is the acellular portion of clotted blood). Forty-five percent of the calcium ions in the blood can diffuse through cell walls; the rest are bound to proteins in the plasma.

Hypocalcemia is a blood calcium level that is below normal. In hypocalcemia the nervous system becomes hyperexcitable, and muscles cannot relax, which may result in muscle tremors, spasms and tetany. Muscles are hyperexcitable in hypocalcemia because low concentrations of calcium outside the cell lead to a lower concentration of positively charged cations outside the cell, which lowers the threshold for muscle contraction. Causes of hypocalcemia include calcium deficiency, vitamin D deficiency, chronic diarrhea, a deficiency of parathyroid hormone, pregnancy and lactation. Thyroid surgery may inadvertently damage or excise the parathyroid glands and result in hypocalcemia.

An abnormally high concentration of calcium in the blood is called **_hypercalcemia_**. Hypercalcemia is less common than hypocalcemia. Possible causes of hypercalcemia include a parathyroid tumor and an overactive parathyroid gland. In hypercalcemia the threshold level for nerve conduction is elevated. As a result muscle and nervous activity is depressed and muscles are weak. Symptoms may include sluggish reflexes, emotional disturbances and cardiac arrest.

Parathyroid hormone (PTH) is secreted by four small parathyroid glands, which are embedded in the posterior surface of the thyroid gland. Low blood calcium levels stimulate the release of PTH, and PTH raises the blood calcium level by negative feedback. PTH acts by stimulating osteoclast activity, which dissolves bone and releases calcium into the blood. PTH also acts by inhibiting the activity of osteoblasts. Parathyroid hormone also acts on the kidneys to reduce calcium excretion and increase phosphorus excretion in the urine. It also promotes a step in the synthesis of **_calcitriol_** (active vitamin D) in the kidneys. **_Vitamin D_** acts to elevate the blood calcium chiefly by increasing calcium absorption in the GI tract and reducing calcium loss in the urine. It also has a stimulating effect on osteoclasts. Although Vitamin D is traditionally classified as a vitamin, it could also be classified as a hormone.

There are at least twenty hormones, vitamins and growth factors that affect bone, not all of which are well understood. Bones grow especially rapidly at puberty. This is due to the influence of growth hormone, thyroxin, insulin, sex and other steroid hormones, and other growth factors. Estrogen has more effect on osteoblasts than testosterone, so girls reach their full height earlier than boys. Boys grow taller because their epiphyseal plates close later, and closure of the epiphyseal plates stops longitudinal bone growth. Precocious puberty and the ingestion of steroids can lead to permanently stunted growth due to premature closure of the epiphyseal plates.

Bone Disorders
A fracture is a broken bone. The following are descriptions of various **_types of fractures._**
Stress--: one that has been created by trauma.
Pathologic--: a break in abnormal bone -- may be caused by osteoporosis or the presence of a tumor.
Closed--: the skin is intact (also called a **_simple_** fracture).
Open--: the skin is broken and bone protrudes (also called a **_compound_** fracture).
Incomplete--: a fracture partway across a bone. The pieces of bone remain joined.

Greenstick--: an incomplete fracture in which the bone is broken on one side and bent on the other.
Hairline--:   a fine crack in a bone.
Comminuted--: a bone fractured into three or more pieces.
Displaced--: the bony pieces are out of alignment.
Nondisplaced--: the bony pieces are in alignment.
Impacted--: one fragment is driven into the spongy bone or medullary cavity of another fragment.
Depressed--: broken bone is pushed inwardly. This type of fracture occurs in the skull, pelvis and chest.
Linear--: the fracture is parallel to the long axis of the bone.
Transverse--: the fracture is perpendicular to the long axis of the bone.
Oblique--: the fracture is diagonal to the long axis of the bone.
Spiral--: the fracture is in the form of a spiral around the long axis. This occurs as a result of a twisting action.
Epiphyseal--: a break through an epiphyseal plate. These are common fractures before the epiphyseal plates close.
Compression--: a pathologic fracture most commonly involving the collapse of the body of a vertebra.
Colles--: a fracture involving the distal radius and ulna. This is a common fracture in falls, especially in patients with osteoporosis.
Pott's--: a fracture at the end of the tibia or the fibula or both. This is a common sports injury of the lower leg and ankle.
Avulsion--: the complete severance of a body part such as a finger.

Stages of healing of a fracture include **(1)** the formation of a hematoma due to broken blood vessels; **(2)** the formation of soft, highly vascular tissue called ***granulation tissue***. Fibroblasts move into this tissue, and osteogenic cells in the periosteum and the endosteum differentiate into osteoblasts and chondroblasts. **(3)** A soft callus of cartilage is formed by chondroblasts. By six weeks osteoblasts will have converted the soft cartilaginous callus into a hard bony callus. **(4)** Remodeling of the callus occurs over the next six months as spongy bone is replaced with compact bone. By then osteoblasts have rejoined the broken ends of the fractured bone, and osteoclasts have dissolved useless fragments of bone.

Right: Types   of
fractures
 (1) Greenstick
 (2) Linear
 (3) Transverse
 (4) Oblique
 (5) Spiral
 (6) Open
 (7) Comminuted
 (8) Impacted
 (9) Colles
(10) Potts

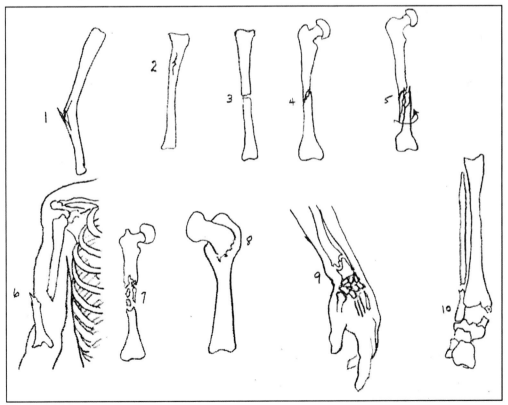

Methods of treating fractures include **(1)** **_closed reduction_**, which is reducing the fracture without a skin incision. **(2)** **_Open reduction_** is where the bone is surgically exposed. Plates, screws and pins are sometimes used with open reduction. **(3)** **_Traction_** is stretching an extremity to approximate the ends of a fracture for proper alignment. Traction is used primarily in children with fractures of the femur. **(4)** **_Electrical stimulation_** suppresses the effects of parathyroid hormone and serves to speed the healing of slow healing fractures. **(5)** **_Immobilization_** is necessary in treating fractures in order to keep the bony fragments in alignment. Immobilization may involve splinting and wrapping or casting.

Osteoporosis is the most common bone disease in America. In this disease bones lose both organic fibers and mineral salts; they become weak and brittle. Osteoporosis is more common in thin, elderly females of northern European ancestry. Outward symptoms include kyphosis, which is an outward deformity of the thoracic spine (a dowager's hump). These patients lose height as their vertebral columns collapse, and back pain is a common problem. High calcium intake, estrogen replacement and drugs like Fosamax are useful, but these treatments are not entirely satisfactory treatments for osteoporosis. Blacks are more resistant to osteoporosis, possibly because their bones are denser genetically. This is reflected in their higher specific gravity (most blacks do not float in fresh water).

Rickets and osteomalacia occur due to a lack of vitamin D. Skin exposure to sunshine is a necessary factor for the synthesis of vitamin D. The lack of melanin in the skin of Europeans may have evolved due to the lack of sunshine in northern climes. Rickets is the childhood variant of vitamin D deficiency, and it results in skeletal deformities. Vitamin D deficiency in adults results in osteomalacia, which involves softening of poorly calcified bones.

Scurvy is due to a deficiency of vitamin C (ascorbic acid), which is necessary for protein synthesis. The bony effects of scurvy are due to a deficiency in the formation of collagen fibers, which results in frequent fractures. Scurvy was epidemic on British sailing ships in the seventeenth and early eighteenth centuries because British sailors were fed a refined diet nearly void of vitamin C. Ascorbic acid was first isolated by Szent Gyorgyi in 1928, but James Lind, a British ship's surgeon, had recognized the ability of oranges and lemons to prevent scurvy as early as 1753.

Paget's disease is due to an abnormal proliferation of osteoclasts and secondary stimulation of osteoblasts. It leads to deformities and can be painful. An increasing hat size in adults is suggestive of Paget's disease. Elderly men are the group most often affected.

Osteomyelitis is an infection in the bone marrow. This is usually a bacterial infection, and it often requires extended periods of time on IV (intravenous) antibiotics. Diabetics and patients on chemotherapy are especially vulnerable to osteomyelitis.

Osteogenesis imperfecta is a genetic disorder of collagen synthesis that results in brittle bones, frequent fractures, blue sclera and deformed teeth. It is also known as "brittle bone disease."

An **_osteoma_** is a benign tumor of bone.

An **_osteochondroma_** is a benign tumor containing both bony and cartilaginous tissue.

An **_osteosarcoma_** is a malignant tumor (cancer) of bone. One cause of bone tumors is exposure to strontium 90, a radioactive isotope that was unleashed into the atmosphere of southern Utah following atomic bomb testing in Nevada over fifty years ago. Strontium 90 has a half life of 28 years. It collected in the bones of exposed individuals, and it slowly released beta particles. Strontium has a valence of +2 (two electrons are in its outer ring) just like calcium, which explains why it has a tendency to collect in bone.

A **_chondrosarcoma_** is a malignant but usually slow growing cancer of hyaline cartilage.

Study Guide
1. Know what makes up the skeletal system (bones, cartilage, joints and ligaments).
2. Know the types of bones according to shape and mode of development (long, short and irregular).
3. Review the make-up of bones, including spongy bone, compact bone, diploë, cancellous bone, osteons, Haversian (central) canals, canaliculi, osteocytes, lacunae, osteoblasts, osteoclasts, marrow, trabeculae, medullary cavity, periosteum, perichondrium and nutrient foramina.
4. Learn how the growth of bones occurs. Know the terms involved including endochondral ossification, intramembranous ossification, metaphysis, diaphysis, epiphysis, epiphyseal plate, articular cartilage, osteogenic cells, endosteum, hyaline cartilage template, and appositional growth.
5. Know what makes up the matrix of bone, and know the compounds that comprise the ground substance of bone.

6. Know the make-up of the matrix and the ground substance of cartilage.
7. Understand the actions of osteoblasts and osteoclasts on bone, and how they respond to the level of calcium in the blood.
8. Understand how bony ossification occurs as a positive feedback process.
9. Know the characteristics of the types of marrow (red, yellow and gelatinous).
10. Know the causes and symptoms of low and high blood calcium levels, and the ways these levels are normalized by negative feedback processes.
11. Know how vitamin D is activated, and how it affects calcium metabolism.
12. Know the physiologic effects of parathyroid hormone.
13. Recognize descriptions of the various types of fractures.
14. Understand the stages involved in the healing of fractures.
15. Recognize the ways that fractures may be treated.
16. Have a general understanding of the following disorders of bone and cartilage: rickets, osteomalacia, Paget's disease, osteomyelitis, osteogenesis imperfecta, osteoma, osteochondroma, osteosarcoma, and chondrosarcoma.

Chapter Eight

The Skeleton

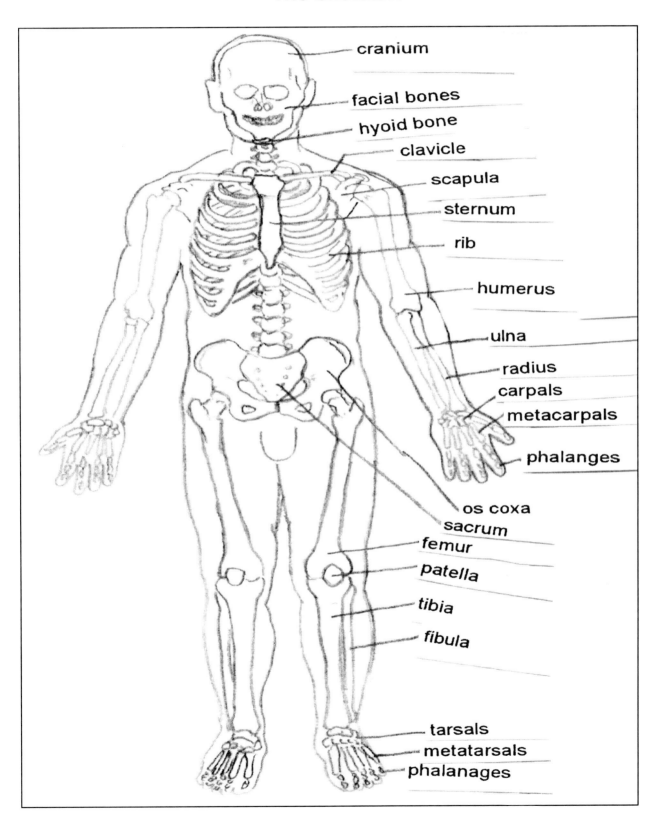

cranium

facial bones

hyoid bone

clavicle

scapula

sternum

rib

humerus

ulna

radius

carpals

metacarpals

phalanges

os coxa

sacrum

femur

patella

tibia

fibula

tarsals

metatarsals

phalanages

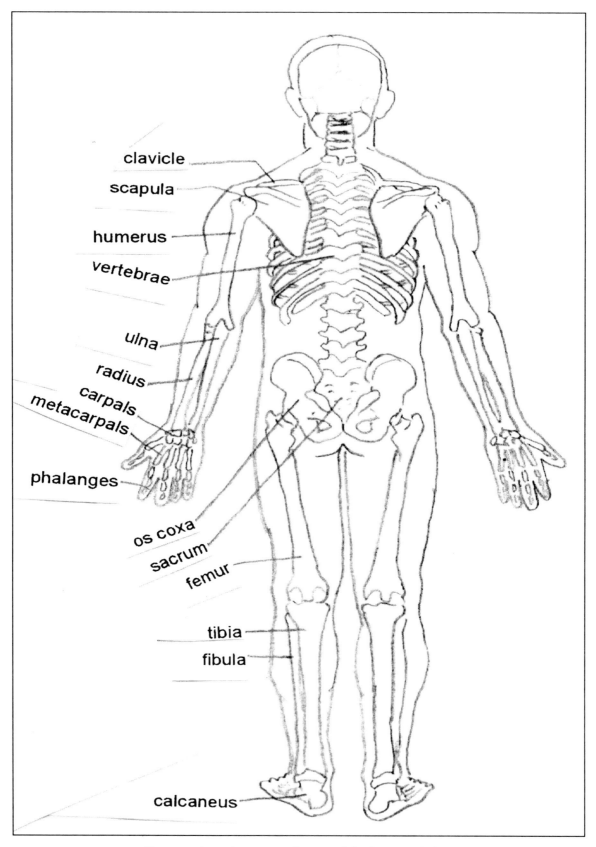

clavicle

scapula

humerus

vertebrae

ulna

radius

carpals

metacarpals

phalanges

os coxa

sacrum

femur

tibia

fibula

calcaneus

Above and previous page: Bones of the human skeleton.

An adult human has approximately 206 bones. The number of bones varies slightly among individuals because of differences in the fusion of bones, an inconsistent numbers of small wormian bones in the cranial suture joints, and inconstancy in the formation of sesamoid bones in the tendons.

Projections from the surface of bones go by many names.
A _**process**_ is a general term for a projection from the surface of a bone.
A _**spine**_ is a short, sharp projection.
A _**condyle**_ is a smooth rounded surface that articulates with another bone.
An _**epicondyl**_e is a projection on a condyle.
The _**head**_ is a hemispheric end of a bone that articulates with another bone.
The _**neck**_ of a bone is a constriction below the head.
A _**crest**_ is an elevated ridge of bone.
A _**line**_ is a smaller elevation than a crest.
A _**facet**_ is a smooth, flat face.
A _**trochanter**_ is a large protuberance on a bone.
A _**tubercle**_ is a smaller protuberance on a bone.
A _**ramus**_ is a branch.

Depressions and holes in bones also go by many names which are listed.
A _**foramen**_ is a hole.
A _**sinus**_ is a cavity.
A _**canal**_ is a tubular passageway.
A _**meatus**_ is an opening into a canal.
A _**fossa**_ is a shallow depression.
A _**sulcus**_ is an elongated depression or groove.
A _**notch**_ is a deep cut.
A _**fissure**_ is a long deep cleft.
An _**alveolus**_ is a pit or socket.
A _**fovea**_ is a small pit.

The _**cranium**_ is the casing for the brain. The _**calvarium**_, or skull-cap, is the top and sides of the cranium. The _**skull**_ is the cranium plus the facial bones. Not all skulls are shaped alike. Male skulls tend to be larger and heavier with more prominent brows. Most racial groups have an elongated skull (dolichocephaly), but the skulls of American Indians, Eskimos and Siberians have a more rounded contour.

The skull contains cavities including the _**cranial cavity**_, which encloses the brain; the _**orbits**_ or eye sockets; the _**nasal cavity**_; the _**buccal cavity**_ or mouth; the _**middle ear cavity**_, which is continuous with the _**mastoid air cells;**_ and the _**paranasal sinuses**_, which are air filled pockets lined by a mucous membrane. The paranasal sinuses include the _**frontal sinus**_, the right and left _**maxillary sinuses**_, the _**ethmoid sinus**_ and the _**sphenoid sinus**_. Most of the skull bones are double, that is, one is on the right and its likeness is on the left. Some skull bones are single due to fusion with their counterpart on the opposite side. Those include the frontal, occipital, sphenoid, ethmoid, maxilla and mandible. The vomer forms as a single midline bone.

The bones of the _**calvarium**_ include the _**frontal**_ bone, _**parietal**_ bones, _**temporal**_ bones, and the _**occipital**_ bone. Those four bones plus the _**sphenoid**_ bone and the _**ethmoid**_ bone enclose the brain and make up the _**cranium**_. The _**frontal bone**_ is the bone of the forehead. It forms most of the roof of the orbits and the anterior part of cranial floor. The supraorbital margin of the frontal bone is an arched ridge beneath the eyebrows. The _**supraorbital foramen**_ is an opening in the supraorbital margin through which the supraorbital nerve enters the face.

**The right and left parietal** bones are behind the frontal bone. They form two prominent bulges on the top of cranial cavity

**The occipital** bone forms the posterior part of cranial floor and walls. The _**foramen magnum**_ is a large hole through the occipital bone at the base of the skull through which the spinal cord passes. The occipital condyles are oval convex processes on either side of foramen magnum that articulate with depressions on the first cervical vertebra. The external occipital protuberance and the superior nuchal line are located on the back of the calvarium just above the foramen magnum. Muscles of the upper back and neck form the nuchal ligament, which attaches to the occipital bone at the nuchal line.

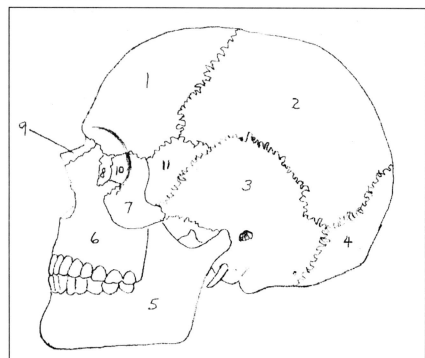

Right: Bones of the human skull.

Top: Lateral view.

Bottom: Inferior view.

(1) frontal
(2) parietal
(3) temporal
(4) occipital
(5) mandible
(6) maxilla
(7) zygoma
(8) lacrimal
(9) nasal
(10) ethmoid
(11) sphenoid
(12) palatine
(13) vomer

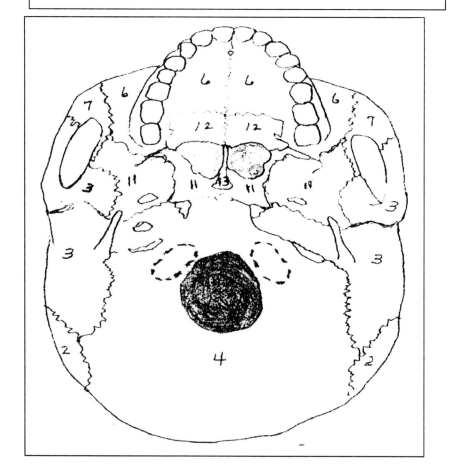

The *two temporal bones* form the lateral areas of the cranium and part of cranial floor. Each temporal bone contains a *an inner ear, a middle ear* and a *mastoid process* with air cells, which are located just behind the ear. The *styloid process* is a slender spike of bone extending downward and forward from the undersurface of the temporal bones anterior to mastoid process. It is easily broken off in laboratory specimens. Two muscles, stylohyoid and styloglossus, originate on the styloid process and assist in swallowing. The *external auditory meatus* is the opening to the external ear canal. It is located in the temporal bone just above the styloid process. The *zygomatic arch* forms the lateral part of the cheek between the orbit and the ear. It is formed by parts of the *temporal* and *zygomatic* bones. The *mandible* articulates with mandibular fossa of the temporal bone.

The bones of the cranium are held together by *suture joints,* which look like the pieces of a jigsaw puzzle. They are fibrous joints that are nearly fused. *Wormian bones* are small variable bones within a suture joint. They are more prevalent among American Indians and some Asiatics. The *coronal* suture is the joint between the parietal bones and the frontal bone; the *lambdoidal* suture is the joint between the parietal bones and the occipital bone; the *sagittal* suture is the joint between the right and left parietal bones; and the *squamous* suture is the joint between the temporal bone and the parietal, occipital and sphenoid bones.

The different bones of the cranium form separately and later grow together. Delayed fusion of the cranial bones permits cranial compression during the birthing process and growth of an infant's brain. *Fontanels* are soft spots in an infant's skull that represent areas where the bones have not yet grown together.

The *ethmoid bone* is a complex irregular bone that makes up part of the anterior portion of the cranial floor, the medial wall of orbits and part of the roof of the nose. The ethmoid bone lies anterior to the sphenoid bone and posterior to nasal bones. The ethmoid bone makes up portions of the cranial cavity including the *cribiform plate* and the *crista galli.*   Olfactory nerves (sensory nerves for smell) pass through numerous small holes in the cribiform plate. The *crista galli* is an attachment point for the meninges (membranous linings over the brain and spinal cord). The middle and superior nasal *conchae* (*turbinates*) are parts of the ethmoid bone. They are thin scrolls of bone in the nasal cavity. (The inferior turbinate is a separate bone). The *ethmoid sinus* is a collection of air cells located above and lateral to the nasal cavity. The perpendicular plate of the ethmoid forms the upper part of *nasal septum*.

The *sphenoid bone* is a complex irregular bone occupying the central portion of the cranial floor behind the nose and orbits. The central part of the sphenoid is called the *body*. The *greater wings* of the sphenoid are lateral projections from the body that form part of the lateral wall of the orbit. The *lesser wings* of the sphenoid are thin, triangular projections from the upper part of body that form the posterior part of the roof of the orbit. The *sella turcica* ("Turk's saddle") is a saddle-shaped depression that contains the *pituitary gland.* The *anterior and posterior clinoid processes* of the sphenoid surround the sella turcica. The *sphenoid sinus* is an irregular, air-filled space within the body of the sphenoid. The *optic foramina* are openings through the sphenoid between the orbits and the cranial cavity; the optic foramina contain the optic nerves (second cranial nerves). The *superior orbital fissues* are slit-like openings into each orbit between the greater wings and the lesser wings of the sphenoid. The superior orbital fissures contain blood vessels, the third and fourth cranial nerves, and a branch of the fifth cranial nerve.

The bones of the face that are not part of the cranium include **(1)** the right and left *nasal bones,* which form the upper bridge of the nose; **(2)** the *vomer*, which forms the lower part of nasal septum; **(3)** the right and left *maxillae*, or upper jaw bones, which contain the maxillary sinuses and the upper teeth. The maxillae also make up part of floor of orbit, the anterior part of the palate (roof of mouth), and the floor and part of lateral walls of the nose. **(4)** The right and left *palatine* bones form the posterior portion of the hard palate, part of the wall of the nasal cavity and part of the floor of the orbit. **(5)** The right and left *zygomatic* bones (*zygomas*) form part of the floor and sidewall of the orbits and the anterior portions of the zygomatic arches. **(6)** The right and left *lacrimal* bones are thin bones about size and shape of a fingernail. They form part of the medial wall of the orbit and the lateral wall of the nasal cavity. The lacrimal bones contain the lacrimal sacs (tear sacs) and upper portions of the nasolacrimal ducts (tear ducts). **(7)** The *mandible* is the lower jawbone. It is formed by the fusion of its right and left halves, which make it the largest and strongest bone of the face.   The mandible contains the lower teeth. The parts of the mandible include the mental protuberance (chin), the body, the ramus, the coronoid process and the condylar process. The powerful muscles of mastication (the temporalis, pterygoids and masseter muscles) attach to the mandible, which is the only bone of the head that is independently movable. The mandible contains the lower teeth.

The neck contains a small U-shaped bone just above the larynx called the **_hyoid_** bone. The larynx is made up of hyaline cartilage. The hyoid bone is distinctive because it has no articulations with any other bone. It is held in place by ligaments and the tendons of small muscles that open the jaw, move the soft palate and depress the base of the tongue. Forensic pathologists can diagnosis death by strangulation by observing a fracture of the hyoid.

The vertebral column, sternum, ribs and pelvis make up the **_axial skeleton_**. The bones of the appendages (arms and legs) make up the **_appendicular skeleton_**.

The following drawings point out different characteristics of the vertebrae.

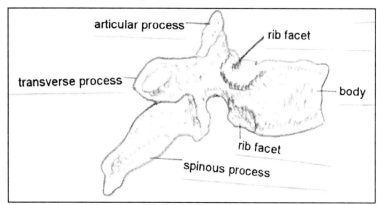

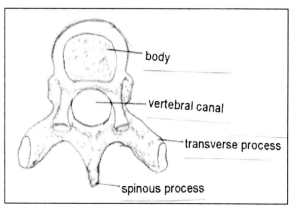

Above: Thoracic vertebra, lateral view.

Above right: Thoracic vertebra from above.

Right: Lumbar vertebra, lateral view.

Below right: Lumbar vertebra from above.

Below: Cervical vertebra from above.

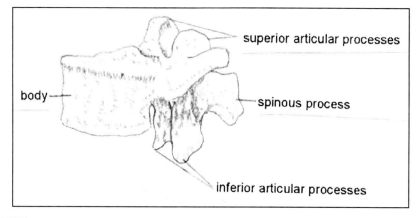

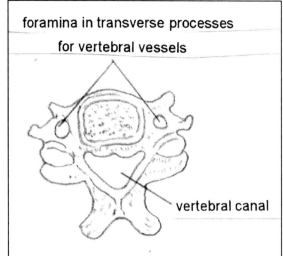

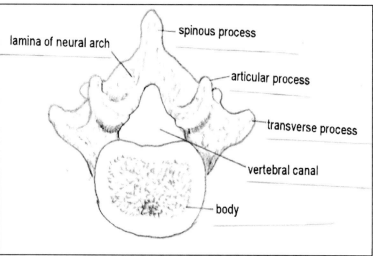

Right: The   vertebral
column, lateral view.

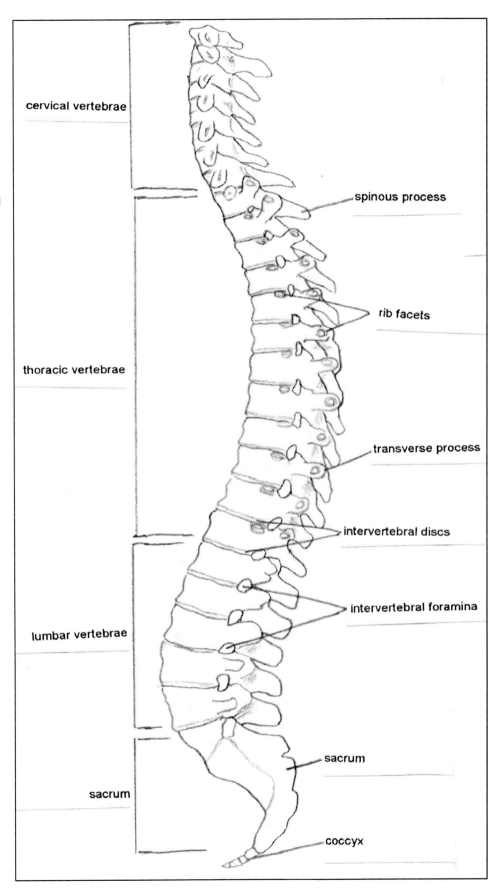

cervical vertebrae

spinous process

rib facets

thoracic vertebrae

transverse process

intervertebral discs

intervertebral foramina

lumbar vertebrae

sacrum

sacrum

coccyx

Right: The   vertebral
column, dorsal view.

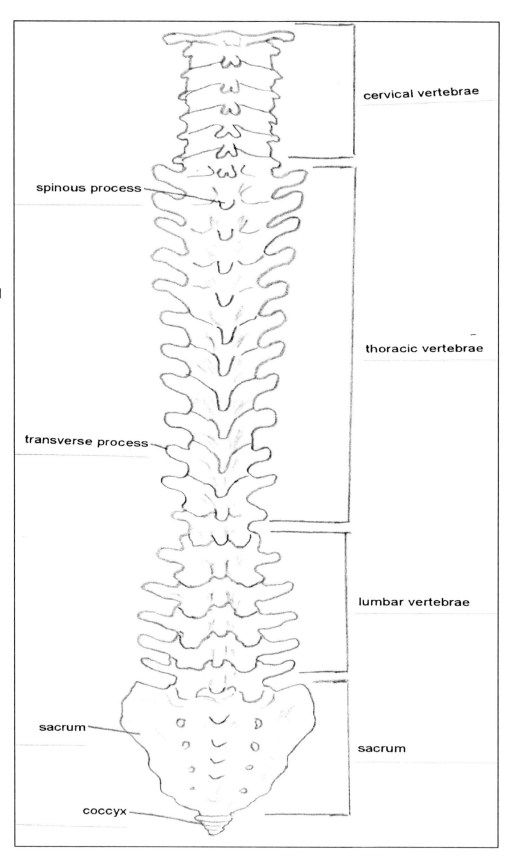

cervical vertebrae

spinous process

thoracic vertebrae

transverse process

lumbar vertebrae

sacrum

sacrum

coccyx

The ***vertebral column*** (spine) is a chain of thirty-three ***vertebrae,*** some of which are fused. Vertebrae extend from the occipital bone to the coccyx (the tail bone). The vertebrae are irregular bones. They gradually increase in size and strength as they descend, which corresponds to the weight they must bear. Each vertebra forms a ring (the ***vertebral ring***), around the ***vertebral canal*** (spinal canal). The ***spinal cord*** passes through the vertebral canal. On the vertebral ring are processes including **(1)** the posterior ***spinous process***, which is ***palpable*** (can be felt through the skin); **(2)** the ***transverse processes***, to which muscles attach; **(3)** the superior and inferior ***articular processes***, by which the vertebrae articulate with each other, and **(4)** processes for rib attachments. The anterior portion of a vertebra is composed of the ***body***, which is a stout disc of bone that provides most of the support for the vertebral column. ***Intervertebral discs*** are discs of ***fibrous cartilage*** between the bodies of vertebrae. The ***nucleus pulposus*** is a gelatinous area in the center of the intervertebral discs. Herniation of the nucleus pulposus is a "slipped disc."

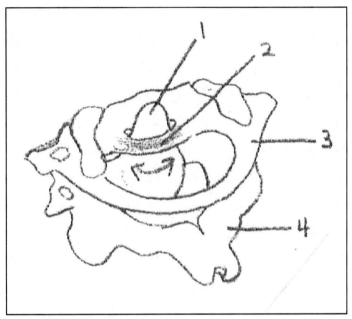

Right: The atlas and axis vertebrae.
(cervical vertebra #1 and #2). The arrows
show how the atlas moves around the
odontoid process of the axis as one turns
his head.

(1) Odontoid process (dens) of the axis.
(2) Transverse ligament.
(3) Atlas.
(4) Axis.

There are ***seven cervical vertebrae*** in the neck. The first cervical vertebra is a delicate ring called the ***atlas***. The articulation between the atlas and the occipital bone allows for the up and down motion of the head. The second cervical vertebra is called the ***axis***. Rotary movement of the head is made possible by the rotation of the atlas around the ***odontoid process (dens)*** of the axis. The seventh cervical vertebra has a prominent spinous process, which allows an examiner to identify the number of a specific vertebra. Cervical vertebrae are distinctive because they contain ***vertebral foramina*** in their transverse processes for the passage of the vertebral arteries to the brain and vertebral veins from the brain.

There are ***twelve thoracic or dorsal vertebrae***. They are distinctive because facets for rib attachments are on the transverse processes and bodies of thoracic vertebrae.

There are ***five lumbar vertebrae***. The lumbar vertebrae are considerably larger than those above. Most cases of herniated discs occur in the lumbar area.

There are ***five sacral vertebrae***, which are fused in adults to form one bone -- the sacrum.

The ***coccyx*** is the vestige of a tail in humans. The number of coccygeal vertebrae varies, but is usually four. The vertebrae of the coccyx are small and serve little purpose except for muscle attachments. The coccygeal vertebrae are fused in adults.

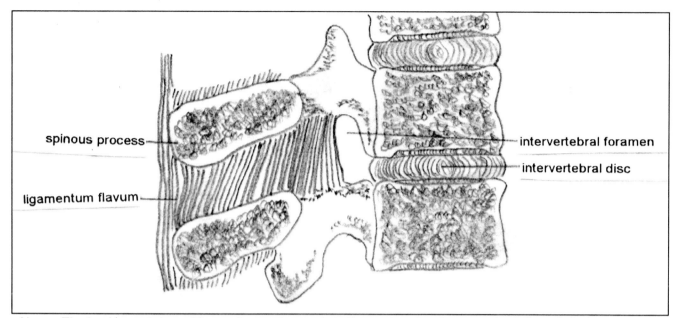

Above: The lumbar vertebrae. The nucleus pulposus is in the center of an intervertebral disc. Spinal nerves exit the vertebral canal through the intervertebral foramina.

There are **_twelve pairs of ribs_**, one pair being attached to each of the thoracic vertebrae. The top seven pairs of ribs attach by their cartilage to the sternum anteriorly; they are called **_true ribs_**. The other five pairs of ribs are called **_false ribs_** because they do not connect directly to the sternum. The eighth, ninth, and tenth ribs attach to the cartilage of the rib above (eventually to the cartilage of the seventh rib). The two bottom pairs of ribs are called **_floating ribs_** because they have no anterior attachments.

The **_sternum_** is the breastbone; it articulates with the rib cartilages. The superior part of the sternum is the **_manubrium._** The manubrium articulates with the clavicle (collar bone). The central part of the sternum is called the **_body_**. The inferior portion of the sternum is cartilaginous and is called the **_xiphoid process_**.

The **_clavicles_** (collar bones) connect the arms to the trunk by way of their connection to the sternum. The clavicles are the most frequently fractured bones in the body. Each clavicle articulates laterally with the **_acromion process_** of the scapula.

Each **_scapula_** (shoulder blade) articulates with the clavicle and humerus on that side of the body. The scapulae are heavy triangular shaped bones with no connection to the axial skeleton except via the clavicles. The **_acromion and coracoid processes_** are two prominent processes on the anterior lateral superior aspect of each scapula. Both of these processes serve as attachment areas for muscles and ligaments. The **_glenoid cavity or fossa_** is the shoulder joint. It is a concavity in the scapula where the head of the humerus articulates with the scapula. The **_spine of the scapula_** is located posteriorly and serves as a site for muscle attachments.

The **_humerus_** is the large bone of the arm. The **_head of the humerus_** articulates with the scapula in the glenoid cavity (fossa). Distal to the head of the humerus are the **_greater and lesser tubercles_**, which serve as sites for muscle attachments. The **_neck_** of the humerus is that portion between the head and the tubercles. The humerus contains two rounded **_condyles_** at the elbow that articulate with the ulna and the radius. Each condyle has a protuberance called an **_epicondyle_**. When the forearm is extended, the **_olecranon_** process of the ulna fits into the olecranon fossa of the humerus posteriorly.

The **_radius and the ulna_** are the bones of the forearm. The **_head of the radius is at the elbow_** and **_rotates_** around the ulna, producing **_supination and pronation_**. The **_head of the ulna is located at the wrist_**. The **_styloid processes_** are projections of bone at the medial and lateral aspects of the wrist. The medial styloid process is part of the ulna, and it is located at the base of the fifth finger. The lateral styloid process is part of the radius and is at the base of the thumb.

There are eight *__carpal__* bones in each wrist, which are arranged in a proximal and a distal row of four bones each. Beginning with the proximal row at the thumb, the carpals are the *__scaphoid__* (navicular of the wrist)__*, lunate, triquetum*__ (triangular), and *__pisiform.__* The pisiform is a *__sesamoid__* bone that grows in the tendon of the flexor carpi ulnaris muscle; it articulates only with the triquetum. Beginning at the thumb the distal row of carpal bones are the *__trapezium__* (greater multangular), *__trapezoid__* (lesser multangular), *__capitate__* and *__hamate.__* The only *__saddle joint__* in the body is formed by the joint between the trapezium and the first metacarpal. A mnemonic for the carpal bones is "Sally left the party to take Charlie home." Older names for the scaphoid (navicular), triquetum (triangular), trapezium (greater multangular) and trapezoid (lesser multangular) remain in use.

There are five *__metacarpal__* bones in each hand, one for each digit. Metacarpals form the knuckles when the fingers are flexed. The *__phalanges (singular, phalanx)__* are the bones of the fingers and thumbs. There are two phalanges in each thumb and three in each finger. Although the metacarpal and phalangeal bones are small, they are classified as long bones because of their shape and the way in which they develop. An interesting observation is the discrepancy in length of the second and fourth fingers between males and females. The fourth fingers of most males are longer than their second fingers. The second and fourth fingers are more equal in length in females, and the second digit is more often the longer.

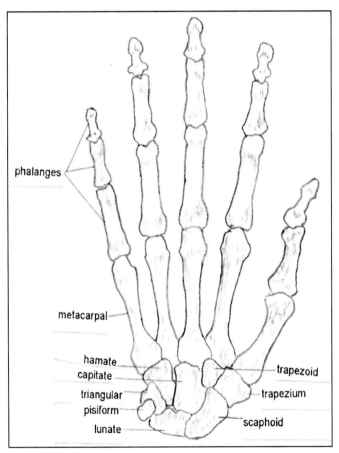 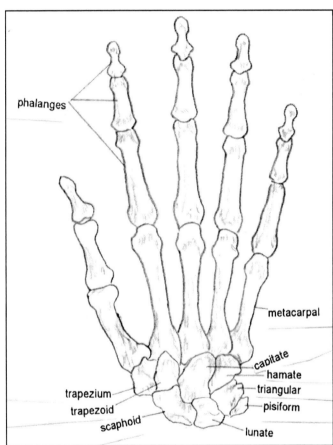

Palmar surface of right hand   Dorsal surface of right hand
Above: The bones of the wrist and hand.

The bony *__pelvis__* is a bowl shaped area formed by a complete ring of bone. It is a fused bone made up of the *__ilium, ischium, and pubis__* from both sides of the body. The pelvis is fused with the sacrum at the sacroiliac joints. The greater or false pelvis is located superior to the lesser or true pelvis; the greater pelvis is the larger of the two. *__Os coxa__* is another name for the pelvic bone. The *__ilium__* is the upper part of the os coxa; it contains the iliac crest, which is palpable in the lower flank. The *__ischium__* is located posteriorly and is the bone that bears the weight of the body when in the sitting position. The *__pubis__* is located anteriorly. The right and left pubic bones are fused at the ***pubic symphysis***, creating the ***pubic arch***. The obturator foramina are large openings near the bottom of the os coxa. They are formed by the pubis and the ischium. They are the largest foramina in the body; they contain the obturator vessels.

There are anatomical differences between the female pelvis and the male pelvis. The female pelvis is shallower and wider and is tilted more forward. The female sacrum is shorter and wider. The male pelvis is narrower, deeper, and more vertical, and the bones are more massive. The ***pelvic outlet*** is the inferior opening of the pelvis; it is larger in the female. The ***pelvic inlet*** is the superior opening to the pelvis; it is round to oval in the female and heart-shaped in the male. The ***acetabulum*** (hip socket) is rotated laterally in the female and anteriorly in the male. The acetabulum is more centered over the body's center of gravity in the male. The pubic arch makes an angle greater than 100 degrees in the female, but less than 90 degrees in the male. These differences in structure reflect differences in function; the female pelvis is structured for childbirth; the male pelvis is structured for speed and endurance in running.

The ***acetabulum*** is the cavity into which the head of the femur fits. The acetabulum is made up of parts of all three pelvic bones (ilium, ischium and pubis).

Right: The bones of the foot.
 This view is of the plantar surface of the right foot.

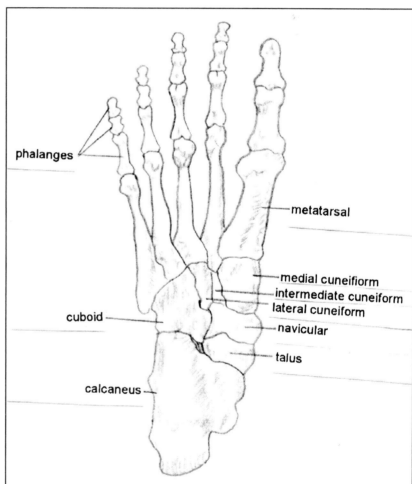

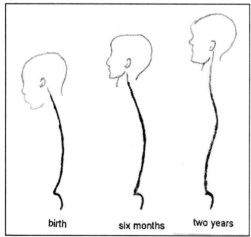

Above: Spinal curvatures at different ages.

The ***femur*** is the bone of the thigh. It is the largest and strongest bone in the body. The head of the femur fits into the acetabulum. The ***neck*** and the ***greater and lesser trochanters*** are distal to the head. The trochanters serve as sites for muscle attachments. The femur contains a lateral and a medial ***condyle*** at the knee. These are large, rounded protuberances that serve as articular (joint) surfaces.

The ***patella*** is the kneecap. It is a sesamoid bone in the tendon of the quadriceps femoris muscle.

The **_tibia_** and the **_fibula_** are the two bones of the leg. The tibia is the medial of the two and is more massive than the fibula. The tibia articulates with the femur at the knee and the talus in the ankle, and it is, therefore, the weight bearing bone of the leg. The two bony prominences at the ankle are the **_medial malleolus_** of the tibia and the **_lateral malleolus_** of the fibula.

There are seven **_tarsal_** bones in each ankle. The **_talus_** articulates with the tibia. The **_calcaneus_** forms the heel. The other tarsal bones are the **_navicular_**, the **_cuboid_**, and the **_medial, intermediate and lateral cuneiform bones._**

There are five **_metatarsal_** bones in each foot, one for each toe. There are two **_phalangeal_** bones in the big toe (hallux) and three for each of the other toes. The metatarsal and phalangeal bones are classified as long bones.

The tarsal and metatarsal bones are arranged so that they form three **_arches_** in the foot -- two longitudinal and one transverse. Arches provide spring to the step and reduce fatigue. The bones are held into an arch shape by ligaments and tendons.

Man has been aided by several changes to his skeleton that have occurred in evolution. These changes occurred slowly over millions of years in prehuman species that no longer exist. Man's closest living relatives today are the apes (chimpanzees and great apes). Apes and other primates are forest dwellers. The precursors of Homo sapiens underwent evolutionary changes that reflect movement out of the forest and into the savannah (grasslands). These changes occurred slowly in species of primates who were ancestors of early man but are now extinct.

One difference between man and other primates is the shape of the spine. The spine of apes, infants and young children is "C" shaped with only one curve. By early childhood the spine has taken on an "S" curvature with curvatures in the cervical area, thoracic area and lumbar area. The cervical curvature plus a more forward positioning of the foramen magnum have allowed man to hold his head upright rather than tilting forward; man's face became flatter as a result. The lumbar curvature moved his center of gravity posteriorly, allowing his body to be upright with a minimum of muscular effort, which facilitates walking, running and standing. A **_kyphosis_** is an excessive dorsal curvature in the thoracic spine, exemplified by a "dowager's hump." A **_lordosis_** is an excessive ventral curvature, usually in the lumbar spine. A **_scoliosis_** is an abnormal lateral curvature of the spine.

The enlargement of the hallux (big toe) of man was associated with a change in function from grasping to pushing off for fast starts. The metatarsal and metacarpal bones of man are straight. In apes they are curved to allow for grasping and hanging from tree limbs.

Changes in the femur and pelvis give man a smoother and more efficient stride and a more upright posture. The femur of man is angled medially, and the knees are closer together and more centered under the center of gravity than in other primates. This allows man to stand with his knees locked for long periods, which results in decreased muscular effort while standing. The ilium (and consequently the origin of the gluteus maximus muscle) is rotated posteriorly, which allows contraction of the gluteus maximus muscle to move the thigh backward. This gives a more efficient walk. In apes the gluteus maximus moves the thigh laterally, resulting in a shuffling gate. The upper extremities of other primates are longer than their lower extremities, and the forelimbs are used in walking, or they are held over their heads and out of the way.

Chevalier de Lamarck (1744-1829) was a French biologist who put forth an early theory of evolution. Lamarck concluded that physical traits develop in order to adapt to environmental factors, and these traits are passed on to offspring. According to Lamarck, giraffes developed long necks in response to their attempts to reach leaves high on trees. After Gregor Mendel and Charles Darwin published their works, Lamarckian theory fell out of favor and was regarded as nonsense. We now accept that evolutionary change occurs due to spontaneous mutations that provide an advantage for the organism.   However, Lamarck was partially correct, because advantages gained from mutations reflect pressures exerted by the environment.

Humans have made some evolutionary changes from earlier primates that have created problems. The human pelvis has become shortened and is more bowl-shaped; the pelvic outlet is narrower, and human fetuses have considerably larger brains and larger heads than other primates. These evolutionary changes have made birthing more difficult, more painful, and more dangerous to the mother and the fetus.

Study Guide

The skeleton should be studied by referencing a model.
1. Know the definitions on page 85 of this chapter.
2. How many bones do you have?
3. Know the sinuses and air cavities of the skull.
4. Know the bones of the cranium and those of the face. Know where to find the following: the sphenoid bone and its sella turcica; the ethmoid bone and its cribiform plate; the occipital bone and its foramen magnum; the sinuses; the orbits; the vomer bone; the temporal bone and its external auditory canal, mastoid process and styloid process; the mandible; the frontal bone; the parietal bone; the zygomatic arch; the maxillary bone; and the lacrimal groove.
5. Locate the hyoid bone.
6. Define the axial skeleton and the appendicular skeleton.
7. Study a cervical vertebra. Locate the body, vertebral foramen, superior and inferior facets, spinous process, and the transverse process with its foramen for vertebral arteries.
8. Recognize the differences between cervical, thoracic and lumbar vertebrae including the presence of transverse foramina in cervical vertebrae, the presence of costal (rib) facets on thoracic vertebrae, and the gradual increase in size from cervical to thoracic to lumbar vertebrae.
9. Recognize the unique features of the atlas and the axis.
10. Know what is meant by a true rib, a false rib and a floating rib, and which ribs are of each type.
11. Recognize the sacrum, the coccyx, and the three bones that make up the os coxa or hip bone.
12. Recognize the bones of the upper extremity including the clavicle, scapula, humerus, ulna, radius, and the bones of the wrist and hand.
13. Be able to name and point out the carpal bones and the bones of the hand.
14. Know the definition of a sesamoid bone, and identify two sesamoid bones in the body.
15. Recognize landmarks on the scapula including the spine, glenoid fossa, coracoid process and acromion process.
16. Locate the three parts of the sternum (manubrium, body and xiphoid process).
17. List the differences between the male pelvis and the female pelvis.
18. Know where to find the acetabulum, patella, femur, tibia and fibula.
19. Identify the tarsal bones and the bones of the foot.
20. Know the following bony landmarks: medial malleolus, lateral malleolus, hallux, pollix, greater trochanter, lesser trochanter, crest of the ilium, pubic symphysis, olecranon fossa, olecranon process, styloid process of the radius, and the styloid process of the ulna.
21. Know what forms the arches of the foot.
22. Know the meaning of kyphosis, lordosis and scoliosis.
23. Understand the evolutionary changes that allowed the ancestors of early man to begin to walk erect for long distances.
24. Which bone is fractured most frequently?
25. Which bone is typically fractured by strangulation?
26. Which bone is the most helpful in identifying the sex of a skeleton?

Chapter Nine

Joints

Orthopedics is the medical specialty dealing with bones and joints. Orthopedics means to "straighten the child," and early orthopedists concentrated on children with spinal deformities.

An **articulation** is a **joint**, or a place where two bones meet. The prefix **"arth-"** refers to joints as does the word **"articular."** **Arthritis** is inflammation of a joint, and **arthrology** is the study of joints. **"Rheumatic"** refers to joints and muscles. **Kinesiology** is a division of biomechanics and is the study of movement by the musculoskeletal system.

Many joints have common names including the shoulder, hip, elbow and knee. All joints have scientific names according to the two bones they connect.

Joints of the body are divided into categories. **Diarthrotic** joints are those that are freely moveable in one or more planes; **amphiarthrotic** joints are slightly moveable, and **synarthrotic** joints are capable of little or no movement.

Another means of classifying joints is by the tissues that make up the joint. Thus a joint may be classified as **fibrous**, **cartilaginous**, **bony** or **synovial**.

Synostoses are **synarthrotic bony** joints where articulating bones of early childhood have fused, and technically it is no longer a joint. The right and left halves of the mandible and the right and left halves of the frontal bone are examples.

Synchondroses are **synarthrotic cartilaginous** joints. The epiphyseal plates of long bones and the costosternal joints are examples of synchondroses. The costosternal joints are hyaline cartilage articulations between the ribs and the sternum. The pubic symphysis, sacroiliac joints, and the intervertebral discs are cartilaginous joints of fibrocartilage. Synchondrotic joints are capable of slight movement. The pubic symphysis relaxes and increases in width during pregnancy. Following birth, this joint returns to normal. Pregnancy also causes the sacroiliac joint to become more mobile.

Fibrous joints are capable of little or no movement, and most are classified as **synarthrotic** joints. Fibrous joints include the suture joints of the skull, the tooth sockets (**gomphoses**), and **interosseous membranes**. Interosseous membranes, or **syndesmoses**, are amphiarthrotic fibrous joints that are found between the shafts of the radius and the ulna and between the shafts of the tibia and the fibula.

A **synovial** joint is a joint that is surrounded by a **synovial cavity**. Most synovial joints are **diarthrotic;** some are amphiarthrotic. Synovial joints include the freely moveable joints of the body including the shoulder, elbow, wrist, hip, knee, ankle, feet, hands, and the articulation of the vertebrae. A synovial cavity is surrounded a fibrous, connective tissue capsule called the **joint capsule**. The inner lining of the joint capsule is the **synovial membrane**, a thin, serous, connective tissue membrane that secretes **synovial fluid** into the cavity. The synovial membrane is **connective tissue**, not epithelial tissue, and it lacks a basement membrane. **Synovial fluid** is viscous and slippery, and it is rich in the glycosaminoglycan, **hyaluronic acid**. The health of a joint can be determined by the viscosity of the synovial fluid. Healthy synovial fluid is viscous and will "string out" when picked up. This is called the **"string test."** Synovial fluid is also rich in glycoproteins and albumin. Albumin is secreted by the liver and is the most abundant protein in plasma. Synovial fluid provides nourishment to the **articular cartilage** that covers the ends of long bones. Synovial fluid also removes waste material from cartilage, and it contains phagocytes for cleaning up debris.

Cartilage contains no blood vessels, therefore, it is slow to repair itself, and it is susceptible to chronic deterioration. Exercising exerts repetitive compression and release to articular cartilage of the knees and hips, which allows the articular cartilage to breathe and get rid of wastes. Articular cartilage deteriorates more rapidly in couch potatoes.

A *meniscus* is a pad of *fibrocartilage.* Menisci are found in the knee, sternoclavicular joint and temporomandibular joint. The intervertebral discs are especially large menisci. Menisci absorb shock and pressure, and they guide the movement of bones. Menisci in the knee keep the tibia from moving laterally in relation to the femur.

Ligaments and *tendons* stabilize joints; both are composed of dense regular connective tissue.
Ligaments bind bone to bone, and tendons bind muscle to bone.
A *bursa* is an enclosed sack containing synovial fluid and lined by a synovial membrane. Bursae are found in clefts between muscles and around tendons at sites where muscles and tendons ride over bony prominences and ligaments. They allow muscles and tendons to glide smoothly over these areas.
Tendon sheaths are cylindrical synovial membranes that are wrapped around tendons and allow them to move smoothly. They are present in the wrist, hand, ankle and foot.

Freely moveable joints exhibit *flexion,* which is a decrease in the angle of a joint, *extension*, which is an increase in the angle of a joint, and *hyperextension*, which is extension of a joint beyond 180 degrees.
Joints have different *ranges of motion* depending on their anatomy. The range of motion of a joint is affected by **(1)** the structure and action of the muscles, **(2)** the articular surfaces of the bones, and **(3)** the strength and tautness of the ligaments, tendons and joint capsule. When ligaments are unusually long and slack, the person may be said to be "double jointed."

Synovial joints are classified into the following six different types:
(1) A *ball-and-socket* joint exhibits a smooth hemispherical head of one bone fitting into a cuplike depression (cavity or fossa) of another bone. For example, the head of the humerus fits into the glenoid fossa, and the head of the femur fits into the acetabulum. The most freely moveable joints in the body are ball-and-socket joints. Ball and socket joints are the only joints that are multiaxial (move in all three planes). The shoulder and the hip are ball-and-socket joints.

(2) A *condyloid* joint is similar in function to the ball-and-socket joint, but it is much less moveable. In the condyloid joint an oval convex surface on one bone fits into a depression of the other bone. Condyloid joints are biaxial, meaning they are capable of movement in two planes. Examples are the temporomandibular joint and the metacarpophalangeal joints at the base of the fingers.

(3) There is only one *saddle* joint in the body -- that is the trapeziometacarpal joint at the base of the thumb. This joint is biaxial (capable of movement in two planes). It allows humans to have an opposable thumb, which is necessary for picking up small objects with dexterity. A saddle joint can be pictured by placing a Pringle's potato chip convex side up and covering it with another chip placed convex side down and rotated ninety degrees.

(4) *Hinge* joints are monaxial, meaning that they are capable of movement in only one plane. In a hinge joint a bone with a convex surface fits into a concave depression on another bone. Examples are the elbow (the humeroulnar joint), the knee (the tibiofemoral joint), and the interphalangeal joints of the fingers and toes.

(5) *Pivot* joints allow one bone to rotate around another. One bone of a pivot joint has a projection that is surrounded by a circular ligament that is attached to the other bone. Examples are the atlantoaxial joint (C1-C2 vertebrae) and the radioulnar joint at the elbow. In the atlantoaxial joint the atlas pivots around the odontoid process of the axis. This movement allows you to turn your head from side to side. In the elbow the head of the radius rotates within the annular ligament, which is attached to the ulna. This movement allows you to supinate and pronate your forearm.

(6) *Gliding* joints are capable of limited movement whereby one bone slides over another. They are monaxial and their movement is limited. Examples include the intercarpal, intertarsal and intervertebral joints. Gliding joints are classified as amphiarthrotic.

Movements of the body are produced by muscular action on bones, and those movements obey the laws of physics. A **_lever_** is an elongated rigid object that rotates around a fixed point. A lever consists of the fixed point, which is called the **_fulcrum,_** an **_effort arm_**, and a **_resistance arm_**. In the skeletal system the fulcrum (fixed point) is represented by a diarthrotic joint. Using the flexing effect of the biceps brachii on the elbow joint as an example, the elbow is the fulcrum, the point of insertion of the biceps brachii on the radius is the effort arm, and the distal end of the forearm is the resistance arm (the part of the body being moved). The position of the three parts of a lever varies among the joints, and all three classes of levers exist in the body. When the fulcrum is in the center as in a seesaw, it is a first class lever. The resistance arm is in the center in a second class lever. The effort arm is in the center in a third class lever. The example using elbow flexion is a third class lever because the effort arm (biceps insertion) is in the center.

The **_temporomandibular joint_** is a condyloid joint with properties of a hinge joint and a gliding joint. It has a small articular disc (meniscus) of fibrous cartilage. A deep yawn will sometimes cause the condyle of the mandible to slip forward and out of the joint. You must press down on the molar teeth and push the jaw backward to replace the mandibular condyle into the joint. A malocclusion of the teeth and constant grinding of the teeth can cause excessive wear of the articular cartilage and chronic pain in this joint. That condition is called the temporomandibular joint syndrome or TMJ syndrome.

The **_shoulder_** joint (scapulohumeral or glenohumeral joint) is a ball-and-socket joint. It is the most freely moveable joint in the body due to the shallowness of the glenoid cavity and looseness of the joint capsule. A ring of fibrocartilage called the **_glenoid labrum_** surrounds the joint. The glenoid labrum deepens the glenoid cavity and helps to hold the head of the humerus in place. The **_rotator cuff_** consists of muscles, tendons and ligaments that support the shoulder joint. The rotator cuff includes **(1)** three glenohumeral ligaments and the coracohumeral ligaments, and **(2)** the supraspinatus, infraspinatus, subscapularis and teres minor muscles and their tendons. All four of the muscles of the rotator cuff have their origins on the scapula and their insertions on the humerus. A tear in one or more of the ligaments, muscles or tendons that make up the rotator cuff is called a torn rotator cuff, and it results in shoulder pain and weakness. Picking up a child by one arm can cause this type of injury. The long tendon of the biceps brachii muscle circles over the shoulder joint and helps to hold the humerus in the glenoid cavity, but the tendon of the biceps brachii is not part of the rotator cuff.

Right: A dorsal view of the shoulder. The shoulder joint is a ball and socket joint. The head of the humerus fits into the glenoid fossa of the scapula. The glenoid fossa is deepened by a ring of cartilage called the glenoid labrum. The joint is strengthened by the ligaments, muscles and tendons of the rotator cuff.

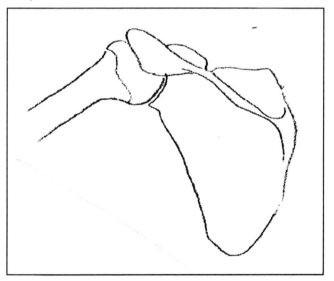

The head of the femur fits into the acetabulum of the pelvic bone (os coxa) to form the hip joint. The hip joint is deepened by the **_acetabular labrum_**, a ring of fibrous cartilage around the acetabulum. The iliofemoral, ischiofemoral and pubofemoral ligaments connect the pelvis to the femur and strengthen the hip. The blood supply to the head of the femur is vulnerable to injury because it is derived from vessels in the **_round ligament_** (ligamentum teres), which traverses the hip joint to enter the apex of the head of the femur. One cause of damage to the artery in the round ligament with secondary necrosis of the femoral head is holding newborns upside down by their feet. Permanent deformity frequently results from this disorder, which goes by several names including aseptic necrosis of the femoral head, coxa plana, and Legge-Perthe's disease.

The **_knee_** or tibiofemoral joint is the largest and most complex diarthrotic joint in the body. It is a hinge joint with a slight ability to rotate and glide laterally. Anteriorly the capsule of the knee joint is made up of the **_patella_** (knee cap), the tendon of the quadriceps femoris (patellar tendon), and ligaments. Other strong ligaments are the **_lateral and medial collateral ligaments_**, and the **_anterior and posterior cruciate ligaments_**. These ligaments and other smaller ligaments of the knee prevent displacement of the femur on the tibia. The ligaments of the knee are susceptible to injury by hyperextension and excessive displacement. When you stand erect and lock your knees, the ligaments of your knees are taut. It takes little muscular effort to maintain this position, and the ability to lock your knees is an important aspect of human bipedalism. Bipedalism was an important evolutionary advancement for man because it provided a more efficient, smoother gait, which made long distance running and walking possible.

Right: An anterior view of the right knee with the patellar tendon cut and retracted.
The knee is primarily a hinge joint, but it also has properties of a gliding joint.
(1) Lateral collateral ligament.
(2) Fibula
(3) Femur
(4) Posterior cruciate ligament
(5) Anterior cruciate ligament
(6) Medial collateral ligament
(7) Patella
(8) Tendon of quadriceps femoris muscle (cut and retracted)
(9) Tibia

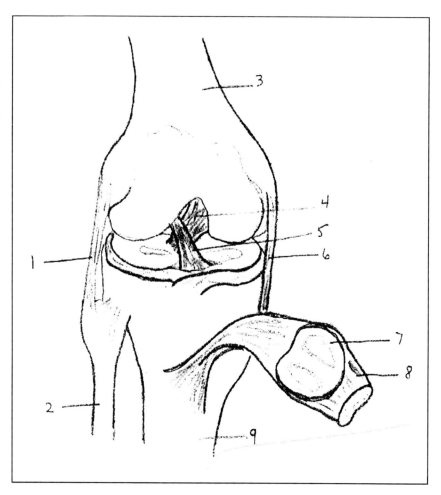

The articular surfaces of adjacent **_vertebrae_** are separated by **_gliding synovial_** joints. The bones of the vertebral column are held together by various ligaments. These ligaments assist in maintaining an upright posture and in returning the spine to extension after it is flexed. The **_ligamentum flava_** are strong elastic ligaments that connect the lamina of adjacent vertebrae. Other ligaments that connect the vertebrae and support the vertebral column are the supraspinal ligament, the nuchal ligament, the interspinal ligaments and the intertransverse ligaments.

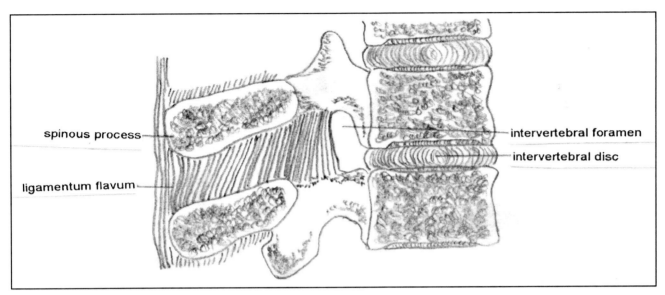

Above: an intervertebral joint. The ligamentum flavum is one of the strong, elastic ligaments that hold the vertebrae in place.

The ***ankle*** or talocrural joint includes the articulation between the ***talus and the tibia***, and the articulation between the ***talus and the fibula***. The talotibial articulation is the weight bearing joint of the ankle. The ***malleoli*** of the tibia and the fibula overhang the ankle and prevent most side-to-side motion. ***Ligaments*** of the ankle include the anterior and posterior tibiofibular ligaments, the deltoid ligament medially, and the lateral collateral ligament.   The ***calcaneal tendon*** is also called the ***Achilles heel;*** it is the combined tendon of the ***gastrocnemius and soleus*** muscles of the calf, which inserts on the ***calcaneus*** bone. An ankle sprain is a torn ligament of the ankle resulting from excessive eversion (turning out) or inversion (turning in) of the foot.

The most common disorders of joints are ***osteoarthritis*** and ***rheumatoid arthritis***. Osteoarthritis is a common condition in elderly people. It involves a gradual degeneration of the articular cartilage. Rheumatoid arthritis is an autoimmune inflammatory disease that is caused by an abnormal antibody that attacks synovial joints.   Other autoimmune inflammatory joint diseases include Marie-Strumpell arthritis or ankylosing spondylitis, which attacks the intervertebral joints, and juvenile rheumatoid arthritis, which attacks the joints of children.

When medications lack efficacy or show toxicity, joint replacement by a metal or plastic prosthesis may be done if the situation demands. This surgical procedure is called an ***arthroplasty***.

Study Guide
1. Know the meanings of the following joint classifications: diarthrotic, amphiarthrotic, and synarthrotic.
2. Know what is meant by these types of joints: fibrous, interosseous membrane (syndesmosis), gomphosis, synchondrosis, symphysis, suture and synovial.
3. Study a synovial joint carefully and note its components including the joint capsule, synovial membrane, synovial fluid and articular cartilage.
4. Know what a meniscus is, where menisci may be found, and the type of cartilage in a meniscus.
5. Be able to define ligament, tendon, bursa, tendon sheath, range of motion, flexion, extension, and hyperextension.
6. Be able to identify and give an example of each type of synovial joint (ball and socket, saddle, condyloid, hinge, pivot and gliding).
7. Know the meaning of the fulcrum, resistance arm and effort arm as they relate to joints.
8. Which joint is the most freely movable joint in the body?
9.   Know where to find the following: acetabular labrum, glenoid labrum, round ligament, medial and lateral collateral ligaments, anterior and posterior cruciate ligaments and the rotator cuff.

Chapter Ten

Muscular Tissue

The **_universal characteristics_** of muscle cells are
(1) **_Excitability._** Muscle cells respond to an electrical stimulus across the cell membrane.
(2) **_Conductivity._** The muscle cells' response to a stimulus is in the form of a wave.
(3) **_Contractility._** Muscle fibers are **_unique_** in that they shorten when stimulated.
(4) **_Extensibility._** The relaxed muscle cell can stretch to as much as three times its contracted length.
(5) **_Elasticity._** After stretch the muscle cell recoils to its original length.

Muscle tissue exists in three forms, skeletal, smooth, and cardiac. Most of the focus of this chapter pertains to **_skeletal muscle._**

Skeletal Muscle

Skeletal muscles are usually attached to one or more bones, but they are sometimes attached to skin, connective tissue or cartilage. Their contractions are **_voluntary_** (under conscious control).

Muscle fascicles are bundles of muscle fibers that are grossly identifiable as strands of muscle. A **_muscle fiber,_** or myofiber, **_is a skeletal muscle cell_**, which is also called a **_myocyte._** Each muscle cell is multinucleated and represents the fusion of multiple stem cells called **_myoblasts_**. Skeletal muscle fibers are thread-like and may be up to thirty cm. long. **_Myofibrils_** are longitudinal bundles of myofilaments that fill most of the muscle cell. **_Myofilaments_** are parallel threads of muscle proteins that are arranged into units called **_sarcomeres._** Myofilaments exhibit **_striations_** of alternating dark and light bands under a microscope.

A **_sarcoma_** is a malignant tumor of connective tissue or muscle tissue. Connective tissue and muscle tissue are derived from mesoderm. A malignant tumor of skeletal muscle is a **_rhabdomyosarcoma_**; a benign tumor of skeletal muscle is a rhabdomyoma. A malignant tumor of smooth muscle is a **_leiomyosarcoma_**; a benign tumor of smooth muscle is a leiomyoma.

The following is a list of words you should know.
Sarco--: a prefix pertaining to muscle or flesh.
Lemma--: a suffix meaning "husk."
Sarcolemma–: the plasma membrane of a muscle cell.
Sarcoplasm–: the cytoplasm of a muscle cell.
Glycogen–: a polymer of glucose.
Myoglobin–: a muscle protein complex that binds oxygen.
Myofiber–: a muscle cell or myocyte.
Myofibril–: bands of myofilaments.
Myofilament–: a thread of muscle proteins.
Transverse ("T") Tubule–: an opening of the SER (smooth endoplasmic reticulum) through the sarcolemma. T tubules conduct electric impulses that produce muscle contraction in skeletal muscles.
Thick filament–: myosin.
Myosin–: a contractile muscle protein.
Thin filament–: actin.
Actin–: a contractile muscle protein.
Sarcomere–: a unit of a myofilament that is contractile. A sarcomere is the area between two Z discs.
Titan (Connectin)–: the elastic protein in a sarcomere.
Elastic Filament--: titan.
Tropomyosin–: a regulatory muscle protein.
Troponin–: a component of tropomyosin that binds with calcium.
Contractile Proteins–: actin and myosin.
Regulatory Proteins–: tropomyosin and troponin.
Sarcoplasmic Reticulum (SR)–: the endoplasmic reticulum of a muscle cell.
Terminal Cisternae–: dilatations in the smooth endoplasmic reticulum that store calcium ions.

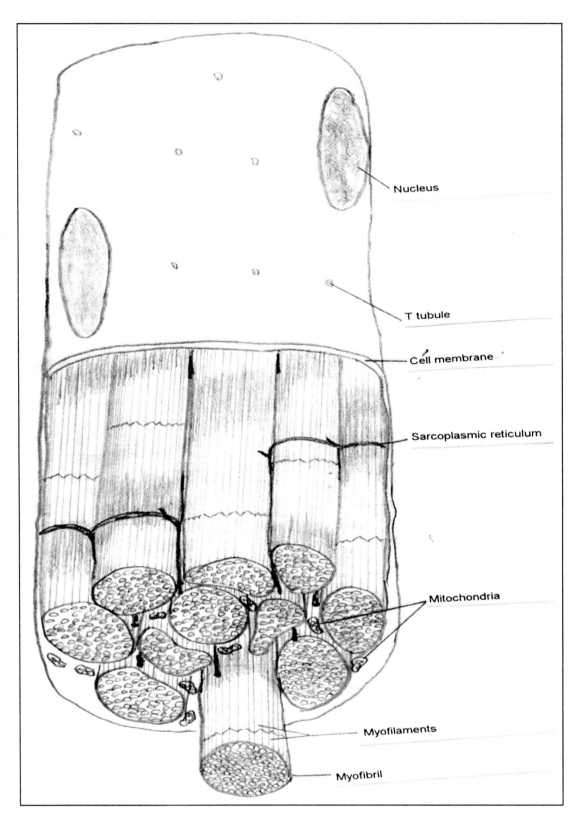

Nucleus

T tubule

Cell membrane

Sarcoplasmic reticulum

Mitochondria

Myofilaments

Myofibril

Above: A muscle cell is a muscle fiber containing myofibrils. A myofibril is made up of multiple parallel chains of sarcomeres. A myofilament is a single chain of sarcomeres. Visible in this Illustration are the sarcolemma, "T" tubules, mitochondria, the sarcoplasmic reticulum and sarcomeres.

The ***sarcolemma*** is the plasma membrane of a muscle cell. It is perforated with openings of tunnels called ***transverse (T) tubules***, which form a network throughout the cell. T tubules connect with dilated areas known as ***terminal cisternae*** of the ***sarcoplasmic reticulum.***   The sarcoplasmic reticulum is the smooth endoplasmic reticulum of a muscle cell. T tubules carry electric impulse to the cisternae, which are storehouses for calcium ions. Bundles of ***myofilaments*** called ***myofibrils*** fill the sarcoplasm of a muscle cell. Also in the sarcoplasm are ***glycogen*** inclusions for energy storage, ***myoglobin*** molecules for binding oxygen, and ***mitochondria*** for ATP production.

Myofilaments exhibit striations of light and dark bands named ***"I" bands, "A" bands, "H" bands and "Z" discs***. ***"A" bands*** are dark and represent the thick filaments, which are composed of myosin. ***"I"*** bands are light and represent the thin filaments of actin and connectin, but not myosin. ***"H"*** bands are relatively light bands in the center of the thick filaments (A bands). They are composed of myosin but not actin because the actin fibers do not reach to the center of the A band. ***"Z"*** discs are thickened elastic filaments of the protein, ***titan***, which is also called ***connectin.*** Z discs anchor the actin and connectin filaments, and they connect two sarcomeres together. ***A sarcomere*** is the area of a myofilament that is located between two Z discs. Z discs connect myofilaments to the cytoskeleton.

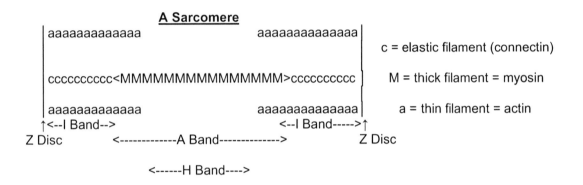

A Sarcomere

```
    aaaaaaaaaaaaa              aaaaaaaaaaaaa |
                                             |   c = elastic filament (connectin)
                                             |
    cccccccccc<MMMMMMMMMMMMMMM>cccccccccc     |   M = thick filament = myosin
                                             |
    aaaaaaaaaaaaa              aaaaaaaaaaaaa |   a = thin filament = actin
    ↑<--I Band-->               <--I Band----->↑
    Z Disc          <-------------A Band------------->       Z Disc

              <------H Band---->
```

Multiple myosin molecules are intertwined in the ***thick filaments.*** Protuberances on the myosin molecules called ***"heads"*** can bend back and forth. Two intertwined actin strands make up a ***thin filament.*** The actin molecules contain ***active sites*** that are capable of binding with the heads of the myosin molecules. Myosin and actin are called ***contractile proteins***. ***Tropomyosin*** is a protein complex that is in linked to actin. ***Troponin*** is a part of tropomyosin. ***When troponin bonds with calcium***, a change in structure of the tropomyosin complex occurs, and ***active sites*** on the actin filaments become ***exposed***, which allows myosin heads to bind with the active sites of actin. Tropomyosin and troponin regulate contraction, and they are called ***regulatory proteins***.

Motor Neurons and the Neuromuscular Junction.
(The word "motor" means "movement.")
Skeletal muscle must be stimulated by a nerve impulse in order to contract. Loss of its nerve connection results in muscle paralysis (paresis). Motor neurons are located in the brain stem, spinal cord or ganglia. Their axons constitute a ***motor nerve.*** Motor nerves travel to muscles where they initiate muscle contractions.

A motor unit is the axon of one motor neuron and all the muscle fibers it innervates. Each muscle fiber is innervated by only one motor unit; however, each motor neuron typically innervates numerous muscle fibers as a consequence of ***axonal branching***. The muscle cells of motor units tend ***not*** to be close together; rather they are ***dispersed*** in a wide area of the muscle. Therefore, stimulation of one motor unit results in a weak, but generalized, contraction. Contractions can be sustained because different motor units alternate contracting and relaxing. Alternation is essential in postural control. One axon may innervate anywhere from three to one thousand muscle fibers. In the eye muscles only three muscle cells are excited by each axon, which results in fine motor control. About one thousand muscle cells are innervated by each motor axon in the gastrocnemius muscle. Thus the stimulus from one axon to the gastrocnemius can provide a strong contraction, which is necessary for a quick start or jump.

A *synapse* is a junction between two nerve cells or between the axon of a nerve cell and a muscle cell. The *neuro-muscular junction (NMJ)* is a synapse between the axon of a nerve cell and a muscle cell. The cells do not actually touch; there is a tiny cleft between them called the *synaptic cleft.* The *motor end plate* is a depressed area on the sarcolemma of the muscle cell that is exposed to the synaptic cleft. The end (synaptic bulb) of the nerve fiber secretes vesicles filled with *acetylcholine* (ACh), a type of *neurotransmitter,* into the cleft. Acetylcholine binds to receptors on the sarcolemma (plasma membrane) at the motor end plate of the muscle cell.

$$CH_3 \qquad\qquad O$$
$$| \qquad\qquad\qquad ||$$
$$H_3\,C - N - CH_2 - CH_2 - O - C - CH_3$$
$$|$$
$$CH_3$$

Formula for acetylcholine (ACh)

A *Schwann cell* (neurilemmacyte) surrounds the entire neuro-muscular junction and insulates it from the surrounding tissue fluid.

Cholinesterase, (specifically acetylcholinesterase), is an enzyme in the synaptic cleft that breaks down acetylcholine, and is thereby able to curtail the muscle contraction.

Right: The neuromuscular junction. The motor nerve axon is surrounded by a Schwann cell sheath. The synaptic knob contains vesicles of a neurotransmitter such as acetylcholine, which are secreted into the synaptic cleft. Receptors to acetylcholine in the plasma membrane of the muscle cell respond by opening ligand-gated channels for the admission of sodium ions into the muscle cell. That is the first stage of muscle contraction.

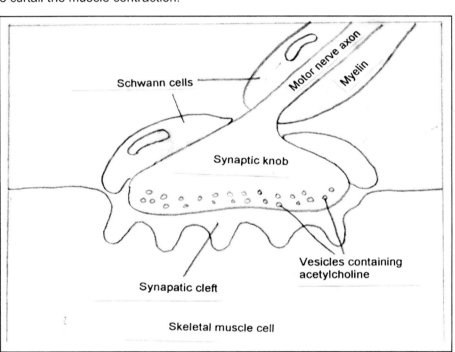

Schwann cells

Motor nerve axon

Myelin

Synaptic knob

Vesicles containing acetylcholine

Synapatic cleft

Skeletal muscle cell

The Phases of Muscle Contraction

(1) Excitation. In the excitation phase a nerve impulse travels to the synaptic bulb, and ACh is released by the nerve ending into the synaptic cleft. ACh binds to receptors on the sarcolemma. *The excitability* of nerve and muscle cells is explained by the presence of a charge differential across the plasma membrane. In the resting state the inside of the membrane is negative to the outside. The *outside has a much higher concentration of sodium*, and *the inside has a much higher concentration of potassium*. The extracellular concentration of Na+ is 144 mEq/L; the extracellular concentration of K+ is 4.5 mEq/L. The intracellular concentration of Na+ is 10 mEq/L; the intracellular concentration of K+ is 141 mEq/L. Other ions with negative charges inside the cell (proteins, nucleic acids, bicarbonate and phosphate ions) and ions with positive charges outside the cell (Ca++) account for the charge differential across the plasma membrane. *The resting potential* of the plasma membrane of a muscle cell is about -90mV (-70 mV for nerve cells). This compares to 1.5 volts for a flashlight battery and 12 volts for an automobile battery. *Excitation* begins with a *change* in the voltage across the plasma membrane. When ACh attaches to a receptor on the cell membrane, it causes *ligand gates* to open in the membrane. Then

sodium rushes into the cell by diffusion, and the inside of the cell quickly changes from -90 mV to (up to) +75 mV (+35 mV for nerve cells). The change to positive in the electric potential will occur only if a sufficient number of sodium ions enter the cell to reach the **_threshold potential of -55 mV_**. When the charge across the plasma membrane reaches zero, sodium gates begin to close, and potassium gates begin to open. Potassium cations rush out of the cell by diffusion and by being repelled by the newly arrived positive Na+ cations. Loss of intracellular K+ turns the inside of the plasma membrane to negative again. These changes first occur at the motor end plate and constitute what is called the **_end plate potential_** (EPP). The EPP causes **_voltage-gated_** sodium ion channels in the sarcolemma adjacent to the NMJ to open and later to close as occurred at the motor end plate. First sodium enters the cell and makes the inside of the plasma membrane positive; then K+ exits the cell returning the inside of the membrane to negative. **_The action potential_** is the quick up and down shift in the electric potential across the plasma membrane as the inside of the cell turns from -90 mV to +75 mV, then returns to -90 mV. Action potentials in the sarcolemma adjacent to the NMJ (neuromuscular junction) trigger a wave known as a nerve impulse to travel down the cell membrane.

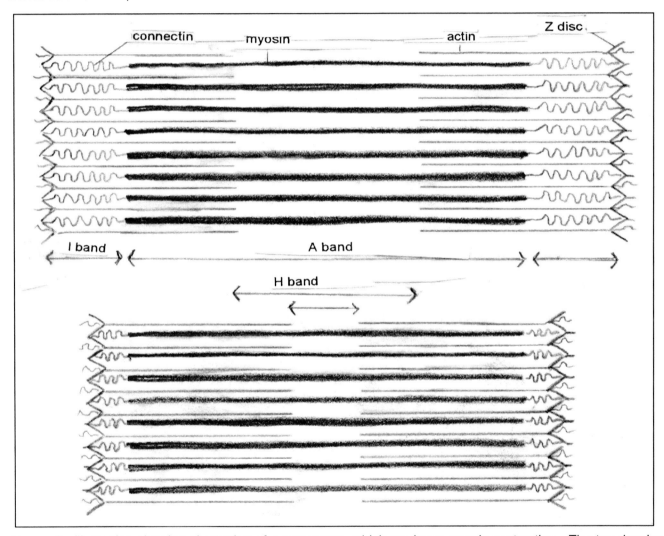

Above: An illustration showing shortening of a sarcomere, which produces muscle contraction. The top drawing shows a relaxed sarcomere. The bottom drawing shows a contracted sarcomere; the thin filaments have been pulled together by bending of the myosin heads. The A band, I band and H band are visible in a microscope. Note that neither the myosin filaments in the thick filaments nor the actin filaments of the thin filaments change in length. Contraction is produced by the actin filaments being pulled closer together, thus shortening the "H" band. The elastic filament (connectin) can stretch and recoil, but that is not the reason a muscle contracts. Muscle contraction is produced by shortening of the sarcomeres created by an increased overlap of myosin and actin filaments.

(2) The ***coupling of excitation and contraction phase*** follows the excitation phase. In the coupling phase the action potential is carried down the sarcolemma like ripples on a pond. When it reaches the T tubules, it dives into the cell via the sarcoplasmic reticulum. It reaches the cisternae, which are storehouses for calcium. The nerve impulse causes calcium ions to pour out of the cisternae into the sarcoplasm surrounding the myofibrils. The calcium ions bind to troponin, which is part of the tropomyosin complex. The ***latent phase*** includes the excitation phase and the coupling phase.

(3) The third phase is called ***the contraction phase***. It begins after calcium has bound to troponin. Calcium binding causes the tropomyosin complex ***to change shape***, which exposes ***active sites*** on the thin filaments (actin molecules). "Heads" of the myosin molecules utilize ATP to move backward into an extended, high energy position. Then the myosin heads bind to active sites on actin. Next, the myosin heads release ADP + phosphate and revert to the flexed, low energy position. This movement is tantamount to paddling a canoe, and it is called the "power stroke." The myosin head tugs actin along with it, which shortens the sarcomere by bringing the thin filaments closer together. This sequence is repeated over and over, each time bringing the thin filaments of the sarcomere closer together. The myosin heads act sequentially. In other words only half of the myosin heads are released from actin at one time. The other half is bound to actin and holding it in place. The whole process of contraction is like pulling up an anchor rope hand over hand.

(4) The last phase of contraction is the ***relaxation phase***. In this phase nerve impulses cease, and ACh stops being released into the synaptic cleft. Acetylcholinesterase degrades the ACh present in the synaptic cleft. Calcium disassociates from troponin and is pumped back into the cisternae by active transport. The tropomyosin complex reverts to its original shape, which occludes the active sites on actin. This prevents the heads of myosin from binding with active sites on actin. Muscle tension eases.

When agents known as ***cholinesterase inhibitors*** are encountered, ACh is not degraded in the synaptic cleft, and a sustained production of nerve impulses occurs. The result is a spastic paralysis or uncontrolled tetany. Cholinesterase inhibitors include some pesticides, nerve gases and medications. Excessive exposure to these agents can be fatal.

Tetanus is a disease caused by a toxin produced by the bacteria, *Clostridium tetani*. *C. tetani* is most commonly encountered as an infectious agent in deep, unclean wounds. Tetanus toxin blocks glycine, an inhibitory neurotransmitter in the spinal cord.   The result is muscle over stimulation with spasm and tetany in skeletal muscles. Spasm of the jaw muscles in patients with tetanus resulted in the common name for the disease -- "lockjaw."

Botulism is a disease caused by a toxin produced by *Clostridium botulinum*, a bacteria species of the same genus as *C. tetani*. *C. botulinum* exists in the soil. The bacteria are not harmful when ingested, but the ingestion of a tiny amount of toxin can be fatal. Botulinum toxin is most frequently encountered in canned foodstuffs that have been inadequately sterilized or improperly stored. Botulinum toxin causes paralysis by blocking the release of ACh at the neuromuscular junctions. Botulinum toxin is the active ingredient in "Botox," a drug that is injected in minute amounts for cosmetic purposes. Botox causes a localized muscle paralysis that reduces skin wrinkling; its effect lasts for months.

Curare is a drug originally found in blowguns used by South American natives. It causes a flaccid muscle paralysis due to blockage of ACh receptor sites at the motor end plate.

Succinyl choline is a drug that is capable of substituting for ACh on receptor sites. When succinyl choline is given IV, it briefly causes generalized muscle fasciculations or twitching; then it blocks the receptor sites from binding ACh for several minutes, producing a depolarizing muscle paralysis. Succinyl choline is not affected by acetylcholinesterase, but it is broken down by cholinesterase in the plasma. The effect of ***curare*** is longer lasting than the effect of succinyl choline. Both have proved useful in anesthesia because the muscle relaxation they produce greatly facilitates insertion of a tube into the airway. Neither drug affects consciousness, so they are given after a short acting barbiturate or other sedative has induced sleep. Both have been used, without sedation, as a form of torture in wartime. Intermittent use of these drugs has proved to be a useful means of extracting information because the prisoner loses muscular activity, but his consciousness is not affected, which is an extremely frightening experience.

The Length-Tension Relationship of a Muscle

If a muscle is nearly fully contracted when it receives a nerve impulse, it can only respond with a weak contraction because the sarcomeres can't get much shorter than they already are. If a muscle is overly stretched when it receives a nerve impulse, initially it can respond only with a weak contraction because few actin and myosin molecules are overlapped, and few cross bridges can form. Therefore, ***a muscle contraction will be strongest if the muscle is in a state of partial contraction*** when the nerve impulse arrives.

After death, muscle contraction called ***rigor mortis*** occurs in about three or four hours. Rigor mortis occurs because the deteriorating sarcoplasmic reticulum releases calcium, which triggers the contraction phase. Relaxation does not occur until two or three days later when the myofilaments have decayed.

The Behavior of Whole Muscles

A ***threshold voltage*** is the minimum voltage required to produce a contraction.

A ***twitch*** is a quick cycle of contraction and relaxation produced by a threshold voltage.

The ***latent period*** (about 2 milliseconds) is the time required for excitation, coupling, and the tensing of elastic filaments before muscle shortening can occur. This corresponds to the excitation and coupling phases and the beginning of the contraction phase.

The ***contraction phase*** is the time period when muscle shortening occurs.

The ***relaxation phase*** is the time period when the muscle loses tension and returns to its resting length.

The Variability of Contractility Strength in the Laboratory

A higher voltage stimulus results in the stimulation of more nerve fibers and a stronger contraction. A higher voltage excites more motor units; the result is called ***spatial summation***.

The strength of a contraction following a threshold voltage stimulus is dependent on the ***frequency*** of the impulses (stimuli/second). Increasing the frequency of nerve impulses will produce a stronger contraction. This is known as ***temporal summation***.

From 0-10 stimuli/second results in equal twitch contractions with full recovery between contractions.

From 10-20 stimuli/second results in recovery to the relaxed baseline between twitches, but each twitch is stronger than the previous twitch, and subsequent twitches develop more tension in the muscle. This is called ***treppe*** (pronounced "treppa"). Treppe is theorized to result from the build up of calcium ions in the sarcoplasm.

From 20-40 stimuli/second causes each stimulus to arrive before the previous twitch is relaxed. Muscle contraction gradually increases to ***incomplete tetanus***. A muscle in incomplete tetanus is in a fluttering, strong contraction with minimal relaxation between stimuli.

Complete tetanus (tetany) occurs ***with 50*** or more stimuli/second. There is no relaxation between stimuli in complete tetany, and a strong, smooth contraction exists. Complete tetany rarely, if ever, occurs in the body because twenty-five stimuli/second are rarely exceeded.

In isotonic contractions there is no change in muscle tension, but the muscle shortens or lengthens. ***Concentric isotonic contractions*** are those that involve the shortening of a muscle. ***Eccentric isotonic contractions*** are those that involve the lengthening of a muscle. When a barbell or a heavy box is lifted and lowered, the lifting phase involves a concentric isotonic contraction, and the lowering phase involves an eccentric isotonic contraction. ***An isometric contraction*** is one in which the muscle develops tension without changing its length.

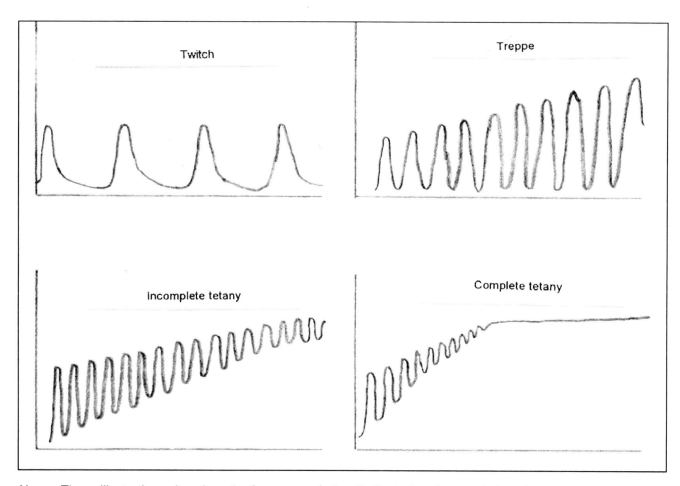

Above: These illustrations show how the frequency of stimuli affects the characteristics of a muscle contraction. In these drawings **time** is represented in the abscissa, and **strength of contraction** is represented in the ordinate. Muscle twitches occur at 0-10 stimuli/second. Treppe occurs from 10-20 stimuli/second. Incomplete tetany occurs at 20-40 stimuli/second, and complete tetany occurs with stimulation rates near 50 stimuli/second. The contractions of treppe, incomplete tetany and complete tetany are stronger than could be produced by a lower frequency of contraction. The increase in strength at higher frequencies of stimuli is termed **temporal summation.**

Sources of ATP

The heads of a myosin molecule must bind with a molecule of ATP in order to extend backward to a position where they can bind an active site on actin. Anaerobic (without oxygen) glycolysis provides two molecules of ATP per each molecule of glucose. Aerobic (with oxygen) respiration produces a theoretical maximum of 36 molecules of ATP per each molecule of glucose. Aerobic respiration requires oxygen to function; anaerobic glycolysis does not. **_Myoglobin_** is a protein in muscle cells that can bind oxygen and store it for future use.

The phosphagen system consists of **_creatine phosphate_** (CP) and **_ADP_**. CP and ADP are used to store high energy phosphate bonds and to synthesize ATP. CP can transfer its high-energy bond to ADP to produce ATP. Two ADP molecules can react and produce one molecule of ATP and one molecule of AMP. One kilogram of muscle typically contains 5 millimoles of ATP and 15 millimoles of CP. This amount of stored high energy phosphate bonds is the amount necessary for one minute of brisk walking or six seconds of fast sprinting. After the existing ATP, the phosphagen stores and the oxygen stored in myoglobin have been exhausted, most of the energy must come from anaerobic fermentation. Anaerobic fermentation can supply enough ATP for 30-40 more seconds of maximum activity after which time aerobic pathways take over ATP production. Aerobic respiration is allowed when the circulatory system has increased the blood flow to muscles and the respiratory system has replenished the oxygen content in the blood. Oxygen consumption by the muscles levels off after 3-4 minutes; ATP production keeps up with demand after that time. Anaerobic fermentation causes the accumulation of lactic acid, a compound that produces fatigue. Lactic acid production ceases when aerobic respiration takes over.

After oxygen availability becomes adequate, the limiting factor to muscle activity is fatigue, which may have several causes including
(1) The muscle stores of glycogen become depleted, and there is a reduction in the blood glucose level.
(2) Fluids and electrolytes (primarily sodium and potassium) are lost through sweating.
(3) A shortage of ATP causes the Na+ and K+ pumps fail to maintain membrane potentials and excitability.
(4) The accumulation of lactic acid produces fatigue and inhibits enzymes involved in ATP synthesis and muscle contraction.
(5) The supply of ACh in the synaptic knobs of motor nerves becomes depleted.

The maximum oxygen uptake is the maximum rate at which an individual can utilize oxygen and produce work. It varies with individuals and usually peaks at age 20. It is higher in trained athletes.

An oxygen debt occurs after exercise. Heavy breathing continues for a period following exercise. During this period (1) oxygen reserves in hemoglobin and myoglobin are replaced; (2) oxygen levels are replenished in the plasma, extracellular fluid, and air of the lungs; (3) ATP and CP stores are rebuilt, and (4) lactic acid is converted to glucose or pyruvic acid in the liver, kidneys and cardiac muscle.

The increased heat produced by muscle activity results in a higher metabolic rate, which requires more oxygen until the body cools down.

Carbohydrate loading is the ingestion of copious quantities of starches and sugars for a period of time before a game or a match. Carbohydrate loading fills the muscles with glycogen, but it also adds water and, therefore, weight to muscles (about 2.7 gm of water for each gram of carbohydrate). Aerobic respiration in active muscles not only involves glucose metabolism, it heavily involves the oxidation of fatty acids and proteins. Glucose, fatty acids and proteins are broken down into molecules that can be metabolized to produce ATP. Fatty acid catabolism must be accompanied by carbohydrate catabolism to keep the cycle operating properly. Without concomitant glycolysis, the fatty acids are incompletely metabolized to acidic ketones, which leads to acidosis (too much acid in the blood).

Slow and Fast Twitch Fibers
Not all muscle fibers are physiologically alike. There are two basic types, slow twitch and fast twitch.
(1) ***Slow twitch*** (also called slow oxidative, red, or type one) fibers are smaller and have ***more mitochondria, more capillaries*** and contain ***more myoglobin***. Slow twitch fibers are adapted to ***aerobic respiration,*** and they are resistant to fatigue. Slow twitch fibers are especially useful in marathon runners. The postural muscles of the back and the soleus muscle of the leg contain a majority of slow twitch fibers. Contractions following stimulation are delayed by about 100 milliseconds in slow twitch fibers.
(2) ***Fast twitch*** (also called fast glycolytic, white, or type two) fibers are larger and are rich in enzymes for ***anaerobic glycolysis*** and the ***phosphagen system***. Fast twitch fibers are high in ***glycogen***, and their sarcoplasmic reticulum releases calcium ions more quickly. Contractions following stimulation may occur as fast as 7.5 msec in fast twitch fibers. They produce more lactic acid, and they fatigue easily. They are especially useful in stop and go sports like basketball and running the one hundred yard dash. In one study of the quadriceps femoris muscles of marathoners, sprinters, and non runners the following ratios of fast twitch and slow twitch fibers was found:

	Percentage of Slow Twitch Fibers	Percentage of Fast Twitch Fibers
Marathon Runners	82%	18%
Non-runners	45%	55%
Sprinters	37%	63%

(3) A few professional athletes have been found to have *intermediate twitch* fibers, which combine some of the characteristics of slow and fast twitch fibers. Intermediate twitch fibers respond quickly, and they are also resistant to fatigue.

Nearly all muscles have both slow and fast twitch fibers. Red muscles like the soleus and the muscles of the back have predominately slow twitch fibers. White muscles like the gastrocnemius contain a majority of fast twitch fibers.

There is a genetic determination for the ratio of slow and fast twitch fibers in any given muscle. West Africans have more fast twitch, white fibers, and they excel in basketball and the 100 yard dash. Members of a small East African tribe living in Kenya and Ethiopia have won seventeen straight New York marathons and nearly half of all the world's marathons, although their total population is very small. The muscles of members of this tribe have been shown to contain a high percentage of the slow twitch, fatigue resistant, red fibers.

Resistance training increases strength, but it does not increase endurance. The cells and the muscles enlarge in diameter and more myofilaments are formed. Mitosis does not occur, but a large fiber may divide longitudinally.

Endurance training increases endurance, but not strength. The number of mitochondria in the muscle fibers increases, the amount of glycogen stored in muscles increases, and the number of capillaries in the muscles increases. These changes occur especially in those muscles with a large number of slow twitch fibers.

Cardiac Muscle

Like skeletal muscle, cardiac muscle is striated; however, cardiac muscle cells are shorter; they are branched, and they usually contain only one nucleus. Cardiac muscle cells are joined together at junctions called *intercalated discs,* which are gap junctions between cardiac muscle cells. The contractions of cardiac muscle cells are *involuntary*; the nerve supply comes from the *autonomic nervous system*. Stimulation from the autonomic nervous system will affect the heart rate and the strength of contraction.

Cardiac muscle is *autorhythmic*, meaning that it contracts from internal stimuli initiated by pacemaker cells in the *sinoatrial (SA) node*. The SA node is a group of specialized myocytes located in the right atrium of the heart. The *atrioventricular (AV) node* is located in the interatrial septum, and it is able to take over as the pacemaker if the SA node malfunctions. Due to the presence of these nodes, Cardiac muscle does not require an external nerve stimulus to contract, and a dissected heart will continue to beat if placed in nutrient rich saline.

A *myocardial infarction* is the death of cardiac muscle cells resulting from an occlusion of a cardiac artery. *Angina pectoris* is chest, left arm or left shoulder pain resulting from ischemia (insufficient blood supply) to cardiac muscle cells due to partial closure of a cardiac artery.

Smooth Muscle

Smooth muscle differs from skeletal muscle by having only one nucleus per cell. Smooth muscle cells have a fusiform shape, and they are much shorter than skeletal muscle cells. Smooth muscle cells lack striations, sarcomeres and Z discs. In smooth muscle the thin filaments of actin are attached to protein clumps called dense bodies, which link actin to the cytoskeleton and the sarcolemma. Myosin is present between the actin filaments, and the two motor molecules produce contraction by reacting chemically similar to the way they do in skeletal muscle. Smooth muscle cells lack T tubules and they contain little sarcoplasmic reticulum; the calcium ions needed for contraction come from the extracellular fluid. The nerve supply to smooth muscle is from the *autonomic nervous system*, and sometimes it is nonexistent. Control of contractions is *involuntary* and does not depend entirely on nervous system stimulation; the muscle may respond to chemical or physical stimuli for example. In the GI tract pacemaker cells exist that can spontaneously depolarize and initiate a wave of contraction called *peristalsis.* Peristaltic waves propel what is eaten through the digestive tract.

Disorders of Muscular Tissue

Muscular dystrophies are a group of related familial diseases wherein skeletal muscles degenerate and are replaced by adipose tissue. In these diseases *dystrophin* is defective or lacking. Dystrophin is a protein that binds actin to the cell membrane. Without dystrophin cell membranes become torn, which leads to cellular necrosis. Skeletal muscle cells do not undergo mitosis, and a gradual loss of muscle cells occurs. Most of the muscular dystrophies are named according to their age of onset or by the muscle groups they affect first. The most common form is the childhood type, also known as _**Duchenne's dystrophy**_. This variety is associated with a sex linked pattern of inheritance (the defective gene is on the X chromosome); therefore, it occurs primarily in males who inherit the defective gene from their mothers who are carriers. Symptoms begin in early childhood, and death usually overtakes the victim by age twenty. Other varieties of muscular dystrophy are associated with an autosomal dominant type of inheritance and an onset later in life. Several variants exist including a _**facioscapulohumeral**_ type that first involves the muscles of the face, shoulder and arm; a _**distal**_ type that first involves the muscles of the hands and feet; a _**progressive ophthalmoplegia**_ type that first involves the eye muscles, and _**a peroneal muscle**_ _**atrophy**_ type that first involves the lateral muscles of the leg. In addition there is an unrelated _**myotonic**_ form of muscular dystrophy that is inherited as an autosomal dominant trait.

**Myasthenia gravis** is a disease of the neuro-muscular junction. Although males and younger people may contract the disease, it most commonly affects older females. In myasthenia _**antibodies attack the neuro-**_ _**muscular junction**_ and bind the acetylcholine receptors. The _**receptors are destroyed**_ and the motor end plate becomes less and less sensitive to ACh. The disease typically involves the eye muscles and muscles of the face initially with double vision (diplopia) and drooping eyelids (ptosis) being common presenting symptoms. Progression of the disease leads to difficulty in walking, swallowing and breathing. Progression may be quite slow; however, the disease is often eventually fatal. Treatment for myasthenia usually involves drugs that inhibit cholinesterase. The inhibition of acetylcholinesterase in these patients permits high concentrations of ACh to remain in the neuro-muscular junction, which promotes ACh binding to undestroyed receptors. The result is that action potentials are more likely to happen; patients are aware of less muscle weakness after taking these drugs.

Tumors originating in myocytes are relatively uncommon, but they are not rare. A rhabdomyosarcoma is a malignant tumor of skeletal muscle cells; a leiomyosarcoma is a malignant tumor of smooth muscle cells. A rhabdomyoma is a benign tumor of skeletal muscle cells, and a leiomyoma is a benign tumor of smooth muscle cells.

Study Guide
1. Define myofilaments, myofibrils, muscle fibers and muscle fascicles.
2. Know the universal characteristics of muscle cells.
3. Which characteristic is unique to muscle cells?
4. Know the definitions given in this chapter.
5. Understand the role of calcium in muscle contraction.
6. Study an illustration of a sarcomere. Identify the following: actin, myosin, connectin (titan), and "Z" disc. Picture how a contracted sarcomere differs from one that is extended.
7. Locate the heads of myosin, active sites on actin, tropomyosin complex and troponin on the sarcomere.
8. Define the regulatory proteins and the contractile proteins of muscle contraction.
9. Know what is meant by a motor unit. Some motor units have a great deal of divergence (branching); some have very little. Give examples with the range of divergence.
10. Define a neuromuscular junction (NMJ). Know how it functions, and know its parts including the synaptic knob, the synaptic vesicles, the synaptic cleft and receptors.
11. Know what Schwann cells (neurilemmacytes) are and where they are located.
12. Know the location and function of acetylcholinesterase.
13. Be able to describe the four phases of muscle contraction (excitation, coupling of excitation and contraction, contraction and relaxation). In your answer include the release of acetylcholine, the binding of ACh to a receptor, the opening of ion channels in the plasma membrane, the conduction of the impulse through the "T" tubules, the release of calcium by the cisternae, and the roles of troponin, tropomyosin, actin and myosin.
14. Describe the effects of cholinesterase inhibitors on the NMJ and on the body.
15. Know the preexisting state of contraction of a muscle that will produce the strongest contraction.
16. Understand the physiology surrounding rigor mortis.
17. Know the meanings of the following: muscle twitch, treppe, incomplete tetanus (tetany), complete tetanus, temporal summation and spatial summation as they relate to muscle contraction.
18. Define an isotonic contraction and an isometric contraction.

19. What is the function of myoglobin in muscle tissue?
20. Know the contents of the phosphagen system and how they produce ATP.
21. List several causes of muscle fatigue.
22. Understand the physiology of carbohydrate loading.
23. What is meant by an oxygen debt?
24. Know the differences between slow twitch and fast twitch muscle fibers, including their physiology, number of capillaries, use of the phosphagen system, speed of reaction, where they are found, and the amount of stored glycogen. Which is specialized for anaerobic glycolysis, and which is specialized for aerobic respiration?
25. Know the special characteristics of cardiac muscle including autorhythmicity and the intercalated discs.
26. Know the special characteristics of smooth muscle and its relation to the autonomic nervous system.
27. Peruse muscle disorders including the muscular dystrophies and myasthenia gravis.

Chapter Eleven

The Muscles

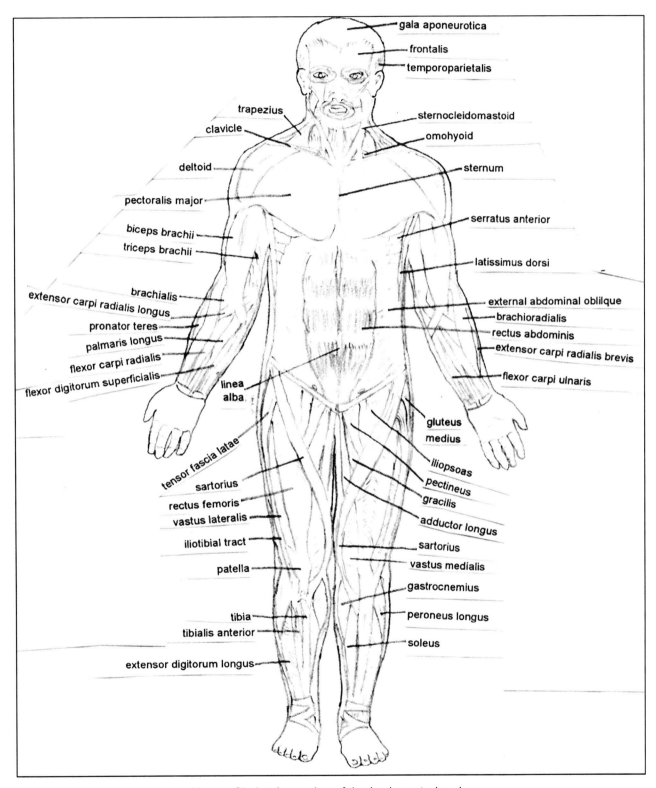

Above: Skeletal muscles of the body, anterior view.

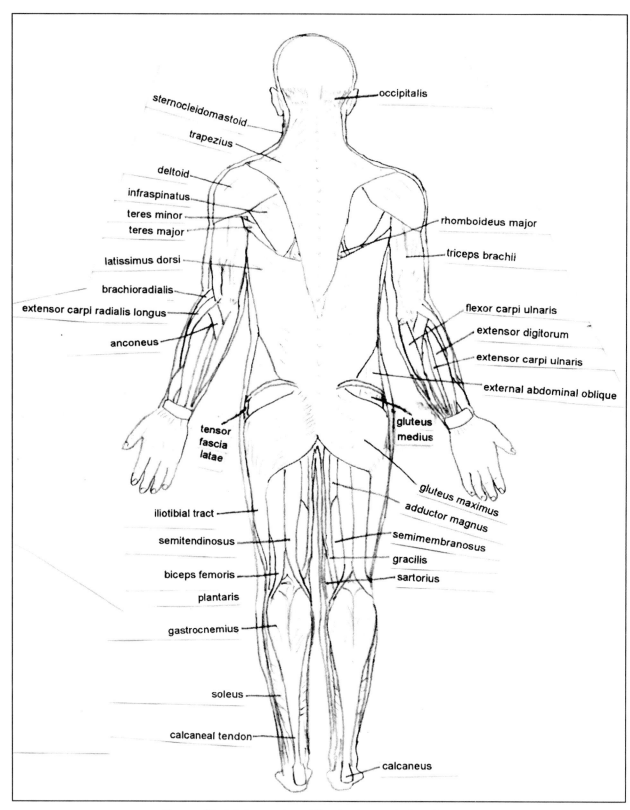

Above: Skeletal muscles of the body, posterior view.

Skeletal muscles serve the total organism in several ways. They provide **_movement_** for the body and its parts; they are necessary in **_communication_** with other people, not only in speech and expression, but also in writing; they control what comes in and goes out of the body through the body's **_sphincters,_** and they produce up to 85% of the **_heat_** generated by the body.

You have approximately 600 skeletal muscles in your body. The number varies slightly among people because some may lack a muscle, whereas others may have an additional muscle. Muscles form body contours, and they account for about 40% of the weight of the body.

There are three layers of connective tissue associated with muscles. They are the **_epimysium_**, the **_perimysium_** and the **_endomysium_**. The epimysium is a dense layer of collagen fibers that surrounds a muscle and separates it from surrounding tissues. Epimysium makes up part of what is called **_fascia,_** which is sheets of connective tissue between tissue body parts. **_Deep fascia_** is found between adjacent muscles and organs. **_Superficial fascia_** is the **_hypodermis_**, a layer of connective tissue beneath the dermis, which contains a considerable quantity of adipocytes. Trauma to a muscle may result in bleeding, and extraneous blood within the epimysium of a muscle can compress and injure nerve fibers and muscle fibers. This is called a **_compartment syndrome;_** it occurs because the epimysium and perimysium have a limited ability to stretch.

The **_perimysium_** is a finer layer of connective tissue containing blood vessels, nerves, collagen fibers and elastic fibers that penetrates the muscle and divides it into bundles of muscle fibers called **_fascicles._**

The **_endomysium_** is a fine layer of connective tissue that surrounds individual muscle fibers. **_A muscle fiber is a muscle cell_**. In skeletal muscle the fibers are thread-like and up to thirty cm. long. Skeletal muscle fibers are **_multinucleated_** cells that are formed by the fusion of many **_stem cells,_** which are called **_myoblasts_**. Each myoblast contributes a nucleus to the muscle cell. A few myoblasts (called **_satellite cells_**) are thinly scattered among muscle fibers, but they have a minimal capacity for regeneration in adults. Muscle fibers contain **_myofilaments_**, which are microscopic strands of motor proteins. Myofilaments are arranged in bundles called **_myofibrils._**

The two ends of a muscle are its **_origin_** and its **_insertion_**. The origin is the stationary end and the end closest to the trunk (proximal end). The insertion is the mobile end and the distal end. Most muscles originate and insert on a bone, but cartilage, skin, connective tissue, and tendons of other muscles also serve as sites of origin and insertion for certain muscles. Sometimes the designation of origin and insertion is arbitrary, such as the rectus abdominis, where both ends are stationary, and circular muscles, which arise and insert at the same locale or within themselves. In naming a muscle the origin is named first, then the insertion. Thus the brachioradialis arises on the humerus and inserts on the radius.

Skeletal muscles frequently have **_tendons_** at their places of origin and insertion. Tendons are **_dense regular connective tissue_** made up of fibroblasts and collagen fibers that run lengthwise. Tendons attach muscle to bone. Tendon fibers are interwoven with the connective tissue of muscle and the periosteum of bone; some tendon fibers extend into the bony matrix.

An **_aponeurosis_** is a broad, flat, sheet-like tendon. Examples of aponeuroses include the **_gala aponeurotica_** of the scalp, the tendon insertion of the **_levator palpebrae_** in the upper eyelid, the origin of the temporalis muscle, the plantar aponeurosis of the sole of the foot, the palmar fascia of the hand, and insertions of the abdominal muscles.

Tendon sheaths are tubular structures of connective tissue that surround some tendons. Tendon sheaths are surrounded by a synovial membrane that secretes synovial fluid. Tendon sheaths are prominent in the wrist and ankle where they allow a tendon to slide freely over a bone and under a retinaculum.

A **_retinaculum_** is a wide band of connective tissue under which tendons pass. Retinaculae in the wrist and ankle keep tendons from elevating off the bones. **_Carpal tunnel syndrome_** results from repetitive wrist and hand movements, which cause swelling. Compression of the median nerve by the retinaculum of the wrist leads to weakness, numbness and tingling of the thumb, forefinger and lateral palmar surface of the hand, and pain on palmar flexion.

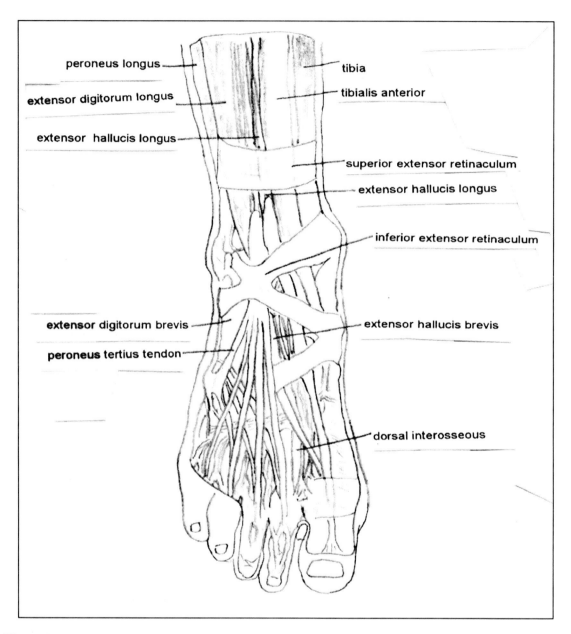

peroneus longus

extensor digitorum longus

extensor hallucis longus

tibia

tibialis anterior

superior extensor retinaculum

extensor hallucis longus

inferior extensor retinaculum

extensor digitorum brevis

peroneus tertius tendon

extensor hallucis brevis

dorsal interosseous

Above: The retinaculae on the dorsum of the ankle are shown in this illustration. Retinaculae are bands of dense connective tissue around the wrist and ankles. They function to keep tendons from elevating off the extremity when the ankle joint or the wrist joint is flexed or extended. They are present on both extensor surfaces and flexor surfaces of the wrists and ankles.

Muscles come in several shapes; the general shape of a muscle is determined by the orientation of its fascicles.

A ***fusiform*** shape is a thick muscle belly with tapering ends. It is exemplified by the biceps brachii and the gastrocnemius. Fusiform muscles are capable of relatively strong contractions.

In a ***parallel*** shaped muscle the fibers run parallel to the length of the muscle. Parallel muscles typically span relatively long distances. The rectus abdominis muscle is an example.

In a ***convergent*** shaped muscle the fibers converge from a broad origin to a narrow insertion. These muscles give strong contractions. The pectoralis major muscle is an example.

Fibers in a ***pennate shaped*** muscle are arranged in the form of a feather. If the bristles of the feather are located on only one side of the stem, it is called ***unipennate***. If the bristles are on both sides of the stem, it is called ***bipennate***, and if there are numerous bipennate stems connected at the insertion of the muscle, it is called ***multipennate***. Examples of unipennate muscles are the palmar interosseous muscles and the semimembranosus muscle of the thigh. An example of a bipennate muscle is the rectus femoris, and an example of a multipennate muscle is the deltoid. Pennate muscles are the strongest type, but they pull at an angle to their tendinous insertion, which reduces the distance that they can move their tendon. Pennate muscles tend to have more fascicles, more muscle fibers and more collagen fibers than other types of muscles.

A ***circular*** muscle is named by the circular direction of its fibers. Circular muscles are present in ***sphincters*** such as the orbicularis oris, orbicularis oculis and anal sphincter.

The ***strength of a muscle contraction*** is influenced by the shape of the muscle. The ***pennate*** arrangement of muscle fibers is able to exert the most tension; the fusiform and convergent arrangements also give strong contractions. ***The circular*** arrangement gives the weakest contraction.

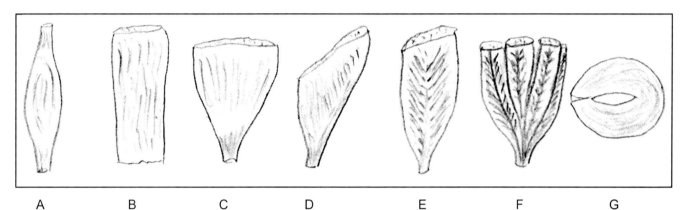

A   B   C   D   E   F   G

Above: Muscles come in different shapes according to the orientation of fibers. (A) fusiform, (B) parallel, (C) convergent, (D) unipennate, (E) bipennate, (F) multipennate, and (G) circular.

The ***agonist*** muscle is the primary muscle that produces most of the force for a joint to move in a specified direction.

A ***synergist*** is a muscle that acts like the agonist to produce a movement. For example brachialis and brachioradialis are synergistic to biceps brachii in flexing the elbow. Or a synergist can assist the agonist by stabilizing a joint, thereby allowing the agonist to work more effectively.

An ***antagonist*** is a muscle that opposes the movement of the agonist by giving an opposite movement. In most cases the agonist and the antagonist contract simultaneously to produce a coordinated movement.

A ***fixator*** is a muscle that prevents a bone from moving and allows another muscle to exert its effect. Fixators are often synergists. They serve to maintain posture and balance. Examples are the scapular muscles, which stabilize the scapula and thereby allow the muscles that move the arm to be effective.

An attempt has been made to name the muscles according to a system. The most common reference names include
digiti--: finger
profundus--: deep
quadriceps--: having four sites of origin
superficialis--: external
pollex, pollicis--: thumb
hallux, hallucis--: big toe
magnus--: large
minimus--: small
maximus--: large
flexor--: decreases the angle of a joint
extensor--: increases the angle of a joint
abductor--: moves away from the midline
adductor--: moves toward the midline

longus--: long
brevis--: short
teres--: round
rhomboideus--: parallelogram shaped
serratus--: serrated, notched
trapezius--: trapezoidal
deltoid--: triangular
indicis--: first finger (forefinger)
transversus--: transverse
oblique--: diagonal
pronator--: elbow rotation so that the palm is back or down
supinator--: elbow rotation so that the palm is up or forward
depressor--: lowers
levator--: elevator (raises)
rectus--: straight
protraction--: thrust forward
retraction--: draw backward
intrinsic--: a muscle having its origin and insertion in the same area (tongue, foot or hand)
extrinsic--: a muscle having its origin removed from the area of its insertion

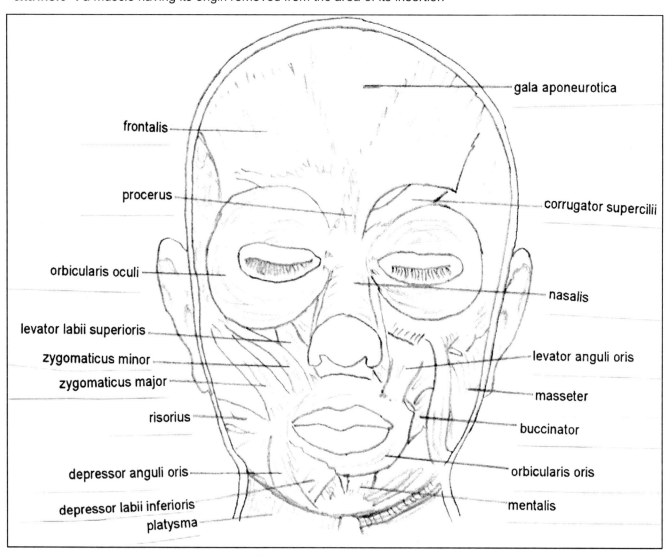

Above: The muscles of the face, frontal view.

Some muscles retain their old names including the **_sartorius_** (which means "tailor") and the **_buccinator_** (which means "trumpeter"). The sartorius muscle of the thigh is useful in the bending position used by tailors to measure garments; it flexes the hip and the knee; it laterally rotates the femur, and it medially rotates the tibia. The buccinator compresses the cheeks, allowing forced expulsion of air.

Muscles are grouped according to locale and the joints they affect. **_Facial muscles_** are the superficial muscles of the face. They provide facial expression by moving the skin of the face. **_Origins_** of the facial muscles may be in the skin, other muscles, or bones of the face. Most facial muscle **_insertions_** are in the skin. The buccinator, orbicularis oris and orbicularis oculi are examples of facial muscles. The facial muscles are innervated by motor fibers in the **_seventh (facial) cranial nerve_**. Paralysis of this nerve is not uncommon because it passes through a narrow foramen behind the ear, (the **_stylomastoid foramen_**). The result of a facial nerve injury is paralysis of the facial muscles on that side of the face, which is called **_Bell's palsy_**. Bell's palsy is disfiguring; the corner of the mouth droops, the lower eyelid droops and the eye waters. Fortunately Bell's palsy is usually temporary.

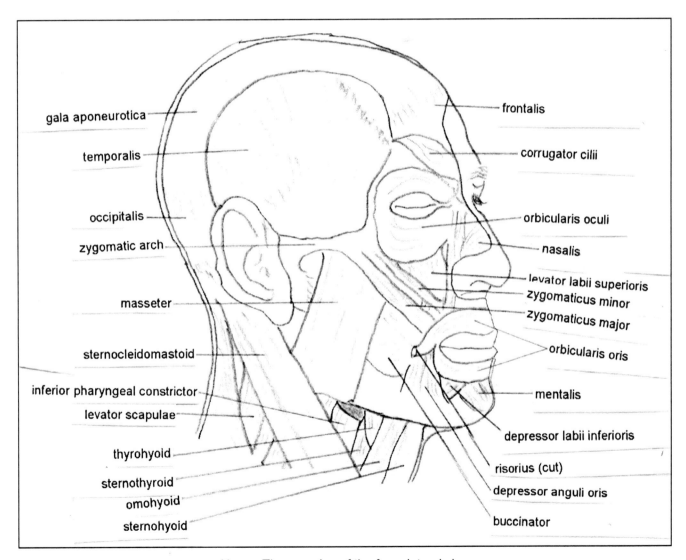

Above: The muscles of the face, lateral view.

The ***muscles of mastication*** are the muscles of chewing and swallowing. They act on the mandible, tongue, pharynx, larynx, hyoid bone, soft palate and epiglottis. The ***elevators of the mandible*** are powerful muscles; they are the ***masseter, temporalis, medial pterygoid and lateral pterygoid*** muscles. These muscles elevate the mandible; the pterygoids also give lateral movement to the mandible. In contrast the depressors of the mandible are several small, weak muscles that open the mouth. Alligator wrestlers are successful because they hold the alligator's mouth closed. The wrestlers can overcome the weak depressors of the mandible, but the powerful elevators of the mandible, which close the mouth, would come into play if the mouth is allowed to open, which could spell disaster for the wrestler. Most ***depressors of the mandible*** originate or insert on the ***hyoid bone***, a small bone of the neck above the larynx. These muscles depress the mandible, and they move the tongue, pharynx and floor of the mouth in swallowing. The thyrohyoid muscle elevates the larynx and moves it to position where it can be covered by the epiglottis while swallowing. The ***tongue*** contains extrinsic muscles and intrinsic muscles. The intrinsic muscles run in vertical, transverse and longitudinal directions. The tongue receives a large amount of innervation relative to its size. This is depicted by a ***homunculus***, which is a picture that relates areas of the brain to peripheral areas that are innervated.

The muscles of the ***head and neck*** are neck flexors and extensors. Neck flexors include the sternocleidomastoid and three scalene muscles. The sternocleidomastoid flexes the neck and turns the head to the opposite side. As its name reflects, the sternocleidomastoid originates on the sternum and the clavicle and inserts on the mastoid process of the temporal bone. The extensors of the neck include the trapezius, splenius capitis and semispinalis capitis. Put your hand on the back of your neck and extend your neck, and you can feel these muscles contract.

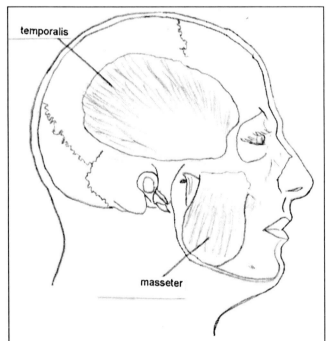
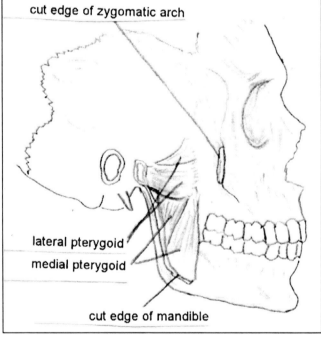

Above: The muscles of mastication include the temporalis, masseter, and the medial and lateral pterygoid muscles.

The muscles of ***respiration*** include the ***diaphragm and the internal and external intercostal muscles***. The ***diaphragm*** separates the thorax from the abdomen; its tendon is central and fibrous. When relaxed, the diaphragm assumes a convex shape with the convexity upwards. When it contracts, it flattens, which increases the volume of the thorax and brings air into the lungs. Vocal teachers are aware that the diaphragm is the primary muscle of respiration, and they teach their students to employ diaphragmatic breathing. The motor nerve to the diaphragm is the ***phrenic*** nerve, which arises from the cervical spinal cord. Any injury above the C3-5 level paralyzes the diaphragm. The ***intercostal muscles*** are located between the ribs. Contraction of the ***internal*** *intercostal* muscles pulls the ribcage down and inward resulting in forced expiration. Contraction of the *external intercostal* muscles pulls the ribcage up and outward resulting in inspiration.

There are four *abdominal* muscles on each side of the body. They serve to protect and support the abdominal organs and to stabilize the vertebral column. The *rectus abdominis* is a long slender muscle near the midline with parallel fibers that run vertically from the pubis to the sternum. The rectus abdominis has four horizontal bands of dense connective tissue called *tendinous intersections*, which can be seen in thin, well-muscled individuals. The other three abdominal muscles are broad, sheet-like muscles that extend over the abdomen and flanks. The fibers of *external abdominal oblique* run downward toward the midline. The fibers of *internal abdominal oblique* run upward toward the midline. *Transversus abdominis* is the deepest of the four; its fibers run in a transverse direction. The abdominal muscles insert by broad, interconnected aponeurotic sheets that extend from the costal margins to the iliac crest. The aponeurotic fibers intersect with those of the opposite side in a midline fibrous band called the *linea alba*, which extends from the xiphoid process to the pubis.

The muscles of the *back* extend, rotate and abduct (bend laterally) the vertebral column. They are designed for maintaining posture -- not for lifting. Consequently the muscle fibers, tendons and ligaments of the vertebral column are subject to strain and tear when they are used to lift heavy objects. Back muscles are seldom individualized, rather they are considered as groups. The *superficial group* includes superior serratus posterior, inferior serratus posterior and erector spinae. *Erector spinae* is a muscle complex that includes iliocostalis, longissimus and spinalis muscles. The *deep group* of spinal muscles includes three muscles that are enclosed in a single muscle sheath (epimysium). They include *multifidus, quadratus lumborum and semispinalis*. Semispinalis is a three-part muscle that includes capitis, cervicus and throacis divisions.

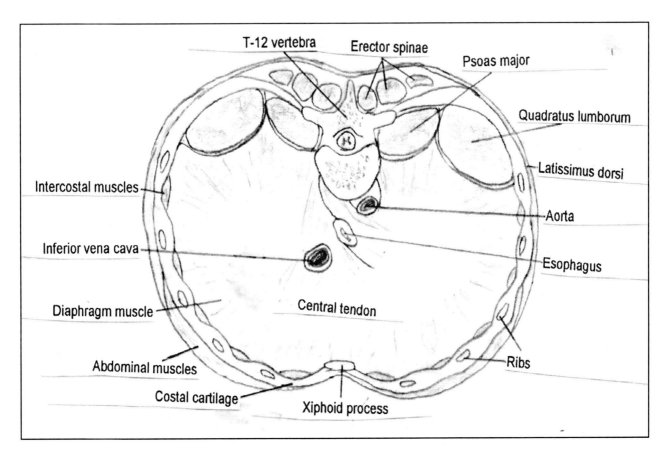

Above: The diaphragm. The diaphragm is a transverse sheet of muscle that separates the thorax from the abdomen. When relaxed, the diaphragm is convex upward. It is flat when contracted. The diaphragm inserts on its central tendon.

The *scapula* is instrumental in providing considerable *movement to the shoulder* (*humeroscapular* joint). Scapular movement is moderated by its attachment to the clavicle. Muscles that *insert on the scapula* rotate, depress, elevate, protract, and retract the scapula. They consist of an anterior group and a posterior group. The anterior group includes pectoralis minor and serratus anterior. The posterior group includes trapezius, levator scapulae, rhomboideus major and rhomboideus minor.

There are nine muscles that cross the shoulder and *insert on the humerus*. Pectoralis major and latissimus dorsi originate primarily on the axial skeleton (sternum and rib cartilage), but pectoralis major also has fibers that originate on the clavicle. Pectoralis major inserts on both the scapula and the humerus. Therefore, it can move the scapula as well as the shoulder joint. Pectoralis major and latissimus dorsi are prime movers that adduct and medially rotate the humerus. Deltoid, teres major, coracobrachialis, **supraspinatus, infraspinatus, teres minor and subscapularis** muscles originate on the scapula and insert on the humerus. The latter four muscles, their tendons, and several ligaments form the *rotator cuff,* which strengthens the shoulder joint. Deltoid in the shoulder, gluteus maximus in the buttocks, and vastus lateralis in the thigh are the sites most often chosen for *intramuscular (IM) drug injections*. *IM injections* are often preferable to injections in the hypodermis because IM injections give more consistent absorption, they are less painful, and they cause less inflammation. Large amounts of a drug may be given IM because the drug will be absorbed into the blood stream gradually. An intravenous injection will usually require slow delivery to prevent drug toxicity. Knowledge of anatomy is necessary prior to giving any IM injection.

The forearm (antebrachium) muscles flex, extend, pronate and supinate the elbow joint. Flexors of the elbow are biceps brachii, brachialis and brachioradialis. *Biceps brachii* has *two scapular origins*. The long head originates on the supraglenoid tubercle and helps to hold the head of the humerus in the glenoid fossa. The short head originates on the coracoid process. Biceps flexes and supinates the forearm. *Brachialis* is deep to the biceps. It arises on the humerus and inserts on the ulna; it flexes the forearm. *Brachioradialis* forms much of the fleshy portion of the pronator surface of the forearm. It is a pure flexor of the forearm that arises on the humerus and inserts on the radius. The extensors of the forearm are *triceps brachii and anconeus*. The pronators of the forearm include pronator teres and pronator quadratus; the former is a small deep muscle near the elbow; the latter is near the wrist. Supinator muscle is a small deep muscle near the elbow; its only action is supination. A *"tennis elbow"* is inflammation of the lateral epicondyle of the humerus where the extensor carpi muscles originate. These muscles extend the wrist, a movement that is crucial in playing tennis.

Muscles that act on the wrist and hand include the *extrinsic* muscles of the forearm and the *intrinsic* muscles of the hand. The *extrinsic* muscles have their origins on the radius, ulna, and condyles of the humerus. They are extensors and flexors of the hand and digits, and they also abduct and adduct the digits and oppose the thumb. The *retinaculae* of the wrist keep tendons from elevating off the wrist when the muscles contract. The palmaris longus tendon is an exception because it passes over the flexor retinaculum. You can see and feel this tendon when you flex your wrist. The palmaris longus inserts into the palmar fascia, which is an aponeurosis of dense connective tissue in the palm.

The tendon of the flexor digitorum superficialis muscle divides before inserting on the middle phalanx of the second, third, fourth and fifth fingers. This division allows the tendons of the flexor digitorum profundus to come through the decussation to insert on the distal phalanges. Intrinsic muscles of the hand originate in the hand; they include four lumbricals, four dorsal interosseous and three palmar interosseous muscles. The interosseous muscles abduct and adduct the digits; the lumbricals flex the metacarpal-first phalangeal joint and extend the interphalangeal joints. The lumbricals are unusual in that their origin is on the tendons of the flexor digitorum profundus muscle. There are fifteen *extrinsic* and eighteen *intrinsic* muscles that act on the hand or wrist.

The *perineum* is a diamond shaped area between the thighs. It is marked by the pubic symphysis anteriorly, the ischial tuberosities laterally, and the coccyx posteriorly. A line drawn between the ischial tuberosities separates the anterior perineum from the posterior perineum. The anterior perineum is the *urogenital triangle*; the portion posterior to the ischial tuberosities is the *anal triangle*. Muscles of the *pelvic floor* are in three layers, superficial, middle and deep. Muscles of all three layers support the pelvic floor. They include the muscles of urination, defecation and copulation. The superficial muscles include those at the base of the penis and around the vagina. The middle group contains the anal and urethral sphincters. The deep group includes the muscles of the *pelvic diaphragm*, which are the levator ani and coccygeus muscles. These muscles support and elevate the

the pelvic floor. A weakened pelvic floor may allow the bladder, rectum or uterus to prolapse. This condition is most frequently seen in females who have delivered many children. A **_cystocele_** is a prolapsed bladder; a **_rectocele_** is a prolapsed rectum.

Right: The primary motor area and the primary sensory area of the cerebral cortex.

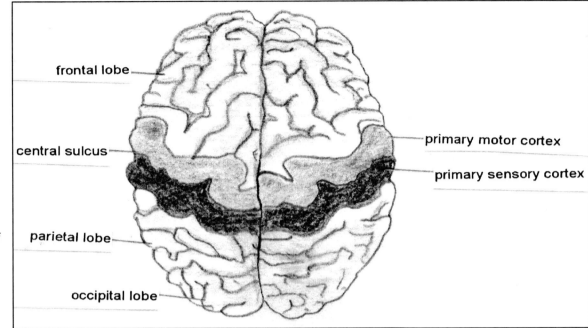

Right: A motor homunculus showing where muscles of different parts of the body are represented in the cerebral cortex.

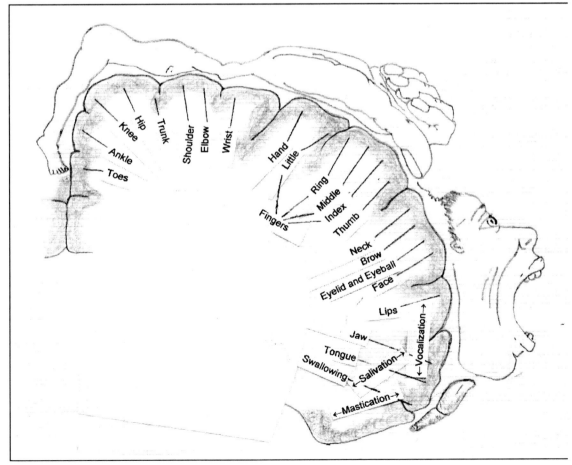

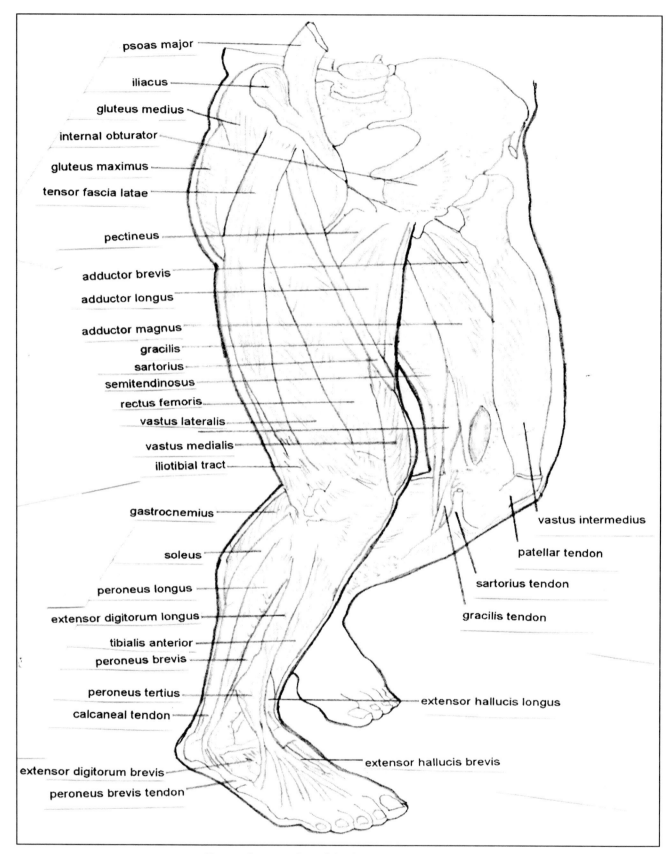

psoas major

iliacus

gluteus medius

internal obturator

gluteus maximus

tensor fascia latae

pectineus

adductor brevis

adductor longus

adductor magnus

gracilis

sartorius

semitendinosus

rectus femoris

vastus lateralis

vastus medialis

iliotibial tract

gastrocnemius

soleus

peroneus longus

extensor digitorum longus

tibialis anterior

peroneus brevis

peroneus tertius

calcaneal tendon

extensor digitorum brevis

peroneus brevis tendon

vastus intermedius

patellar tendon

sartorius tendon

gracilis tendon

extensor hallucis longus

extensor hallucis brevis

Above: the muscles of the lower extremity.

A *hernia* is a protrusion of a loop of bowel through a weak area in the muscular wall of the abdomen. The inguinal canal of males is the most common site for a hernia, but hernias are also seen in the umbilicus and the diaphragm. The *reduction* of a hernia is the act of mechanically replacing it back into the abdomen by hand manipulation. A hernia that is cannot be mechanically reduced is called an *incarcerated* hernia. A hernia that has had its blood supply compromised is a *strangulated* hernia.

Most of the muscles that move the *hip* joint originate on the pelvic bone (os coxae) and insert on the femur; however, two of them, (gracilis and sartorius), insert on the tibia. The powerful flexors of the hip originate on bodies of the vertebrae and adjacent ilium. Extensors of the hip originate on the posterior surface of the pelvis. The muscles of the anterior group are hip flexors that include iliacus, which fills the iliac fossa, and psoas major, which originates on the lumbar vertebrae. *Iliacus and psoas major* are the *main flexors of the hip*. Rectus femoris, which is part of the quadriceps femoris muscle, also flexes the hip. Tendons of iliacus and psoas major converge to constitute the iliopsoas muscle, which inserts on the lesser trochanter of the femur. Psoas major is the muscle that butchers refer to as the filet mignon. The *lateral and posterior* muscles that act on the femur *extend* the hip joint. This movement is paramount in climbing and beginning to run. These muscles include *gluteus maximus*, (the primary muscle of the buttocks), *gluteus medius and gluteus minimus.*

Lateral rotators of the *hip* include six smaller muscles that abduct or adduct the femur. The muscles in this group are obturator internus, obturator externus, gemellus superior, gemellus inferior, piriformis; and quadratus femoris (do not confuse this with the quadriceps femoris!). *Fascia lata,* (the lateral *iliotibial band*), is a tendinous aponeurosis of the tensor fascia lata muscle on the lateral aspect of the thigh. Fascia lata is connected to the deep fascia of the thigh. Deep fascia divides thigh muscles into three groups, an anterior group of knee extensors, a posterior group of knee flexors, and a medial group of hip adductors.

Muscles of the *knee* include *quadriceps femoris*, which is the most powerful muscle of the body. The four parts of the quadriceps muscle include rectus femoris, vastus medialis, vastus lateralis and vastus intermedius. Each has a separate origin and a somewhat different action, but all extend the knee. The four parts of quadriceps converge into one large tendon (the *patellar tendon* containing the patella), which inserts on the tibia. The *tibial tuberosity* is a rough projection on the anterior surface of the tibia where the quadriceps tendon inserts. It is an area of bone that is roughened by thick periosteum and tendon fibers that interconnect and penetrate the bone. The longest muscle of the body is *sartorius*, which originates on the anterior superior spine of the ilium, crosses the thigh from lateral to medial and inserts on the medial aspect of the tibial tuberosity. "Sartorius" means tailor, and the action of the sartorius (hip and knee flexion, lateral femoral rotation, and medial tibial rotation), produces the crouching movement used by tailors in their work. The posterior thigh muscles are the *"hamstring"* muscles. The hamstrings extend the hip and flex the knee; they form the tendons at the back of the knee. Tendons of the hamstring muscles outline the medial and lateral boundaries of the *popliteal fossa* at the back of the knee. The three hamstring muscles are semimembranosus and semitendinosus, which insert medially on the tibia, and biceps femoris, which inserts laterally on the fibula. The hamstrings received their name from the fact that butchers hung their hams by tendons of these muscles. Popliteus is a small muscle around the knee joint that serves to unlock the knee.

Muscles of the *leg* act on the ankle and the foot. They are separated by dense fascia into anterior and posterior compartments. The *anterior* compartment includes four muscles that dorsiflex the ankle and extend the toes. They are tibialis anterior, peroneus tertius, extensor hallucis longus and extensor digitorum longus. All four of these muscles have their tendons held down by a retinaculum over the anterior surface of the ankle. The *posterior* group (the calf muscles) includes superficial, deep and lateral sections. These muscles plantar flex the foot. Medial muscles of the posterior group invert the foot; lateral muscles of this group evert the foot. The *superficial section* of the posterior leg muscles includes gastrocnemius, soleus and plantaris muscles. The tendons of gastrocnemius and soleus converge to make up the *Achilles or calcaneal tendon*, which inserts on the calcaneus bone at the heel. The calcaneal tendon is the strongest tendon in the body. Damage to this tendon impedes plantar flexion, making it impossible to push off with the foot when starting to walk or run. The *deep section* of posterior leg muscles includes three plantar flexors of the foot (tibialis posterior, flexor hallucis longus, and flexor digitorum longus). The *lateral section* of posterior leg muscles includes two muscles that plantar flex and evert the foot (peroneus brevis and peroneus longus). "*Peroneus*" means *fibula*, and some texts refer to the peroneus muscles as "fibularis." "Crural" refers to the leg.

The leg muscles mentioned above constitute the *extrinsic* muscles that act on the foot. The *intrinsic* muscles acting on the foot originate and insert on the bones and tendons of the foot and on the plantar aponeurosis. They include the ***lumbricals and the dorsal and plantar interosseous muscles.*** These muscles dorsiflex and plantar flex the foot; they flex, extend, abduct, and adduct the toes, and they support the arches. The ***plantar aponeurosis*** is a fan-like sheet of dense connective tissue extending from the calcaneus bone to the bases of the toes on the plantar surface of the foot.

A List of the Major Skeletal Muscles

Most people have a more than six hundred skeletal muscles. This section is a list with descriptions of the major muscles and muscle groups.

Facial Muscles
The muscles of facial expression are small muscles that originate on facial bones, other facial muscles, and the dermis. They insert primarily into the dermis. They are innervated by the facial nerve (CN VII), and they produce facial expressions. Paralysis of the facial muscles causes the face to sag, as happens in Bell's palsy. These muscles are in the scalp, forehead, around the eyes, nose and mouth, and in the neck. **Orbicularis oris** encircles mouth; **orbicularis oculis** encircles the eyes; risorius and zygomaticus curl up the corners of mouth into a smile. **Buccinator** is used in blowing and sucking, and it keeps food on top of the teeth. **Platysma** is a superficial muscle in the neck. **Gala aponeurotica** is a sheet of dense connective tissue that extends from the frontalis muscle in the forehead to the occipitalis muscle at the back of the head.

Musculature of the Tongue
The **intrinsic** muscle of the tongue allows for movement of the tongue in speech and in swallowing by pushing food onto the teeth and into the pharynx. The muscle fibers of the intrinsic tongue muscle run in vertical, transverse and longitudinal directions. The intrinsic muscle is innervated by the hypoglossal nerve (CN XII or cranial nerve number twelve). The **extrinsic** muscles of the tongue are used in swallowing. They connect the tongue to the hyoid bone, styloid process of the temporal bone, soft palate and the mandible. They are innervated by the hypoglossal nerves and the spinal accessory nerves (CN XI).

Muscles of Mastication
Four major muscles make up the muscles of mastication. These muscles arise from skull bones and insert on the mandible. They include **temporalis** and **masseter,** which elevate the mandible, and **medial and the lateral pterygoid** muscles, which elevate and provide lateral movement of the mandible. Lateral movement is used to grind food with the molar teeth. **Digastric** muscle is a small muscle that depresses the mandible (closes the mouth). Other small muscles attach to the hyoid bone and the thyroid cartilage of the larynx. They stabilize the hyoid and the larynx, and they assist in swallowing. They include **sternohyoid, sternothyroid, omohyoid, stylohyoid, mylohyoid, geniohyoid, thyrohyoid, and hypoglossus.**

Muscles acting on the Neck
The neck extensors include **trapezius** and muscles of the upper back. Flexors of the neck include the **sternocleidomastoid** and **three scalene** muscles.

Muscles of the Back
The back muscles attach to the vertebral column and to the ribs. They flex, extend, and provide lateral movement of the vertebral column. They are grouped into four groups.
(1) The **semispinalis** group extends the neck
(2) **Multifidus** rotates the vertebral column
(3) **Quadratus lumborum** is located between the ilium and the 12th rib. It provides lateral flexion
(4) The **superficial group,** which includes the **posterior serratus** muscles and the **erector spinae** group. The erector spinae consists of three columns of muscles that extend the vertebral column.

Muscles of Respiration

Breathing requires the use of muscles. The **diaphragm** is the major muscle of respiration; it is a muscular dome between the thoracic and abdominal cavities. Its muscle fascicles extend from the chest wall to a fibrous central tendon. Contraction lowers the central tendon of the diaphragm and produces inspiration by increasing the volume of the thorax. Contraction of the diaphragm also raises the abdominal pressure, which helps to expel urine and feces and facilitate childbirth. Intercostal muscles are located between the ribs. The **external intercostal** muscles produce inspiration by elevating and expanding the chest. The external intercostals extend downward and anteriorly between the ribs. When contracted, they provide inspiration by pulling the ribcage up and outward. The **internal intercostal** muscles provide forced expiration by compressing the chest. They extend upward and anteriorly between the ribs. When contracted they pull the ribcage downward forcing expiration. Normal expiration requires no muscular activity; it occurs due to elastic recoil by the lungs.

Muscles of the Abdomen

Four pairs of muscles make up this group. They are **rectus abdominis, external oblique, internal oblique, and transversus abdominis.** The three latter muscles are broad, sheet-like muscles of the flank and abdomen. The rectus abdominis is a relatively narrow, parallel (vertical) muscle near the midline. The fibers of the four abdominal muscles run in different directions. Each functions to support and protect the viscera, stabilize the vertebral column, and to help in respiration, urination, defecation and childbirth.

Muscles of the Pelvic Floor

Muscles of the pelvic floor are divided into three layers, superficial, middle and deep. These muscles support the pelvic outlet. They include the sphincter muscles of urination, defecation and copulation. This area is the **perineum.** The perineum is defined as the diamond-shaped area bounded anteriorly by the pubic symphysis, laterally by the ischial tuberosities and posteriorly by the coccyx. A line drawn between the two ischial tuberosities divides the diamond shape of the perineum into an anterior triangle, which is the **urogenital triangle**, and a posterior triangle, which is the **anal triangle**. The perineum is penetrated by the anal canal, urethra and vagina.

Muscles Acting on the Scapula

Muscles that act on the scapula originate on the axial skeleton and insert on the scapula or the clavicle. They provide scapular rotation, elevation, depression, protraction and retraction.   Muscles that insert on the clavicle serve to brace the shoulder by limiting scapular movement. An anterior group of these muscles includes **pectoralis minor and serratus anterior**. Pectoralis minor arises from ribs 3, 4 and 5 and inserts in the coracoid process of the scapula. It lifts the ribs and protracts and depresses the scapula. The serratus anterior arises from ribs 1-9 and inserts on the medial border of the scapula. It abducts, rotates and depresses the scapula; it is a primary muscle used in throwing.

The posterior group includes **trapezius, levator scapulae, rhomboideus major and rhomboideus minor**. These muscles rotate, retract, protract, elevate and depress the scapula.

Muscles Acting on the Humerus

Nine muscles cross the shoulder joint to insert on the humerus. They arise from the axial skeleton, the clavicle and the scapula, and they include the prime movers of the humerus in flexion and extension. Seven muscles arise on the scapula and insert on the humerus. They are **deltoid, coracobrachialis, teres major, subscapularis, teres minor, infraspinatus and supraspinatus.** The rotator cuff stabilizes the shoulder joint. It is formed by the subscapularis, supraspinatus, infraspinatus and teres minor muscles, their tendons, and by several ligaments.

Deltoid has numerous actions on the humerus including abduction, flexion, extension, medial rotation and lateral rotation. **Latissimus dorsi** is a flank muscle that extends, adducts and rotates the humerus. It is called the "swimmer's muscle" because it produces strong downward strokes of the arm. Latissimus dorsi originates on the vertebrae, ribs and ilium, and it inserts on the humerus. **Pectoralis major** flexes the shoulder and adducts and rotates the humerus. It originates on the ribs, sternum and clavicle, and it inserts on the humerus.

Muscles that act on the Forearm, Wrist and Hand

The muscles that act on the elbow serve to flex, extend, pronate and supinate the forearm. They arise on the scapula and the humerus, and they insert on the radius and ulna. The principal flexors are biceps **brachii, brachialis and brachioradialis.** The biceps brachii has two origins on the scapula -- the long head and the short head. The long head passes over the top of the shoulder joint, which helps to stabilize the shoulder. **Triceps brachii** is the only muscle on the back of the arm. It is the primary extensor of the elbow. It arises on the humerus and the scapula, and it inserts on the ulna. **Supination** of the forearm is provided by the biceps brachii and the supinator muscle. **Pronation** is provided by the pronator teres and pronator quadratus.

Muscles of the anterior part of the forearm serve to flex the wrist and fingers. They arise on the humerus, radius and ulna. **Carpi** muscles insert on the carpal or metacarpal bones. **Digitorum** muscles insert on the bones of the fingers. **Pollicis** muscles insert on the bones of the thumb. Names for muscles of the wrist and hand include the terms "ulnaris" and "radialis," which refer to an origin on the ulna or the radius. Other terms for forearm muscles include profundus (deep), superficialis (superficial), brevis (short) and longus (long). The tendon of flexor digitorum superficialis splits and inserts on the sides of the middle phalanges. The tendon of flexor digitorum profundus comes through the opening of this split tendon and inserts on the distal phalanges.

Extensors of the wrist and hand are in the posterior compartment of the forearm. They arise on the humerus, radius and ulna, and they insert on carpal bones, metacarpal bones, or phalanges.

A **retinaculum** encloses tendons of the wrist except for the **palmaris longus** tendon, which is superficial to the flexor retinaculum and inserts on the palmar fascia. The palmaris longus muscle is absent in ten percent of the population.

Intrinsic muscles of the hand have their origins and their insertions on bones or tendons in the hand. They include **lumbrical** muscles, **dorsal interosseous** muscles, **palmar interosseous** muscles and several muscles that act on the thumb. The **thenar eminence** is the fleshy muscle mass at the palmar base of the thumb. The thenar eminence contains the bodies of flexor pollicis brevis, abductor pollicis brevis and opponens pollicis. The **anatomical snuff box** lies over the trapezium bone at the base of the thumb posteriorly. It is the space between the tendons of extensor pollicis longus medially, and the tendons of extensor pollicis brevis and abductor pollicis longus laterally. You can identify your anatomical snuff box by abducting and extending your thumb maximally.

Muscles that Act on the Hip

Muscles acting on the hip include an anterior and a posterior group. The anterior group includes **iliacus and psoas major,** which merge into a single tendon, the iliopsoas. Iliacus arises on the ilium, and psoas major arises on the lumbar vertebrae. Iliopsoas inserts on the femur; it is the main flexor of the hip. Psoas minor is also a flexor of the hip.

The posterior muscles acting on the hip include **gluteus maximus, gluteus medius, gluteus minimus, quadratus femoris and piriformis muscles.** These muscles arise on the pelvis and lumbar vertebrae and insert on the femur. They serve to extend the hip, and they rotate, abduct and adduct the femur.

Other muscles that act on the hip joint include **tensor fascia lata, adductor magnus, adductor brevis, adductor longus, gracilis, gemellus, obturator externus, obturator internus, pectineus, and sartorius.** Tensor fascia lata is an abductor of the hip. It inserts on the iliotibial band (fascia lata).

Muscles that Act on the Knee

The strongest muscle in the body is **quadriceps femoris.** This muscle consists of four parts, **vastus lateralis, vastus medialis, vastus intermedius and rectus femoris.** Each part has a different origin on the ilium or the femur and a somewhat different action on the hip, but all extend the knee. The four parts of this muscle merge to form the patellar tendon, which inserts on the tibia. It is the primary extensor of the knee.

The primary flexors of the knee are the **hamstring** muscles. These muscles arise on the pelvic bone and the femur, and they insert on the tibia or the fibula. Tendons of these muscles enclose the **popliteal space** on the posterior surface of the knee. The hamstring muscles include **biceps femoris** laterally, and **semitendinosus and semimembranosus** medially. The biceps femoris inserts on the fibula; the semitendinosus and semimembranosus insert on the tibia.

Popliteus is a small muscle in the knee that serves to unlock the knee from full extension.

Muscles That Act on the Foot

Muscles that act on the foot and ankle originate on the tibia, fibula and femur. Muscles of the leg are separated into anterior and posterior compartments.

The anterior compartment includes **extensor digitorum longus, extensor hallucis longus, peroneus tertius and tibialis anterior.** These muscles serve to extend the toes and dorsiflex the ankle. Peroneus tertius everts the foot; tibialis anterior inverts the foot. The posterior compartment includes three superficial muscles that plantar flex the foot. These are **gastrocnemius, soleus and plantaris**. (Plantaris is sometimes absent). The tendons of gastrocnemius and soleus merge to form the calcaneal tendon.

The deeper muscles of the posterior compartment of the leg are also plantar flexors. They include **tibialis posterior, flexor digitorum longus, and flexor hallucis longus.**

The muscles of the lateral compartment of the leg arise from the fibula. They provide both plantar flexion and eversion to the foot, and they provide lift to the heel and forward thrust. They include peroneus brevis and peroneus longus.

The intrinsic muscles of the foot include nineteen small muscles that flex and extend the toes and support the arches. They arise and insert on the bones and tendons of the foot. They include the **lumbrical and interosseous muscles.**

Athletic Injuries

Muscles, tendons and ligaments are vulnerable to sudden intense muscle contractions and stress. Proper warm-up is helpful in reducing the incidence of these injuries. Some of the most common injuries include
(1) **Shin splints**--: inflamed and painful anterior crural muscles (the dorsiflexors) -- usually caused by excessive running.
(2) **Pulled hamstrings**--: an injury to biceps femoris, semitendinosus, or semimembranosus.
(3) **Tennis elbow**--: an inflamed lateral epicondyle of the humerus at the origin of the extensor carpi muscles.
(4) **Rotator cuff injury**--: a tear of a rotator cuff muscle, tendon or ligament.
(5) **Pulled groin muscle**--: an injured adductor of the thigh.
(6) **Charley horse**--: a muscle strain or a hemorrhage into a muscle, also a painful muscle cramp.
(7) **Rider's bones**--: ossification in a tendon of a thigh adductor caused by prolonged horseback riding.
(8) **Pitcher's arm--:** inflammation in the elbow at the origin of the flexor carpi muscles.
(9) **Compartment syndrome**--: a hemorrhage into a muscle that restricts blood flow to that muscle due to inelasticity of the epimysium and perimysium.

Study Guide

1. Name the ways that muscles serve the body (movement, communication, control of orifices and heat production).
2. How many muscles do you have?
3. Define a myofilament, myofibril, muscle fiber (myofiber) and myofascicle.
4. Define the endomysium, perimysium and epimysium.
5. Define the hypodermis, superficial fascia and deep fascia.
6. Describe the histological differences between the three types of muscle tissue (skeletal, cardiac and smooth).
7. Define aponeurosis, retinaculum, and tendon sheath.
8. Understand the pathology (abnormality) in the carpal tunnel syndrome.
9. Describe each type of skeletal muscle according to the orientation of its fibers (fusiform, parallel, pennate varieties, convergent, and circular). Give an example of each type. Which type is strongest? Which is weakest? Which contracts at an angle to its tendon?
10. Define the origin, insertion and body of a muscle.
11. Define a muscle agonist, synergist, antagonist and fixator.
12. Know the terms used in the muscle system that are included in this chapter.
13. Know the meanings of buccinator and sartorius.
14. Locate the gala aponeurotica.
15. Know the cause and symptoms of Bell's palsy.
16. Know the elevators of the mandible.
17. Know what is meant by a homunculus.

18. Locate your sternocleidomastoid muscle. Identify its origin and its insertion. How does your head move when one and when both sternocleidomastoid muscles contract?
19. What are the muscles of respiration?
20. Name and locate the muscles of the abdominal wall. In which direction do their fibers run?
21. Locate the perineum, the urogenital triangle and the anal triangle.
22. Know the definition and cause of a hernia.
23. Where are the safest and most effective places to perform an intramuscular (IM) injection?
24. Know which muscles make up the rotator cuff.
25. Name three flexors of the elbow.
26. What muscle is the primary extensor of the elbow?
27. What is a tennis elbow?
28. Review the iliacus and psoas major muscles (iliopsoas). What is their action?
29. Name the four parts of the quadriceps femoris. What is the primary action the quadriceps femoris?
30. What is the strongest muscle in the body?
31. Where can you find the fascia lata?
32. Name and locate the hamstring muscles. Define their action.
33. Know where to find the popliteal fossa and the Achilles heel (calcaneal tendon).
34. What is the meaning of the word, "peroneal?"
35. What is the meaning of the word, "crural?"
36. Know which bony articulations accept weight bearing in the knee and in the ankle.

Chapter Twelve

Nervous Tissue

The fundamental properties of nervous tissue are **excitability** (nerve cells detect and respond to stimuli), **conductivity** (nerve cells produce electrical signals that travel to and from the central nervous system [CNS], and **secretion** (chemicals called neurotransmitters are released at synapses, which are nerve cell junctions).

The brain and spinal cord make up the **CNS**. The **peripheral nervous system (PNS)** is composed of peripheral nerves and ganglia. The **neuron** is the cellular unit of the nervous system. The peripheral nerves are made up of the axons of neurons and their surrounding sheaths. The bodies of the neurons are located in the CNS and peripheral ganglia. **Ganglia** are swellings in nerves where cell bodies of neurons are concentrated. Ganglia contain **synapses,** which are junctions between nerve cells. Ganglia may contain **sensory** and/or **motor** nerve fibers. Sensory impulses travel from the periphery to the CNS, and motor impulses travel from the CNS to the periphery. **Interneurons** are neurons in the brain and spinal cord that link sensory and motor neurons. **Tracts** are conduits of **myelinated axons** in the CNS. Tracts in the CNS correspond to nerves in the PNS.

An **afferent** nerve is a **sensory** nerve that carries signals from the periphery to the CNS. **Visceral afferent** nerves carry sensory impulses from the organs of the chest and abdomen; **somatic afferent** nerves carry sensory impulses from muscles, skin, bones and joints.

An **efferent** nerve is a **motor** nerve that carries signals from the CNS to muscles, glands and organs of the body. Nerves to skeletal muscles make up the **somatic motor division**. Most of the impulses of the somatic motor division are **voluntary** (under conscious control), but reflexes such as the patellar tendon reflex (knee jerk) are **involuntary.**

The **autonomic nervous system** is a **visceral motor** system. It is made up of **visceral efferent** nerves that carry impulses to organs, glands and smooth muscle. Autonomic impulses are part of a visceral reflex, and the conscious mind has little or no control over these impulses (they are **involuntary**). The autonomic nervous system is divided into two divisions, the **sympathetic** division and the **parasympathetic** division. The sympathetic nervous system is called the **"fight or flight"** system because stimulation of the sympathetic division creates arousal for action. The pulse increases; the respiratory rate increases; blood flow to the skeletal muscles increases, and digestion slows. The effects of the parasympathetic nervous system generally oppose the effects of the sympathetic system. Stimulation of the parasympathetic system decreases pulse and blood pressure, increases digestion and exerts a calming effect on the body. The parasympathetic system is called the "**rest and digest"** system. Drugs that affect the autonomic nervous system are some of the most important drugs in pharmacology.

A neuron is a large cell, 5-135 microns in diameter. The **body** of a neuron is also called the **soma** or the **perikaryon**. The body contains organelles including Golgi bodies, mitochondria, and endoplasmic reticulum; it also contains inclusions and a cytoskeleton. Mature neurons lack centrioles; they do not undergo mitosis after adolescence. But they are long lived; many survive as long as the individual. It has been found that up to one thousand new neurons are born each day from preexisting stem cells, but the significance of new neurons is in question because the time required for them to be included in the circuitry of the brain is lengthy.

Typical neurons have many extensions called dendrites and a single extension called the axon. **Dendrites receive** messages from other neurons; **axons relay** messages to other neurons, muscle cells or glands. Dendrites are smaller than axons, and they often exist in a tangled network. They usually arise from a few thick processes in the soma. If you visualize the soma as the size of a tennis ball, the dendritic network would form a bushy mass that would fill a thirty seat classroom, and the axon would be up to a mile long with the diameter of a garden hose. There is never more than **one axon** per neuron, but that axon may be as long as one meter (39 inches). The axon arises from a mound in the soma called the axon hillock, and it often has terminal arborizations (branches at the end). An axon ends in a **synaptic knob**. Vesicles of neurotransmitter molecules in the synaptic knob are secreted into the synapse. An axon contains cytoplasm (**axoplasm**) with organelles, and it is surrounded by a plasma membrane called the **axolemma**.

   **Schwann cells,** or _**neurilemmacytes,**_ provide support for peripheral nerves by surrounding nerve fibers of the peripheral nervous system.   The _**neurilemma**_ is the covering around an axon created by Schwann cells. Schwann cells form a multilayered wrapping around the axons of somatic motor nerves and some sensory nerves. This wrapping is called _**myelin**_; it consists of the cell membrane of the Schwann cell. Myelin is about 80% lipid, and it contains all of the ingredients of a cell membrane including phospholipids, glycolipids, cholesterol and glycoproteins. The presence of myelin around an axon greatly increases the speed of an impulse traveling down that axon. A myelinated nerve fiber is _**white**_ because myelin is white. Nerve fibers that lack myelin are gray and are called _**gray**_ fibers. Both white fibers and gray fibers have Schwann cells surrounding their axons, but only the white fibers have the multilayered myelin coating. Somatic motor nerves are myelinated. Autonomic nerves to visceral organs are unmyelinated. The myelination of nerves begins during fetal development and proceeds rapidly in infancy, but it is not complete until late adolescence. The neurilemma makes a tubular structure that is important in the regeneration of nerve fibers after injury because regenerating axons grow through the neurilemma tube. Cells called _**oligodendrocytes**_ provide the myelin sheath in the tracts of white matter in the CNS, but tracts in the CNS lack a neurilemma, and they do not regenerate. A small unmyelinated nerve conducts an impulse at a speed of 0.5 - 2 mps (meters per second). 0.5 mps is about one mile an hour or 1.5 feet a second. The nerve signal may travel as fast as 120 mps (300 mph) in a large myelinated nerve. The larger the diameter of an axon (or nerve), the faster the nerve impulse travels. A giant squid may grow to be 55 feet long, but its nerves are unmyelinated. The reactions of this cephalopod would be quite slow, but it compensates by having the largest nerves in the animal kingdom; they are the diameter of a man's arm.

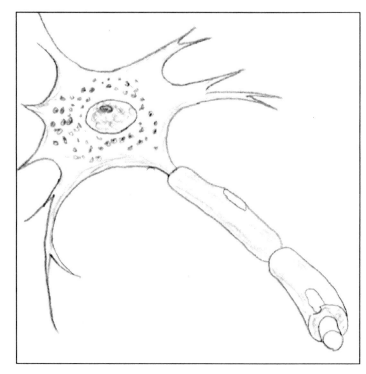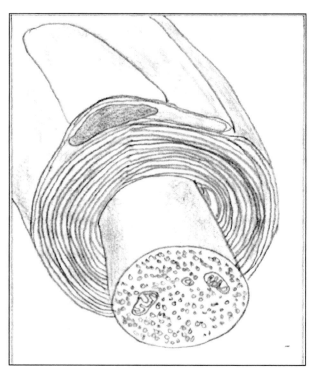

Above: Schwann cells surround all nerve fibers. The Schwann cells of some nerves wrap their plasma membrane around the nerve fiber and create a myelin sheath that encloses the axon and provides faster nerve conduction. The drawing on the left is a neuron with its axon extending toward the bottom right. Schwann cells surround the axon. A magnified drawing of the axon and its myelin sheath is on the right.

All about the Synapse

   A synapse is a junction between two neurons or between a neuron and an effector cell such as a muscle fiber or gland. The _**presynaptic axon**_ does not actually touch the cell membrane of the _**postsynaptic cell**_; they are separated by a _**synaptic cleft**_ that is about 20-40 nanometers between neurons and about 60-100 nm at the neuromuscular junction. The ***synaptic delay*** is the time it takes for the events to occur that allow a nerve impulse to bridge the synapse. This delay amounts to only about 0.5 milliseconds (msec).

The resting membrane potential for a neuron is about -70 millivolts (mv). This figure represents the difference in charges across the cell membrane, the inside of the cell being -70 mv relative to the outside of the cell. This resting potential represents a high concentration of potassium (K+) ions inside the cell and a high concentration of sodium (Na+) ions outside the cell. These concentrations are maintained by the ***active transport*** mechanism of the Na-K pump. The presence of additional anions such as sulfates, phosphates, proteins and nucleic acids in the cell maintains the negative charge inside the membrane. The normal concentrations of Na+ are 144 mEq/L outside the cell and 10 mEq/L inside. For K+ the figures are 4.5 mEq/L outside and 141 mEq/L inside.

The presynaptic axon ends in a ***synaptic knob***, a swollen area of the axon at the synapse, which contains vesicles of a ***neurotransmitter***. When a nervous impulse reaches the synaptic knob, ***voltage-regulated gates*** for calcium ions open, and calcium enters the knob. Calcium causes the vesicles containing a neurotransmitter (such as acetylcholine) to fuse with the axolemma, which then spews the contents of the vesicles into the synaptic cleft by ***exocytosis.***

Right: A diagram of the action potential of nerve conduction. "A" is the time period of the action potential, when the nerve fiber is **absolute**ly refractory to the transmission of another impulse.
"B" is the **relative** refractory period, when an inordinately large impulse is required to begin another action potential. -70 mv is the **resting** potential. -55 mv is the **threshold** voltage required to begin an action potential.

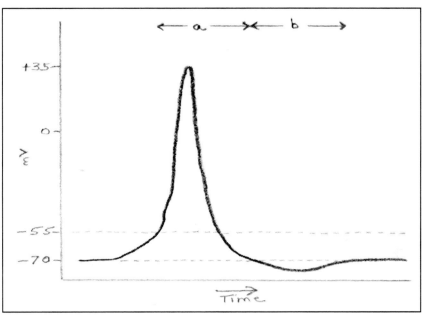

Once in the synaptic cleft, some of the neurotransmitter molecules briefly bind to ***receptors*** in the postsynaptic cell membrane. These receptors are ***ligand-gated sodium channels.*** When a receptor is stimulated by a neurotransmitter, sodium channels open and sodium ions rush into the cell by diffusion. The rapid influx of sodium ions alters the resting potential of -70 mv. If the threshold level of -55mv is reached, a small area of the postsynaptic cell membrane surrounding the receptor depolarizes. This is called a ***local potential.*** The size of the depolarized area and consequently the strength of the local potential depend upon the number of nearby receptors that have been bound to a neurotransmitter. Adjacent to the synapse are areas called ***trigger zones***, which contain numerous ***voltage-gated*** sodium channels. If the area of depolarization created by the local potential is large enough, a nearby trigger zone will reach the threshold level of -55mv. When the threshold is reached, voltage regulated sodium channels open in the trigger zone, and an ***action potential*** begins. Action potentials are manifest by a rush of sodium ions into the postsynaptic cell. The local potential at the synapse must be of sufficient magnitude to reach the threshold level of -55 mv in the trigger zone for an action potential to be created. The processes of ***spatial summation*** and ***temporal summation*** are useful in producing depolarization of the trigger zone past its threshold; they are means by which local potentials are made stronger. Spatial summation involves the addition of other local potentials; temporal summation involves an increased rapidity of firing of a local potential. Firing of an impulse between ten and twenty times a second will produce stronger muscle contractions due to the build up of calcium in the cytoplasm, a phenomenon called *treppe*. Rates higher than twenty impulses per second produce tetany (spasm).

When the membrane potential reaches zero, sodium channels begin to close, and potassium channels begin to open allowing K+ to leave the cell. The membrane potential reaches about +35 mv before the efflux of K+ becomes greater than the influx of Na+; at that time the membrane potential begins to fall dramatically to a hyperpolarizing level of -90 mv.

The affected area of the membrane cannot respond to an additional stimulus while sodium channels are open; this is the **_absolute refractory period._** The **_relative refractory period_** exists during hyperpolarization; during this period only an exceptionally strong stimulus will reach the threshold level.

Once the threshold (-55mv) is reached in the trigger zone, an action potential begins. The impulse is propagated down the cell membrane by the opening of additional voltage-regulated sodium ion gates in the membrane. The impulse cannot travel backward due to the refractory period. Lidocaine, bupivacaine and other local anesthetic drugs act by decreasing membrane permeability to sodium ions. That prevents sodium from entering the nerve cell and eliciting an action potential. The speed of a nervous impulse depends upon **(1)** the diameter of the nerve (impulses travel more quickly through larger nerves), and **(2)** the presence of myelin (which accelerates nervous transmission). In nerves lacking myelin, the impulse travels by sequentially opening voltage-regulated sodium ion gates in the cell membrane.

Schwann cells surrounding a myelinated nerve are about one mm apart. **_Nodes of Ranvier_** are tiny areas lacking myelin between Schwann cells. Voltage-gated sodium channels are concentrated at the nodes of Ranvier. The nerve impulse skips from node to node in the myelinated axon. Sodium enters and potassium exits the nerve only at the nodes. This is called **_saltatory conduction_** of a nerve impulse. The myelinated areas of the nerve between nodes are called **_internodes._**

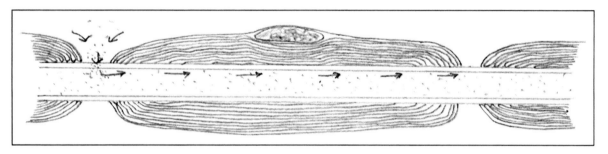

Above: An illustration of saltatory conduction. The impulse arrives from the left and opens sodium channels at the node of Ranvier. Sodium ions enter the axon. Sodium ions inside the axolemma move to the right and open voltage regulated gates at the next node. The movement of sodium ions inside the axolemma can be likened to "musical chairs." The impulse is propagated from node to node by sequentially opening voltage-regulated gates to sodium. Sodium and potassium can diffuse across the axolemma only at the nodes of Ranvier.

Most of the neurons in the CNS are **_multipolar,_** meaning they have one axon and many dendrites. **_Bipolar_** neurons have one axon and one dendrite; they are sensory neurons in the olfactory epithelium of the nose, the retina of the eye and the cochlea of the ear. Sensory neurons may have their somas in either a peripheral ganglion, a paravertebral ganglion, or in the spinal cord. Sensory neurons with their bodies in a ganglion are **_unipolar_** neurons. Unipolar neurons have only one process that extends from the soma. That process is an axon, but it divides into an afferent stem and an efferent stem. **_Anaxonic_** neurons have many dendrites but no axon; they communicate only through their dendrites, which do not initiate action potentials. They are found in the retina of the eye and in the brain.

Many axons are long and distant from their cell bodies, which necessitates a form of transport to and from the cell body and the end of the axon. Proteins, neurotransmitters and other compounds are synthesized in the cell body and must be transported to the axon. Other materials move from the terminal end of the axon to the cell body. Substances are transported up and down the axons by **_axonal transport_**. Anterograde flow is toward the axon. Retrograde flow is toward the cell body. Axonal transport may be **_fast_** (20-400 mm/day), or **_slow_** (0.5-10 mm/day). Slow axonal transport is called **_axoplasmic flow_**. Materials that move by fast transport include organelles such as mitochondria, vesicles, neurotransmitter molecules, amino acids and nucleotides. Some disease causing organisms (pathogens) and toxins also move by fast transport including the Herpes simplex virus, Herpes zoster virus, polio virus, rabies virus, and tetanus toxin.

Right: Not all neurons are alike as shown by this drawing. "A" is a multipolar neuron having many dendrites and one axon. "B" is a unipolar neuron having no dendrites and one axon, which has an afferent (sensory) branch and an efferent branch to the spinal cord. "C" is a bipolar neuron having one dendrite and one axon. Some neurons lack axons and communicate only through their dendrites. Unipolar neurons are found in dorsal root ganglia near the spinal cord. Bipolar neurons are found in the eye, the ear, and the olfactory mucosa of the nose. Multipolar neurons are the most common and are found throughout the nervous system.

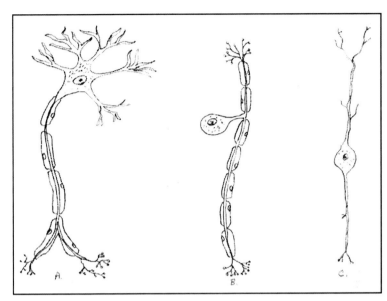

There are several unique histologic features in neurons. **_Nissl bodies_** are small dark staining globules on the rough endoplasmic reticulum of a neuron. They consist of a dense mesh of microtubules and actin filaments. **_Lipofuscin_** is a lipid globule in the cytoplasm of neurons that contains worn out organelles and cellular products. It is found mostly in older people and is thought to be harmless.

A majority of the cells in the CNS are not neurons, rather they are **_glial cells_**. Glial cells found in the CNS include astrocytes, oligodendrocytes, microglia and ependymal cells. **_Astrocytes_** are the most numerous, accounting for 90% of the cells in some areas of the brain. Astrocytes provide a supportive network for brain tissue; they secrete growth factors, and they provide for the healing of injuries by forming scar tissue. Astrocytes form tight junctions with endothelial cells of capillaries, creating a **_"blood-brain barrier"_** that strictly controls what substances get from the blood stream into the brain. Astrocytes metabolize glucose to pyruvate, which neurons use to produce ATP. (ATP production by neurons is restricted to the aerobic respiration of glucose, and neurons are extremely sensitive to a loss of their blood supply and a subsequent lack of oxygen.) Glial cells divide actively, and they are susceptible to cancerous change. Tumors that arise from glial cells are typically malignant (meaning "bad"). They are usually incurable, although their growth rate may be slow. Astrocytoma and glioblastoma multiforme are two malignant brain tumors that arise from glial cells.

Oligodendrocytes (oligodendroglia) are bulbous cells with many processes that surround axons and create the myelin coating of tracts in the CNS. Their counterparts in the PNS are Schwann cells. Oligodendrocytes provide the myelin sheath of white matter tracts in the CNS. But tracts in the CNS have no neurilemma tube, and consequently the nerve fibers they contain cannot regenerate.

Microglial cells are small macrophages that develop from monocytes. Microglial cells concentrate in areas of trauma, stroke and infection where they serve to engulf bacteria and debris.

Ependymal cells are sometimes classified as glial cells. Ependymal cells line cavities in the brain called ventricles, and they line the central canal of the spinal cord. They do not rest on a basement membrane, so they are regarded as connective tissue cells and not epithelial cells. They secrete **_cerebrospinal fluid (CSF)_**, and they have mobile cilia, which provide a current of flow to circulate CSF. **_Hydrocephalus_** (literally "water on the brain") can occur in infants when the circulation of CSF is anatomically blocked. In this situation ependymal cells continue to secrete CSF against a pressure gradient, but because the circulation of CSF is blocked, CSF is not reabsorbed. An infant with untreated hydrocephalus has a gradually enlarging head. Mental retardation occurs because the brain is compressed by the excessive amount of CSF in the cranial cavity. Pseudotumor cerebri is a physiologic condition in adults in which more CSF is secreted than can be absorbed. The cranial cavity of adults cannot expand, and patients with pseudotumor cerebri develop increased intracranial pressure and headaches.

**Schwann cells** are susceptible to neoplastic change. _**Neurofibromatosis,**_ or Von Recklinghausen's disease, is a genetic disorder that is characterized by the development of multiple Schwann cell tumors called neurofibromas or Schwannomas. Neurofibromas are benign and slow growing, but they tend to become numerous and unsightly. Neurofibromatosis is inherited as an autosomal dominant trait. The "Elephant Man" of literature and the Hollywood movie was once thought to have had neurofibromatosis, but it now appears more likely that he had proteus syndrome, a genetic disorder that leads to tumors and overgrowth of skin and bone.

**Multiple sclerosis** (MS) is an immunologic disorder in which abnormal antibodies attack the myelin sheath. MS typically waxes and wanes over the course of many years. Practically any part of the nervous system that is myelinated may be affected including the optic nerve, peripheral somatic motor nerves, sensory nerves and the brain. Loss of vision, speech defects, numbness and paralysis may result. MS occurs primarily in the developed, temperate regions of the world -- North America, Europe and Japan. It is not selective to gender or race. It is suspected that the abnormal antibodies in patients with MS are a response to products of an industrialized society.

**Tay Sachs disease** is a fatal genetic disorder of infants in which a normal lipid called a ganglioside builds up to toxic levels in the myelin sheath. These children develop neurologic symptoms around six months of age, and they rarely live past the age of four. No treatment is effective for this tragic disease; parents and doctors can only watch as the child slowly loses sight and neurologic functions. Tay Sachs disease is an autosomal recessive disorder, and it occurs primarily in Ashkenazi Jews (Eastern European Jews). Many couples choose to have no more children after watching a child succumb to this disease. The carrier state is detectable by laboratory tests.

Neurotransmitters

In 1921 a German pharmacologist by the name of Otto Loewi discovered that a chemical was released by cardiac tissue of frogs when he stimulated the vagus nerve. Both the chemical and electric stimulation of the vagus nerve, (cranial nerve X), slowed the heart rate. The substance that Loewi found was _**acetylcholine (ACh).**_ ACh has been found to be the predominant neurotransmitter in the human body, but there are many others.

Acetylcholine

I. _**Acetylcholine**_ is the most common neurotransmitter in the body, and it is the neurotransmitter involved in _**cholinergic synapses**_. It is broken down by the enzyme, acetylcholinesterase. It usually acts in an excitatory synapse, but it sometimes acts in an inhibitory synapse, such as in cardiac muscle where it slows the heart rate.

II. **Monoamines** are neurotransmitters that are derivatives of the _**aromatic**_ (ring containing) amino acids, _**tyrosine, tryptophan, and histidine**_. Monoamines include the catecholamines (epinephrine, norepinephrine and dopamine), serotonin and histamine. Monoamines are produced by the removal of the carboxyl (acid or COOH) group from an amino acid. The enzyme _**monoamine oxidase**_ breaks down monoamines by oxidative deamination (the addition of oxygen and the removal of the NH2 group)

_(A)_ Monoamines that are _**tyrosine**_ derivatives are called _**catecholamines**_. They include:
   (1) _**epinephrine,**_ which is also known as _**Adrenalin.**_ Epinephrine is released into the blood stream by the _**medulla of the adrenal gland**_ in times of marked stress. It constricts blood vessels, speeds the heart rate and dilates bronchioles.
   (2) _**Norepinephrine**_ is a neurotransmitter in the CNS and the PNS. Synapses where norepinephrine acts as

neurotransmitter are called ***adrenergic synapses***. An adrenergic synapse is less direct than a cholinergic synapse in the process of opening ligand gated sodium channels. Norepinephrine does not directly affect the ligand regulated sodium channels; rather it stimulates the receptor to activate an enzyme that converts ATP to cyclic AMP. The cyclic AMP acts as a ***secondary messenger*** which causes the sodium channels to open.

(3) ***Dopamine*** is a neurotransmitter found in areas of the CNS including the ***substantia nigra*** of the midbrain, which is a nucleus of cells with inhibitory synapses. Damage to neurons in this area produces the tremors and rigidity of Parkinson's disease.

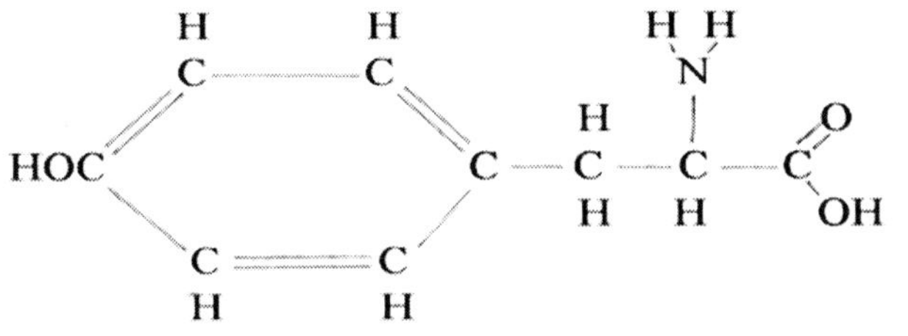

Tyrosine

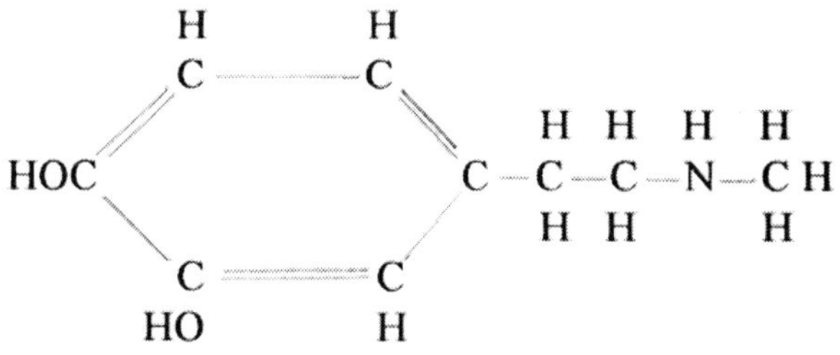

Epinephrine

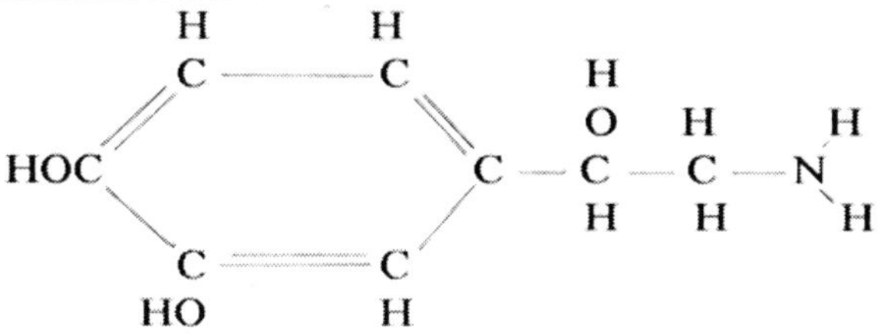

Norepinephrine

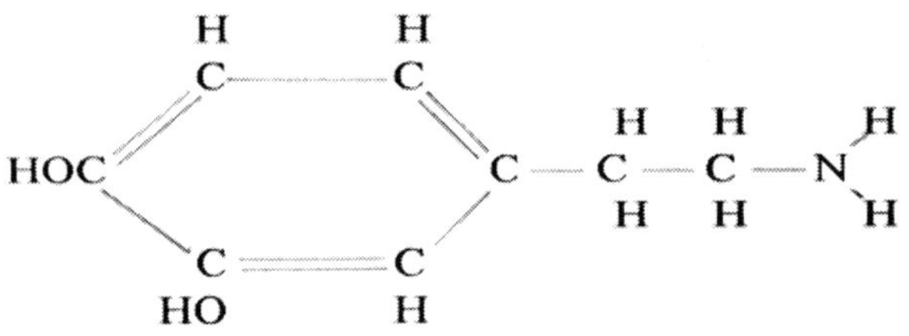

Dopamine

(B) ***Serotonin*** is a derivative of the amino acid, ***tryptophan***. Serotonin is a powerful vasoconstrictor and smooth muscle stimulator that is implicated in ***migraines*** and the ***carcinoid syndrome.*** The latter is an intestinal tumor of serotonin producing cells (argentaffin cells) that results in blood pressure instability and intermittent flushing of the skin. The metabolism of tryptophan and ***niacin*** are linked, and a deficiency of tryptophan can lead to ***pellagra***, a disease of niacin deficiency. Niacin is vitamin B3, a substance that is required for the production of ATP. Pellagra is characterized by ***dermatitis, diarrhea and dementia***. One hundred years ago pellagra was common in the southern states where the diet of some people consisted largely of corn (maize), corn being woefully deficient in tryptophan. Pellagra has also been reported in patients with carcinoid tumors because these tumors convert so much dietary tryptophan to serotonin, which leaves little tryptophan to be converted into niacin. Normally only one percent of dietary tryptophan is converted into serotonin. Patients with a carcinoid tumor may have 60% or more of their dietary tryptophan converted to serotonin. Serotonin is a mood elevator; the antidepressant drug Prozac acts by blocking the reuptake of serotonin by the synaptic knob, thereby allowing serotonin to exert its effect for a longer period. Serotonin is an ***indole amine*** that is broken down by monoamine oxidase to ***5-hydroxy indole acetic acid (5HIAA).*** Certain foods, especially bananas, contain serotonin, and if several bananas are eaten before testing the patient's urine for 5HIAA, the test may lead to a false positive interpretation of high levels of endogenous 5HIAA (and serotonin).

(C) ***Histamine*** is a derivative of the amino acid ***histidine.*** There are two types of histamine receptors, H1 and H2. H1 receptors produce vasodilation and pruritis (itching) in the skin. H2 receptors stimulate the parietal cells of the stomach to secrete hydrochloric acid.

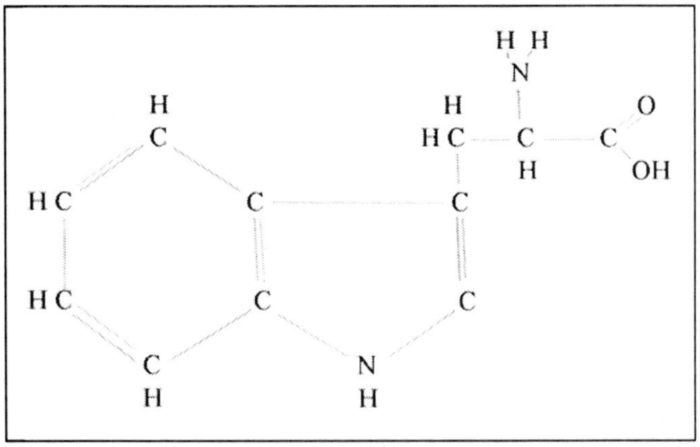

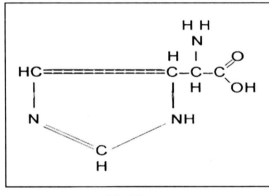

Tryptophan

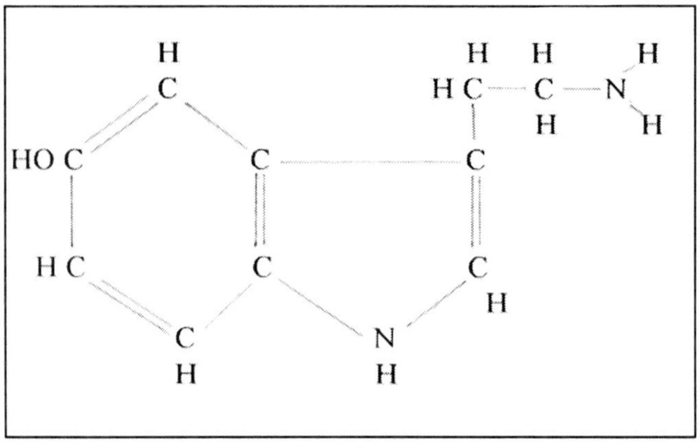

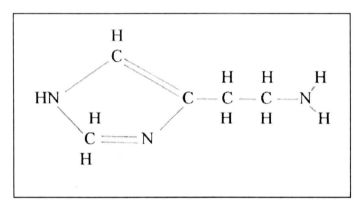

Serotonin

Histidine

Histamine

III. *__Amino acids__* are the building blocks of proteins. Some amino acids function as neurotransmitters.

(A) *__Glycine__* is an amino acid that functions as a neurotransmitter in inhibitory synapses of the spinal cord. Glycine acts by opening K+ channels. The efflux of K+ hyperpolarizes the membrane, thereby making it less sensitive to a stimulus. Tetanus toxin produces tetany by inhibiting the inhibitory effects of glycine.

(B) *__GABA (gamma amino butyric acid)__* is an amino acid that is involved in inhibitory synapses in the brain. It acts by opening chloride (Cl-) channels in the cell membrane; the influx of Cl- ions hyperpolarizes the membrane, thereby making it less sensitive to a stimulus.

(C) *__Aspartic Acid__* is an amino acid that is usually involved in excitatory synapses. The artificial sweetener Aspartame is metabolized to aspartic acid, which can produce hyperactivity and seizures if given in sufficient quantities to susceptible people.

(D) *__Glutamic Acid__* is an amino acid that is usually excitatory. Monosodium glutamate (MSG) is a flavor enhancing food additive that is derived from glutamic acid. MSG produces seizures and hyperactivity when given in sufficient quantities to susceptible individuals.

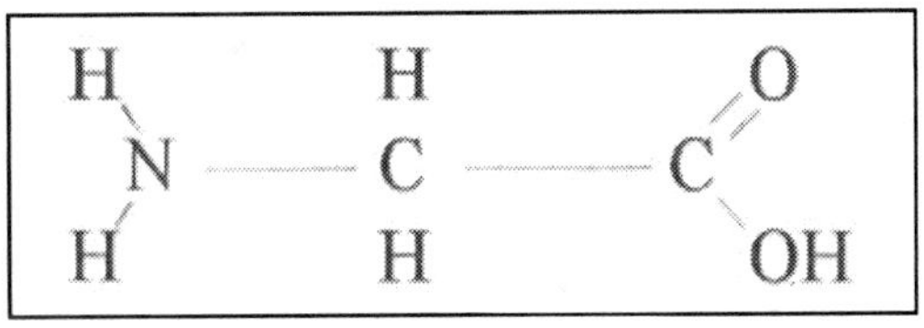

Glycine, the simplest amino acid ("R" is a hydrogen atom)

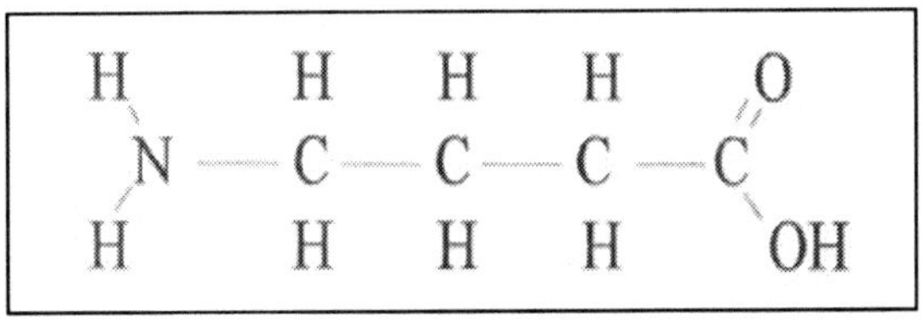

GABA (gamma amino butyric acid

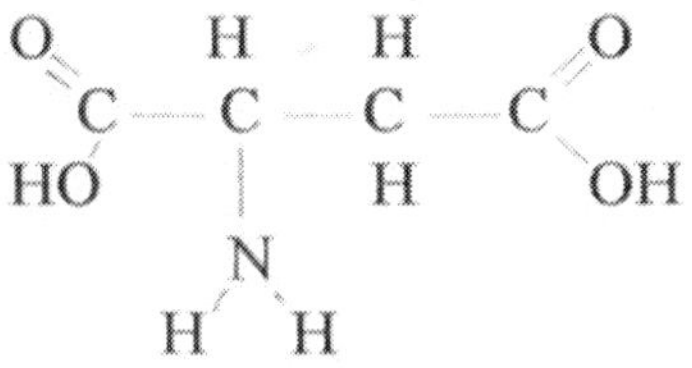

Aspartic acid

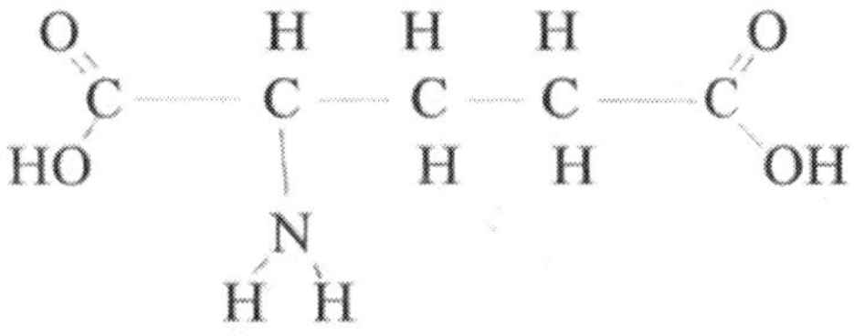

Glutamic acid

IV. **_Neuropeptides_** are neurologically active peptides that contain from two to forty amino acids. They typically act at lower concentrations and for longer periods of time than do the other neurotransmitters. They may affect the brain, creating a myriad of feelings such as food cravings, which may produce eating disorders. Other examples of peptides that serve as neurotransmitters include **_enkephalins, endorphins and dynorphins_**. These compounds are collectively called **_endogenous opioids_** because of their powerful analgesic and euphoric effects on the brain.

Some neuropeptides act as **_neuromodulators_** as well as neurotransmitters. Neuromodulators modify synaptic transmission by such means as influencing the cell to alter neurotransmitter synthesis, alter the number of receptor sites, or affect the breakdown, release or the reuptake of a neurotransmitter. **_GABA_** is an amino acid that can function as a neuromodulator by preventing the opening of voltage regulated calcium gates in the synaptic knob, which restricts the release of neurotransmitters from the presynaptic neuron. **_Nitric oxide (NO)_** is a neuromodulator that stimulates a presynaptic neuron to release more neurotransmitter.

Whether or not a synapse is excitatory or inhibitory **_depends on the receptor, not the neurotransmitter_**. Although ACh and glutamic acid are most often excitatory, their function is inhibitory in some synapses.

All action potentials are the same. It is the sum of the excitatory and inhibitory messages that a neuron receives that determines perception by a neuron. Thus we can determine whether a food tastes salty or sweet. Judgments such as this are determined by which neurons are firing, the frequency of the firing rate, and the total number of neurons firing. All of these things affect interpretation and, therefore, the response to the impulses received.

Learned material can be **_declarative_**, meaning it can be expressed in words, or it may be the **_retention of motor skills_**, such as playing the piano or driving a vehicle. **_We learn these skills by the development of synapses_**.

There are about 14 to 16 billion neurons in the cerebral cortex of your brain. 2.5 billion of the total neurons in the cerebral cortex are pyramidal cells. **_Pyramidal cells_** are responsible for all of your cognitive learning, and they control all the voluntary activity that you do. They do not undergo mitosis, but fortunately for us they are capable of living over a hundred years. It is the **_synapses_** these cells make that are the means by which your brain processes information. Each pyramidal cell typically has 40,000 synapses. A single neuron in the spinal cord participates in about 10,000 synapses. Each **_Purkinje cell_** (a neuron in the cerebellum of the brain) has about 100,000 synapses. There are about **_100 trillion_** total synapses between the neurons of the cerebral cortex. Long term memory entails building these synapses in the cerebral cortex.

Right: Neuronal circuitry exists in several different patterns. In a diverging circuitry the impulse spreads from one neuron to many. In a converging circuitry multiple impulses lead to a single neuron. In a reverberating circuitry, the impulse travels in circles and is long lasting. In a parallel circuitry, impulses travel several different routes from the same source to the same end.

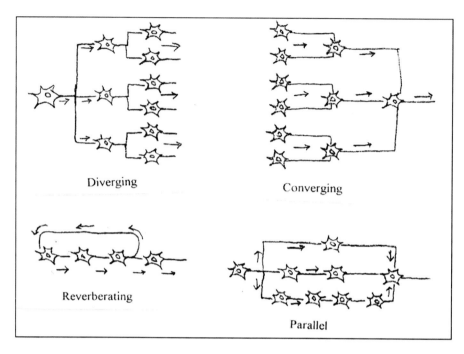

Diverging

Converging

Reverberating

Parallel

Short term memory involves **_reverberating circuits_**, which are recirculating impulses in the brain. Short term memory is lost when the circuit is no longer active. Other circuitry patterns among neurons are classified as (1) **_divergent_**--: where a neuron sends impulses to multiple recipient neurons; (2) **_convergent_**--: where a neuron receives the same message from several neuronal pathways; and (3) **_parallel_**--: where several pathways exist with the same neuronal origin and the same neuronal destination. Pathways in a parallel circuit contain different numbers of neurons, and the messages consequently do not reach their destination at the same time. This results in a received message that is repeated.

In addition to the chemical synapse, which involves a neurotransmitter, there is the **_electrical synapse._** The **_intercalated discs of heart muscle_** are electrical synapses. They consist of **_gap junctions_** between muscle fibers that conduct the nerve impulse quickly from one cell to another. There is no synaptic cleft, no synaptic delay, and no neurotransmitter is involved in an electrical synapse.

Alzheimer's disease is a growing problem in the United States. It affects nearly half the population over age 85. Symptoms may include confusion, memory loss, moodiness, combative behavior, and an inability to walk, talk and care for oneself. In this disease the pyramidal cells of the cerebral cortex die, and the cerebral cortex atrophies. Dendrites become entangled, and plaques of a lipoprotein called **_beta amyloid_** collect in the extracellular space as a result of the breakdown of cells. Some cases of Alzheimer's disease appear to have a genetic basis, but most cases occur at random for unknown reasons.

Parkinson's disease is the result of traumatic, toxic, inflammatory, or other injury to neurons in the **_substantia nigra of the midbrain_**. Neurons in this area contain numerous inhibitory synapses that utilize the neurotransmitter **_dopamine_**. Damage to neurons in the substantia nigra results in increased and uncontrollable muscle contractions, tremors and rigidity. These patients typically have a slow shuffling gait, slurred speech, and a staring expressionless face; they may eventually become unable to write, button their clothes or feed themselves. L-Dopa, a precursor of dopamine, is given to these patients with good effects early in the disease. L-Dopa is able to cross the blood-brain barrier; dopamine cannot. Viral encephalitis is inflammation of the brain caused by a virus, which can lead to damage to the substantia nigra and the development of Parkinson's disease. There was an outbreak of Parkinson's disease in the 1920's and 1930's in patients who had suffered from viral encephalitis in the 1918 influenza pandemic. One of the victims of the 1918 pandemic was President Woodrow Wilson. Wilson had a severe case of influenza with encephalitis during the peace talks in Paris following World War I. Wilson's illness was accompanied by euphoria with headstrong, erratic behavior, which contributed to the failure of the Paris peace talks to provide a just and lasting peace in Europe.

The cause of encephalitis associated with influenza was probably the 'flu virus itself, but some believe that another virus may have been responsible -- that being the virus that caused a concurrent epidemic of Von Economo's lethargica. Because Von Economo's lethargica and influenza both suddenly arose from nowhere to epidemic proportions in 1918 and have not returned, it is suspected that they were caused by the same virus. The question cannot be answered with certainty because the influenza virus was not identified until 1933.

A hereditary form of Parkinson's disease has been found, but such cases are rare. Damage to the substantia nigra resulting in Parkinson's disease is more likely to be associated with inflammation (encephalitis), trauma, or excessive exposure to toxic chemicals.

Study Guide
1. Know the fundamental properties of nervous tissue (excitability, conductivity and secretion).
2. Define the central nervous system (CNS) and the peripheral nervous system (PNS).
3. Identify the following: afferent nerve, efferent nerve, motor nerve, sensory nerve, visceral nerve, somatic nerve, voluntary nerve, involuntary nerve and ganglia.
4. Identify the autonomic nervous system (ANS) and its divisions (sympathetic and parasympathetic).
5. Familiarize yourself with the neuron and its parts including the body, the axon and the dendrites.
6. Understand the role of the Schwann cell (neurilemmacyte), myelin and the nodes of Ranvier.
7. Know what is meant by a multipolar neuron, a bipolar neuron, a unipolar neuron and an anaxonic neuron.
8. Appreciate the difference between fast and slow axonal transport.
9. Know the meaning of the terms Nissl body and lipofuscin.
10. Name the types of glial cells and know the function of each (astrocytes, oligodendrocytes. microglia and ependymal cells).
11. Understand the structure and function of the blood-brain barrier.
12. Know where ependymal cells can be found.
13. Recognize how the following disorders affect the nervous system: neurofibromatosis, multiple sclerosis, hydrocephalus, Tay Sachs disease, Alzheimer's disease and Parkinson's disease.
14. Review the structure and physiology of a synapse including its parts and their individual functions.
15. Know the difference between a ligand-gated channel and a voltage-gated channel.
16. Know what is meant by a second messenger and give an example (cyclic AMP).
17. Understand the absolute refractory period (sodium channels remain open) and the relative refractory period (the membrane is hyperpolarized).
18. Describe saltatory conduction.
19. Name and classify the primary neurotransmitters.
20. Familiarize yourself with the following: monoamine oxidase, catecholamine, acetylcholine, acetylcholinesterase, pseudocholinesterase, epinephrine, norepinephrine, dopamine, serotonin, histamine, glycine, gamma amino butyric acid (GABA), aspartic acid, glutamic acid, nitric oxide, enkephalins, endorphins and dynorphins.
21. Recognize the following disorders and how they relate to neurotransmitters: the carcinoid syndrome, migraines, pellagra and Parkinson's disease.
22. Know that the action of a neurotransmitter on a synapse ultimately depends on the receptor and not on the neurotransmitter.
23. Know the meaning of a declarative skill and a motor skill.
24. Appreciate how many neurons, pyramidal cells, Purkinje cells, and synapses are in various parts of your nervous system.
25. Know the differing patterns of neuronal circuitry that exist in your CNS (reverberating, divergent, convergent, parallel), and where and how they function.

Chapter Thirteen

The Spinal Cord and Spinal Nerves

The ***central nervous system*** consists of the brain and spinal cord. The ***peripheral nervous system*** consists of the peripheral nerves and ganglia.

Anatomically the spinal cord is a rope-like tissue of neurons and tracts within the vertebral canal. It is about as thick as a man's finger. It lies between the ***foramen magnum*** of the occipital bone and the ***medullary cone***, which is the terminus of the cord. The medullary cone is at the L-3 level at birth, but it is at the L-1 level in adults because the vertebral column grows more than the spinal cord. Within the vertebral canal and below the medullary cone is the ***cauda equina*** ("horse's tail"). The cauda equina is a region of spinal nerves that extends from the L-2 level to the bottom of the vertebral canal. Spinal nerves exit the cauda equina at each vertebral level between L-2 and the coccyx. Both the right and left sides of the spinal cord receive sensory nerves and send out motor nerves. Spinal nerves exit the vertebral canal through intervertebral foramina, which are spaces between two consecutive vertebrae. Spinal nerves are named according to the vertebra where they exit. The spinal cord has swellings at the cervical and lumbar areas that correspond to an increased number of neurons that send and receive nerve fibers from the upper and lower extremities.

Right: The lower end of the spinal cord ends in a slight dilation called the medullary cone, which is at the L-1 level in adults. In the vertebral canal beneath the cord is a streamer of spinal nerves called the cauda equina. The cauda equina consists of spinal nerves that exit the lower vertebral column from L-2 to the coccyx. The pia mater is connected to the lower end of the vertebral canal by a fine thread called the filum terminale or coccygeal ligament.

One of the functions of the spinal cord is ***conduction***. It serves as an information highway between the brain and the rest of the body. Not all sensory impulses are sent up to the brain, however. Some sensations make an arc in the spinal cord and produce an involuntary motor response called a ***reflex***. The spinal cord also coordinates nerve signals involved in ***repetitive movements*** such as walking (locomotion), which involves numerous motor neurons that are located in the spinal cord.

In the congenital anomaly known as ***spina bifida***, vertebral arches fail to fuse in a section of the spine. Mild forms may be asymptomatic, but more severe cases involve prolapse of the spinal cord and spinal nerves into a cyst. Such individuals often suffer from paraplegia and lack of bladder control.

Three layers of connective tissue called ***meninges*** surround the brain and the spinal cord. They are **(1)** a thick, fibrous outer layer called ***dura mater***; **(2)** a thin central layer with mesothelium on its inner surface called ***arachnoid***; and **(3)** a fine, delicate layer adherent to the brain and the spinal cord called ***pia mater***.

The dura and the arachnoid are adherent in the vertebral column, and they are called the dura-arachnoid. The epidural space lies between bone and dura mater in

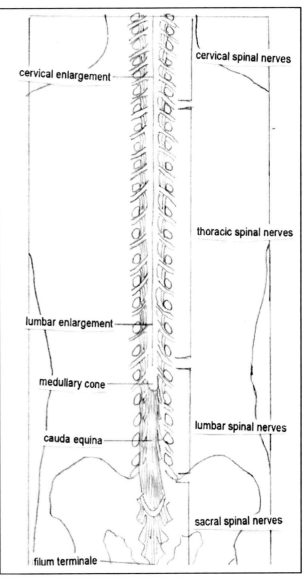

145

the vertebral canal. The epidural space is injected with a local anesthetic to produce an epidural block. Strands called trabeculae extend through the subarachnoid space from the arachnoid to the pia. Cerebral spinal fluid (CSF) fills the subarachnoid space. The cord is anchored to the vertebral column by strands of pia mater. ***Denticulate ligaments*** anchor the cord to the dura at regular intervals, and the ***filum terminale*** anchors the cord to the coccyx. The filum terminale is an extension of pia from the medullary cone to the bottom of the vertebral canal. It is part of the coccygeal ligament that anchors the cord to L-2.

Right: A drawing of a transverse section of the spinal cord.
(1) dorsal horn
(2) ventral horn
(3) lateral horn
(4) dorsal column
(5) ventral column
(6) dorsal root ganglion
(7) ventral root of spinal nerve
(8) dorsal root of spinal nerve
(9) gray commissure
(10) central canal
(11) dorsal ramus
(12) ventral ramus

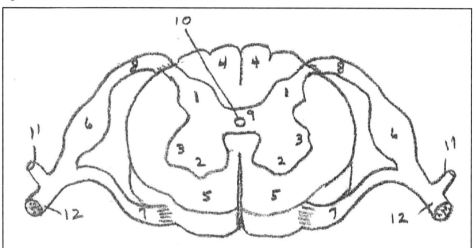

The ***dorsal roots*** of spinal nerves and the ***dorsal horns*** of the cord are ***sensory*** in nature. The ***ventral roots*** of spinal nerves and the ***ventral horns*** of the cord are motor in nature. The ***lateral horns*** contain neurons of the autonomic nervous system. The gray commissure connects the right and left sides of the cord.

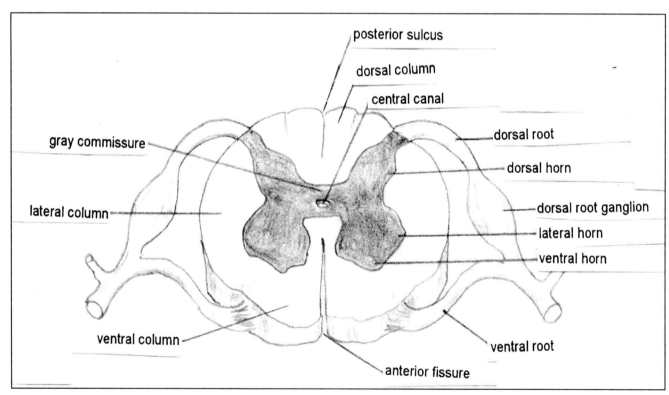

Above: A transverse section of the thoracic spinal cord showing the dorsal, ventral and lateral horns; dorsal root ganglion; central canal; dorsal, ventral and lateral columns of white matter, and a spinal nerve.

146

The **_columns_** contain **_tracts_** of white matter traveling to or from the brain. Columns consist of myelinated axons. The dorsal columns contain sensory axons traveling from the cord to the brain, and the ventral and lateral columns contain motor axons traveling from the brain to the cord. Many tracts **_decussate_** (cross from one side of the body to the other); thus a lesion on the left side of the brain can produce paralysis or sensory defects on the right side of the body and vice-versa.

A **_peripheral nerve_** is composed of multiple nerve fibers, which are bunched into groups called **_fascicles._** A **_nerve fiber_** is the axon of a neuron with its surrounding Schwann cell. The **_epineurium_** is a connective tissue sheath surrounding the nerve; the **_perineurium_** is a connective tissue sheath containing capillaries that surrounds fascicles, and the **_endoneurium_** is a connective tissue sheath surrounding individual nerve fibers. Peripheral nerves can be **_sensory_** (afferent) or **motor** (efferent). Efferent nerves are designated either **_somatic_** (supplying skeletal muscle) or **_visceral_** (supplying organs, smooth muscle and glands). Most nerves contain both sensory and motor fibers and are called **_mixed_** nerves.

Right: A transverse cut of the vertebral column and spinal cord. Shown here are
(1) the epidural space,
(2) the subarachnoid space,
(3) the dorsal root,
(4) a spinal nerve, and
(5) the body of a vertebra.

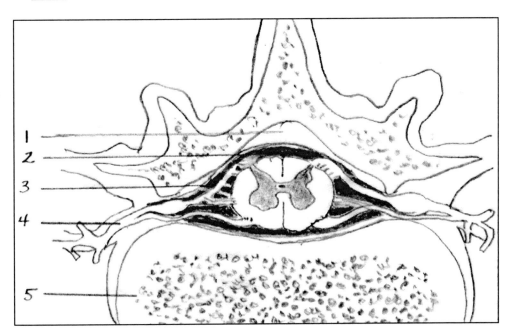

Some nerve fibers of the peripheral nervous system synapse in ganglia. Neurons in **_dorsal root ganglia are sensory_** in nature. They are unusual in that they are **_unipolar_**. Each of these neurons has only one process, which is called the axon. The axon divides near the body of the neuron into an afferent arm and an efferent arm. The afferent arm carries impulses from sensory nerve endings to the efferent arm. The efferent arm carries the impulse to the dorsal horn of the spinal cord. Some nerve fibers pass through the dorsal root ganglia without synapsing; they synapse in the dorsal horn of the spinal cord.

There are 31 pairs of spinal nerves. All are named according to the vertebra above the nerve except the cervical nerves, which are named for the vertebra below the nerve. The first cervical nerves exit above the atlas (C-1), and the eighth cervical nerves exit the vertebral column between C-7 and T–1. Consequently there are eight pairs of cervical nerves but only seven cervical vertebrae. The other spinal nerves include twelve pair of thoracic, five pair of lumbar, five pair of sacral and one coccygeal pair.

Each spinal nerve is formed by the union of a dorsal (sensory) root and a ventral (motor) root. The dorsal roots contain a dorsal root ganglion. The dorsal and ventral roots unite distal to the cord to form a spinal nerve, which soon branches into a **_dorsal ramus_** and a **_ventral ramus._** Both the dorsal ramus and the ventral ramus are mixed (sensory and motor) nerves. The dorsal ramus goes to the muscles and skin of the back. The ventral ramus is the larger of the two; it innervates the extremities and organs of the abdomen and thorax. A small meningeal nerve branches off the spinal nerve proximal to its division into rami.

Nerve plexuses are networks of nerve fibers. Nerves from a plexus supply a particular part of the body. Plexuses receive nerve fibers from several different spinal nerves, and nerve fibers exiting a plexus have regrouped into new nerves. Thus spinal nerve C-5 contributes to both the **_cervical plexus_** and the **_brachial plexus_**, and the median nerve contains input from spinal nerves C-5, C-6, C-7, and C-8.

The **_cervical plexus_** receives nerve fibers from spinal nerves **_C-1 through C-5_**. It sends out nerves that innervate the muscles and skin of the neck, upper shoulders and part of the head and ear. It sends out the **_phrenic nerve_**, which innervates the **_diaphragm with fibers from C-3, C-4, and C-5_**. Any injury to the cord at the C-3 level or above leads to paralysis of the diaphragm and respiratory failure.

Right: The cervical plexus. A nerve plexus is a web-like network of nerves. The cervical plexus supplies nerves   to the neck and upper back. The cervical plexus also supplies the diaphragm via the phrenic nerve, which has roots in spinal nerves C-3, C-4 and C-5. The diaphragm is the primary muscle of respiration. A spinal cord injury above C-4 can lead to respiratory paralysis.

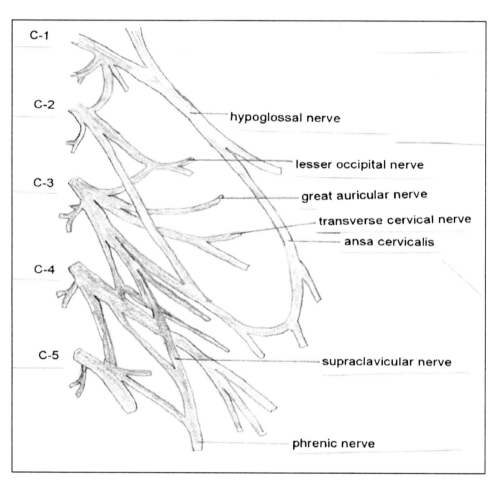

The **_brachial plexus_** receives input from spinal nerves **_C-4 through T-2_**. This plexus supplies the lower part of the shoulder and all of the upper extremity. The brachial plexus is located deep between the neck and axillae. The ulnar nerve, radial nerve, median nerve, musculocutaneous nerve and axillary nerve are five major nerves that exit from this plexus. They supply the muscles of the arm, forearm and hand. The **_ulnar nerve_** is on the side of the little finger (medial); it innervates flexors of the wrist and fingers. The radial and median nerves are on the side of the thumb (lateral).   The **_radial nerve_** supplies extensors of the wrist and elbow; the **_median nerve_** runs through the antecubital fossa (anterior bend of the elbow) to supply the skin of the hand, the thenar muscles and the intrinsic muscles of the hand. The **_musculocutaneous nerve_** supplies the flexors of the elbow (biceps brachii, brachioradialis and brachialis), and the **_axillary nerve_** supplies the deltoid and teres minor muscles.

The **_lumbar plexus_** receives input from spinal nerves **_T-12 through L-4_**. The main nerve emanating from the lumbar plexus is the **_femoral nerve_**. It supplies the muscles and skin of the thigh. Other branches from the lumbar plexus supply the abdominal muscles and most of the skin of the lower extremity.

The *__sacral plexus__* receives input from spinal nerves *__L4 to S4__*. This plexus forms the *__sciatic nerve__*, the largest and longest in the body. The sciatic nerve passes down through the buttocks and into the thighs where it divides into the tibial and common peroneal nerves. The sacral plexus supplies motor fibers to muscles of the buttocks, lower extremity and genitalia.

The *__coccygeal plexus__* innervates the genitalia and muscles of the pelvic floor. The coccygeal plexus receives fibers from spinal nerves S4, S5 and the coccygeal nerve.

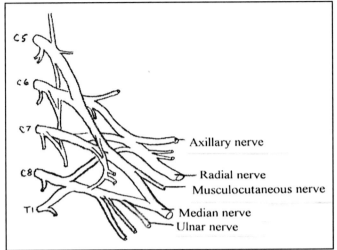

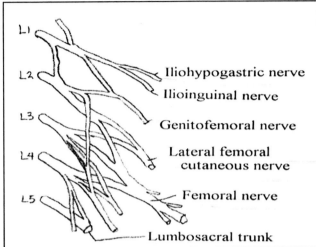

Above: The brachial plexus supplies innervation to the upper extremity.

Above: The lumbar plexus supplies innervation to the abdomen and lower extremity.

Right: A muscle spindle, a sensory nerve ending for detecting proprioception. Intrafusal fibers are muscle fibers that respond to motor stimuli from gamma efferent nerves by contracting. The annulospiral nerve endings detect stretch that is produced by contraction and relaxation of the intrafusal fibers.

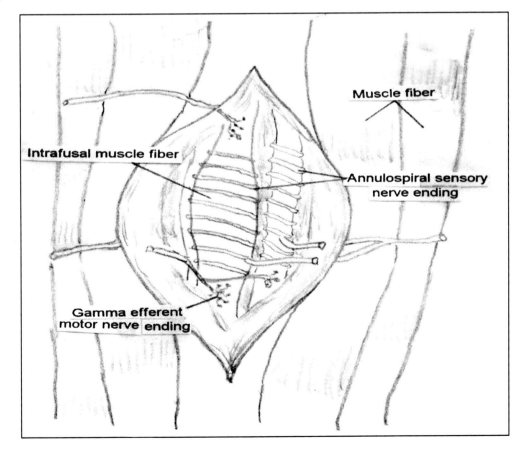

149

Proprioception is appreciation of the position of the body or a portion of the body in space. It allows you to stand and recognize the position of your body in space with your eyes closed. ***Muscle spindles*** are special complex sense organs in skeletal muscle that coil around ***intrafusal fibers,*** which are specialized muscle cells. Intrafusal fibers are innervated by motor nerves called ***gamma efferent*** nerves, and they contract simultaneously with muscle fibers. Sensory nerve endings in muscle spindles respond to contractions of the intrafusal fibers, and they provide the CNS with a sense of ***proprioception.***

Golgi tendon organs are specialized sense organs in tendons near the tendon-muscle junction. Golgi tendon organs are a tangle of knobby nerve endings that sense excessive tension in a tendon brought on by excessive muscle contraction. Stimuli from Golgi tendon organs result in reflex relaxation of muscle contraction in areas of excessive tension, which serves to make a contraction more evenly distributed and protects the tendon from damage.

Right: Dermatomes.
Each spinal nerve receives
sensory input from a specific
area of the skin; these areas
are called ***dermatomes***.
There is overlap between
dermatomes, but the
level of a spinal injury can
be determined according
to the dermatomes that
have become
desensitized following an
injury.

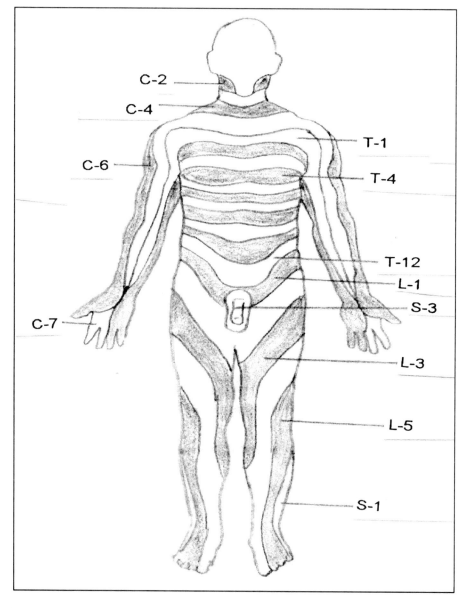

A somatic ***reflex*** is a quick, involuntary and consistent reaction of a muscle or gland to a stimulus. Reflexes are automatic responses and occur without conscious knowledge. A ***reflex arc*** involves a ***stimulus*** to a sense organ and an ***afferent nerve fiber*** that synapses in the dorsal root ganglia or the dorsal horn of the cord. Sometimes ***interneurons*** in the cord are involved in reflex arcs and modify the response. ***Efferent motor fibers*** carry an impulse from the cord to the ***skeletal muscles***, which contract to complete the arc.

The **_stretch reflex_** (tendon reflex) is elicited when a tendon is suddenly stretched. Tendon reflexes are easily elicited in the patellar tendon, calcaneal tendon and the tendon of the triceps brachii. The tendon reflex helps maintain equilibrium and posture, and it prevents falling. Both extensor and flexor muscles are involved in most reflexes including the stretch reflex. The resulting reflex both stimulates muscle contraction and inhibits contraction by antagonist muscles. For example, in the **_patellar reflex_** the quadriceps femoris contracts when it is stretched and the hamstring muscles are inhibited from contracting by interneuronal connections in the cord.

Another reflex is the **_flexor withdrawal reflex_**. This reflex occurs when an extremity such as a foot is suddenly withdrawn from a painful stimulus. In this reflex flexors of the knee and hip contract, lifting the foot. This reflex also stimulates extensor muscles in the other leg, which allows you to stand quickly on one foot.

Poliomyelitis is a disease caused by the poliovirus, which infects motor neurons in the brain stem and ventral horns of the spinal cord. Symptoms include muscle pain, weakness, and loss of reflexes. Paralysis and muscle atrophy follow. Respiratory failure and death can result if the muscles of respiration are affected. Prior to the development of the polio vaccine, the wards of many hospitals were filled with children on iron lungs, which served to expand and contract the chest cavities of polio patients with respiratory paralysis.

Amyotrophic lateral sclerosis (also known as ALS and Lou Gehrig's disease) is a slowly progressive disorder of unknown etiology (cause) that involves degeneration of the motor neurons of the spinal cord. Sclerosis (scarring) results especially in the lateral areas of the cord, and the neurotransmitter, glutamate, accumulates to toxic levels. Symptoms include muscle weakness, which includes the muscles of speaking and swallowing, and fasciculations, which are twitches of fascicles that indicate motor neuron damage. The intellect is unaffected in this disease. One prominent individual who suffered from ALS for many years was Stephen Hawking, a brilliant British physicist who worked and wrote scientific papers despite being almost completely paralyzed.

Spinal muscular atrophy is a genetic disorder that is inherited as an autosomal recessive trait. This disease causes more deaths among children less than two years than any other genetic disease. The defective gene does not synthesize a protein (survival motor protein) that is necessary for the survival of motor neurons. Sensation and intellect are not affected. Symptoms may appear at birth, or they may be delayed until adulthood. One in forty people carry the abnormal gene, and the disease affects one in six thousand newborns. The carrier state is identifiable by a quantitative blood test for survival motor protein.

Shingles is a painful cutaneous eruption caused by the **_Herpes varicella-zoster_** virus. This is the same virus that causes chickenpox (varicella). Following an infection with chickenpox, the virus can remain viable in dorsal root ganglia. When immunity wanes, fast axonal transport brings viral particles to a dermatome of the skin where the painful eruption occurs. A vaccine has recently become available for this infection.

Compression of the axilla may result in **_injury to the radial nerve_**, a branch of the brachial plexus. Axillary injuries can be caused by the use of crutches or by replacing a dislocated shoulder too vigorously. Damage to the radial nerve causes the extensors of the hand, wrist and fingers to become weak or paralyzed. The result is chronic persistent flexion of the wrist and fingers, which is known as a "**_wrist drop_**,"

The **_sciatic nerve_** is the longest, largest and most vulnerable nerve in the body. **_Sciatica_** is sharp, stabbing pain radiating from the buttock to the ankle as a result of sciatic nerve compression. Sciatica may be caused by a herniated disc in the lumbar area, osteoporosis of the vertebrae, arthritis of the spine, pregnancy, hip dislocation, or improper injections in the buttocks. (Always inject in the upper outer quadrant). Sciatica has also been described after sitting too long in a hard chair or driving for long periods on a fat wallet filled with credit cards

Spinal cord trauma paralyzes ten to twelve thousand people every year in the U.S. Young males between the ages of 16 and 30 are at greatest risk due to their occupations and activities. Falls from ladders and roofs, gunshot wounds, stab wounds, automobile accidents, motorcycle accidents and diving accidents are common causes for this type of injury.

A complete transection of the cord results in immediate flaccid (limp) paralysis below the level of the injury. All reflexes and sensation are lost below that level. Bladder and bowel reflexes are lost, which result in urinary and fecal retention. Blood pressure drops, and fever occurs due to an inability to sweat, which is secondary to a lack of stimulation from the sympathetic nervous system. Respiratory failure occurs if the injury is at the C-3 level or above. Later hyperreflexia, incontinence and hypertension occur; somatic reflexes begin to reappear, and a spastic (contracted) paralysis replaces the initial flaccid paralysis.

__Paraplegia__ is loss of muscle movement and muscle atrophy in both lower limbs; it occurs with lesions of the spinal cord between vertebrae T-1 and L-1. *__Quadriplegia__* is the loss of muscle activity in all four extremities; it occurs with high cervical spinal cord injuries. *__Hemiplegia__* is loss of muscle activity in the upper and lower extremities of the same side of the body. Hemiplegia does not result from a complete transection of the spinal cord, but it may result from an injury to the brain.

Study Guide
1. What makes up the CNS?
2. Know that the spinal cord conducts information to the brain and receives information from the brain via tracts.
3. Know that the spinal cord is involved in stretch and other reflexes that help us stand, walk and respond quickly to stimuli.
4. Review the gross anatomy of the spinal cord from the foramen magnum to the medullary cone.
5. What is the cauda equina, and where can it be found?
6. Name and describe the layers of the meninges.
7. Know that the dorsal roots, dorsal horns, dorsal tracts and ganglia are afferent and sensory. Know that the ventral roots, ventral horns and ventral tracts are efferent and motor. Know that the lateral horns are motor and are part of the autonomic nervous system.
8. What makes up a spinal nerve? How many cervical nerves do you have, and how does that compare to the number of cervical vertebrae?
9. Define a dermatome.
10. Define proprioception. What sense organs detect proprioception?
11. Recognize the major ways the following disorders affect the spinal cord and spinal nerves: poliomyelitis, amyotrophic lateral sclerosis (ALS), and shingles (Herpes zoster).
12. Define quadriplegia, paraplegia and hemiplegia. Where would a lesion be located that would produce each of these types of paralysis?
13. Which nerve of the body is the longest and most vulnerable to injury?
14. Compression of the axilla can damage which nerve? What effect would that have?
15. Name the nerve plexuses of the body, and tell what they innervate.

Chapter Fourteen

The Brain

A discussion of the brain requires directions. **_Rostral_** is used in place of anterior (toward the forehead). **_Caudal_** is used in place of posterior. Caudal means "tail;" it describes the direction toward the occiput and spinal cord.

The three major parts of the brain can easily be seen and identified. They are the **_cerebrum_**, the **_cerebellum_** and the **_brainstem_**. The cerebrum contains 83% of the volume of the brain and is the site of conscious activity. However, the cerebellum contains 50% of the neurons of the brain because the coordinated movements directed by the cerebellum require a great deal of neuronal control.

Right: A view of the superior aspect of the human brain. This illustration shows the top of the cerebrum. The cerebellum and the brain stem are not visible in this view.

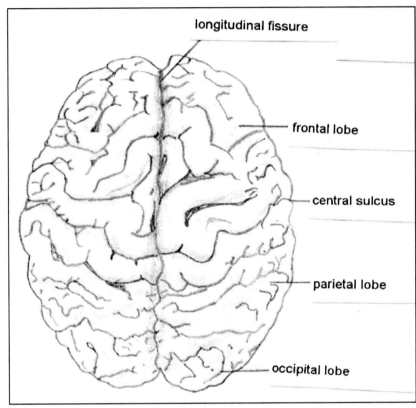

The brains of males and females differ in several aspects, and each sex has areas where it typically excels. Multiple studies have shown a weak but significant correlation between **_brain mass_** and intelligence within each sex. A composite of multiple studies concludes that the correlation of head size and intelligence is about 0.30. Male brains are larger in size and contain more mass than female brains. The average brain of an adult male weighs 1600 grams, and the average brain of an adult female weighs 1450 grams. That difference is largely but not completely tempered when it is adjusted to total body size, yet there appears to be no difference in intelligence between the sexes. The **_number and quality of synapses_** in the cerebrum has been determined to be a more important determinant for intelligence than brain mass or the total number of neurons.

As humans have evolved over the past two million years, the size of the brain has nearly tripled. This increase in size corresponds to the invention of tools and especially with the development of language. However, there are disadvantages to having large brains. One disadvantage is the increased weight of the head, which must be borne by the musculoskeletal system. The evolution of air filled sinuses in the skull helped to reduce the weight of the head. Also the foramen magnum is placed more anteriorly in man than in other primates, which balances the head on the vertebral column. The major price that a species has to pay for a large head is in childbirth. The head of a full term baby today is frequently larger than the birth canal of its mother. This disparity is reflected in the 25% to 30% incidence of Caesarian section deliveries being performed by obstetricians practicing in the U.S. today. Yet Homo sapiens of the twenty-first century A.D. has a slightly smaller cranial capacity than Cro-Magnon man, who lived 35,000 years ago. Our ancestors may have been smarter than we are.

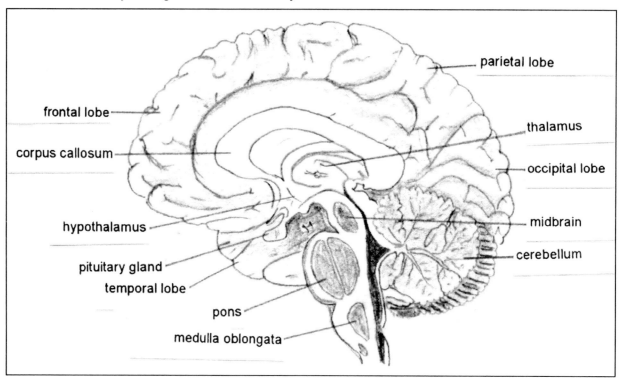

Above: A midsagittal cut through the human brain.

The brain and spinal cord are composed of **_gray matter_** and **_white matter_**. Gray matter consists of neurons, neuroglia (glial cells) and unmyelinated fibers. White matter consists of myelinated nerve tracts that are a conduit from one area of the CNS to another.

The nervous system develops from **_ectoderm_**, as does the epidermis of the skin. Muscles and the various types of connective tissues develop from **_mesoderm_,** and the lining and glands of most of the GI tract and respiratory tract develop from **_endoderm_**. In the development of the embryo the ectoderm forms a **_neural groove_**, which invaginates into a **_neural tube_**. The lumen of the neural tube becomes the **_ventricles_** of the brain and the **_central canal_** of the spinal cord. Three areas of enlargement form on the neural tube; they are **(1)** the **_prosencephalon, or forebrain_**, which develops into the **_telencephalon_** (cerebrum) and the **_diencephalon_** (thalamus, hypothalamus, and epithalamus). The eyes develop as an extension of the prosencephalon. **(2)** The **_mesencephalon (midbrain)_**, and **(3)** the **_rhombencephalon or hindbrain_**, which develops into the **_metencephalon_** (pons and cerebellum) and the **_myelencephalon_** (medulla).

The **_cerebrum, cerebellum, midbrain, pons and medulla oblongata_** can be seen by examining the external surface of the brain. Deeper anatomical structures of the brain are difficult to visualize without an illustration or model.

The obvious structural landmarks of the **_cerebrum_** are **_gyri_** (hills) and **_sulci_** (valleys or grooves). The surface of the cerebrum is divided by **_fissures_**. The **_longitudinal fissure_** separates the cerebral hemispheres; the **_transverse fissure_** separates the cerebrum and the cerebellum; and the **_lateral (or Sylvian) fissure_** separates the temporal lobe from the parietal and frontal lobes. The **_surface_** layer of the cerebrum is composed of gray matter called the **_cerebral cortex._** ("Cortical" is often used to refer to the cerebral cortex.) Masses of gray matter called nuclei and basal ganglia are buried deeply in the cerebrum and other parts of the brain. The white matter is more centrally located in the cerebrum and is in the form of **_tracts._**

Right: A view of the inferior surface of the brain.

frontal lobe

olfactory tract

optic chiasm

pituitary gland

trigeminal nerve

pons

temporal lobe

medulla oblongata

spinal cord

cerebellum

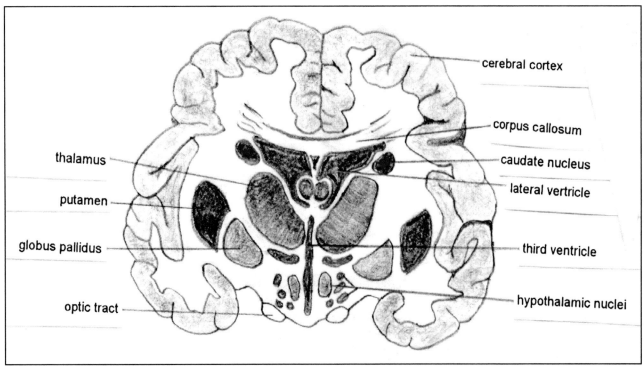

cerebral cortex

corpus callosum

caudate nucleus

lateral vertricle

thalamus

putamen

globus pallidus

third ventricle

optic tract

hypothalamic nuclei

Above: A drawing of a frontal section of the anterior portion of the brain. The cerebral cortex is the external gray layer.

Three layers of meninges cover the brain and the spinal cord. In the vertebral canal the **_dura mater_** is adherent to the arachnoid, but they are separate coverings over the brain. The dura covering the brain is split into two layers, an outer layer that is the periosteum of the cranial bones and an inner meningeal layer. The inner layer contains folds of fibrous connective tissue. Those folds include the **_falx cerebri_**, which extends into the longitudinal fissure between the two cerebral hemispheres; the **_tentorium cerebelli_**, which extends into the transverse fissure between the cerebrum and the cerebellum; and the **_falx cerebelli_**, which is a shallow extension between the cerebellar hemispheres. **_Venous sinuses_** within the cranium are spaces that contain venous blood; they are located between the two layers of dura. The major venous sinuses are: (1) the **_superior sagittal sinus_**, which is at the top of the longitudinal fissure, (2) the **_inferior sagittal sinus_** at the bottom of the longitudinal fissure, (3) the right and left **_transverse sinuses_** in the transverse fissure between the cerebrum and the cerebellum, and (4) the right and left **_cavernous sinuses,_** which connect above the sphenoid bone and below the frontal lobes. The straight sinus, occipital sinus, petrosal sinus and sigmoid sinus are linked to the other sinuses. The sinuses drain into the internal jugular veins and the vertebral veins. The cavernous sinuses are strategically located around the stalk of the pituitary gland (hypophysis), and they are traversed by the carotid arteries, the third and fourth cranial nerves, and branches of the fifth cranial nerve.

The **_arachnoid mater_** is a thin layer under the dura that has wispy connections to the underlying pia mater. A mesothelial layer that is in contact with cerebrospinal fluid covers the inner surface of the arachnoid. The **_pia mater_** is thinner than the arachnoid. It is a membranous one cell layer that closely follows the surface of the cerebral cortex.

A **_subdural hemorrhage_** is a venous hemorrhage that may result following blunt trauma to the head. The blood is poorly reabsorbed because the subdural space is an enclosed space. When red cells in the hemorrhage begin to lyse, the osmolarity in the hemorrhage starts to increase. Water seeps into the hemorrhage by osmosis, and the hematoma gradually increases in size, which compresses the brain and simulates a tumor. Subdural hematomas frequently require surgical evacuation.

A **_subarachnoid hemorrhage_** is a life-threatening emergency that results from the rupture of an artery. Blood rapidly pours into the subarachnoid space. The most likely site of the bleeding is the circle of Willis, an arterial circle surrounding the stalk of the pituitary gland at the base of the cerebrum. Arteries in the circle of Willis are prone to **_aneurysms_**, which are dilated areas of an artery that occur due to a localized weakness in the arterial wall.

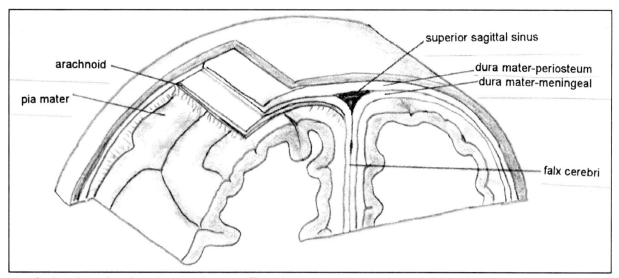

Above: A drawing showing the meninges. The dura mater is made up of two layers, an outer layer that is periosteum and an inner meningeal layer. The two layers of the dura are tightly attached except where they are separated by venous sinuses. The subdural space is between the dura and the arachnoid. The arachnoid is a thin layer with web-like connections to the underlying pia mater. The pia is a membranous one cell layer on the surface of the brain. The subarachnoid space is occupied by cerebrospinal fluid. The dura and arachnoid have mesothelium on their inner surfaces. The pia is a mesothelial layer.

Deep within the brain are four chambers called ***ventricles***, which are connected chambers filled with ***cerebrospinal fluid (CSF).*** The ***two lateral ventricles*** are located deep in the cerebral hemispheres. The ***third ventricle*** is a narrow vertical space under the corpus callosum between the right and left halves of the thalamus. The ***fourth ventricle*** is between the cerebellum and the pons. The ***foramina of Munro*** connect the lateral ventricles with the third ventricle; the ***cerebral aqueduct*** (mesencephalic aqueduct) connects the third and fourth ventricles. The fourth ventricle is continuous with the central canal of the spinal cord. Three small openings connect the fourth ventricle to the subarachnoid space.

CSF is produced by ***ependymal cells***, which make up the internal lining of the ventricles and the central canal of the spinal cord. Each ventricle contains a special aggregation of ependymal cells called a ***choroid plexus***. Most of the CSF is secreted by ependymal cells in the choroid plexuses. CSF is also secreted into the subarachnoid space by ependymal cells in the arachnoid. CSF travels from the lateral ventricles to the third ventricle, then to the fourth ventricle where it exits through three small apertures into the subarachnoid space surrounding the brain and spinal cord. The apertures in the fourth ventricle are the ***foramen of Majendie*** in the midline and a right and left ***foramen of Luschka***. A small amount of CSF is produced by ependymal cells in the central canal of the spinal cord and flows up to the fourth ventricle. CSF is reabsorbed into the blood stream at the ***arachnoid villi***, which are cauliflower-like areas of arachnoid that extend through the dura into the superior sagittal sinus.

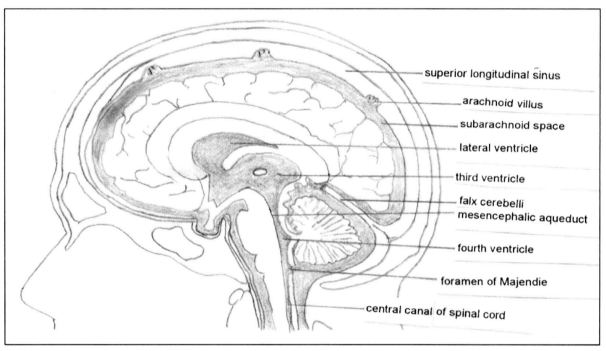

superior longitudinal sinus
arachnoid villus
subarachnoid space
lateral ventricle
third ventricle
falx cerebelli
mesencephalic aqueduct
fourth ventricle
foramen of Majendie
central canal of spinal cord

Above: A drawing showing the locations of CSF. CSF is secreted by choroid plexuses in the ventricles. It flows from the lateral ventricles through the interventricular foramina of Munro into the third ventricle. From the third ventricle it flows through the mesencephalic aqueduct to the fourth ventricle where it receives CSF from the central canal of the spinal cord. CSF exits the fourth ventricle through three tiny foramina and enters the subarachnoid space that surrounds the brain and spinal cord. CSF is reabsorbed into the blood stream from arachnoid villi, which are projections of arachnoid into the superior sagittal venous sinus.

CSF bathes the brain and is constantly being secreted and reabsorbed. About 100-160 cc of CSF is present at any one time, and the CSF turns itself over every 5-8 hours. The brain ***floats*** in CSF, which ***protects*** the brain. CSF also ***supplies nutrients*** and removes wastes. CSF is normally a clear, colorless liquid. It has more sodium and chloride than plasma, but less potassium, calcium and glucose. It has no cells and almost no protein. CSF can be examined following a ***spinal tap***, which is done by inserting a needle into the subarachnoid space of the vertebral column between the spinous processes of two adjacent lower lumbar vertebrae. A few cubic centimeters (cc) of CSF are withdrawn and examined. Any abnormalities in CSF are an aid to diagnosis. For example, a low glucose and high protein content indicate infection (meningitis). Bright red (arterial) blood is present in the CSF following a subarachnoid hemorrhage.

The brain weighs only three to four pounds, but it receives 15% of the cardiac output. Neurons utilize only **_aerobic respiration_** for ATP production, and the brain consumes 20% of the body's glucose and oxygen. A ten second interruption in blood flow results in a loss of consciousness, and a four minute interruption produces irreversible brain damage.

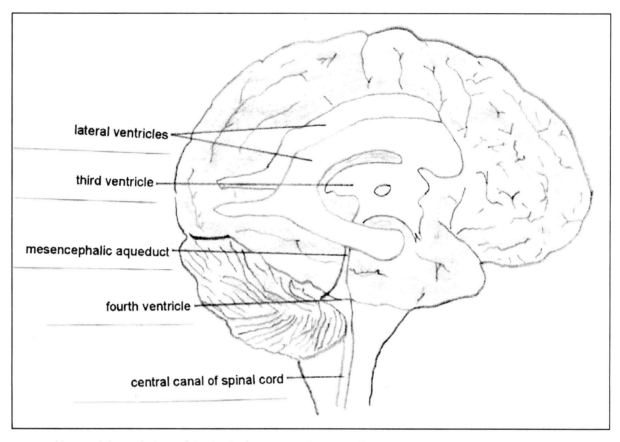

Above: A lateral view of the brain from the right side. The ventricles are pictured in relief.

The **_blood-brain barrier (BBB)_** separates the blood from brain tissue. It consists of **_tight junctions_** between astrocytes and endothelial cells lining the capillaries. Only select molecules can penetrate this barrier, which protects and isolates the brain from undesirable substances. The BBB is highly permeable to water, oxygen, carbon dioxide, and glucose; it is less permeable to sodium, potassium, chloride, urea and creatinine. Ethyl alcohol and caffeine easily penetrate the BBB. Tight junctions between ependymal cells and the blood are present in the choroid plexuses, but they are lacking elsewhere. Consequently the barrier between blood and CSF is not as restrictive as between blood and brain tissue. There are centers in the hypothalamus that monitor blood pH, glucose concentration and osmolarity. The blood-brain barrier is necessarily lacking in these areas, and disease organisms such as viruses may enter the brain at these locations.

Areas of the Brain

The **_medulla oblongata_** is the most caudal area of the brain. It is about three centimeters long, and it is continuous with the pons rostrally and the spinal cord caudally. The medulla, pons, midbrain and diencephalon make up the **_brainstem_**. Caudally the medulla extends to the foramen magnum, which is the dividing point between the brain and the cord. All ascending and descending communications between the brain and the cord must go through the medulla. The dorsal surface of the medulla is the fourth ventricle. The ventral surface of the medulla is visible externally and includes the olive nuclei and the pyramids. The **_olive nuclei_** are surface enlargements with underlying gray matter that monitors blood pressure, heart rate and respiration. Other gray matter nuclei in the medulla monitor vomiting, coughing, sneezing, hiccupping, salivation, sweating, and GI secretions. Nuclei for cranial nerves IX, X, XI and XII are in the medulla. The *__pyramids__* contain the *__corticospinal tracts__*, which are prominent white matter tracts containing motor fibers descending from the cerebrum to the cord.

The *__pons__* is immediately rostral to the medulla. It contains ascending and descending tracts between the cerebrum and the cord, and it contains tracts going to and from the cerebellum. Nuclei of cranial nerves V, VI, VII and VIII are in the pons. These nuclei are concerned with facial sensation and mastication (CN V), eye movements (CN VI), facial expression (CN VII), and hearing and equilibrium (CN VIII). Other nuclei in the pons are concerned with sleep, taste, respiration, swallowing, bladder control and posture.

The *__cerebellum__* is second only to the cerebrum in size. Neurons of the cerebellum are called *__Purkinje cells__*, and they make up 50% of the neurons in the brain. The cerebellum is divided into a right and left hemisphere, and it is separated from the pons by the fourth ventricle. Except for deeply located nuclei, the gray matter of the cerebellum is on the surface and the white matter is deep. The central gray matter of each cerebellar hemisphere contains *__four nuclei__*, a large dentate nucleus, an emboliform nucleus, a small globose nucleus and the nucleus fastigii. All connections between the cerebellum and the rest of the brain go through one of these nuclei to the medulla, pons or midbrain.

__Folia__ are small gyri on the surface of the cerebellum. On sagittal sections cerebellar white matter can be seen to branch into a pattern called *__arbor vitae__*. The cerebellum primarily functions below consciousness to produce skilled *__coordinated movements__*. In spite of the large number of neurons in the cerebellum, loss or damage to the cerebellum is not life threatening. Destruction of the cerebellum leads to *__ataxia__*, which consists of awkward and clumsy movements; walking is exceedingly slow and difficult, and climbing stairs is impossible.

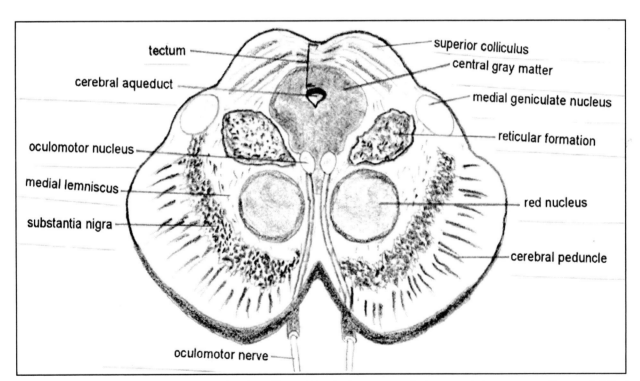

Above: A transverse cut through the midbrain. The midbrain (mesencephalon) contains gray matter nuclei that are responsible for visual tracking, audio tracking, alertness, muscular control and other modalities. White matter tracts connect the midbrain to the cerebrum, thalamus, basal ganglia, pons, medulla, and spinal cord.

The *__midbrain or mesencephalon__* lies between the hindbrain (medulla, pons and cerebellum) and the forebrain (diencephalon and cerebrum). It contains nuclei for cranial nerves III and IV, both of which are concerned with eye movements. Areas in the midbrain include the *__cerebral peduncles__*, which contain the corticospinal tracts; the *tegmentum* with its red nucleus; the *substantia nigra,* which contains many inhibitory synapses, the loss of which results in Parkinson's Disease; the *central gray matter;* the *medial lemnisci,* which contain sensory tracts from the cord; the *tectum,* which overlies the cerebral aqueduct; the *superior colliculi,* which aid in visual tracking; the *inferior colliculi,* which aid in sound tracking; and much of the *reticular formation*. The *reticular formation* extends from the thalamus to the spinal cord and consists of over one hundred nuclei with numerous functions including the establishment of *alertness and sleep* and the provision of balance and posture. Damage to the reticular formation may lead to irreversible coma. Some general anesthetics act by blocking signals in the reticular formation. The reticular formation is also instrumental in *habituation,* which is the ability to ignore repetitive inconsequential noises and other stimuli, and yet retain sensitivity to other sounds and stimuli. Thus one can hear a baby's cry but sleep through traffic noise.

The *diencephalon* is part of the prosencephalon (forebrain), and it is the most rostral part of the brainstem. It consists of the *thalamus, hypothalamus and epithalamus*. In cross section the *thalamus* is a heart-shaped mass of gray matter that is composed of two long ovoid cylindrical structures joined at the base. Its two halves are situated deep in the brain, lateral to the third ventricle and lateral and below the two lateral ventricles. The thalamus acts like a *switchboard* to and from the cerebrum. Nearly all the sensory input to the cerebrum synapses in the thalamus, and the thalamus receives motor input from the cerebrum as well. The *internal and external capsules* are tracts of white matter that connect the thalamus to the cerebral cortex. The thalamus is well connected to the *limbic system,* which is involved in emotions and memory. The thalamus is also involved in arousal, eye movements, taste, smell, hearing, equilibrium, and skin sensations. Both the *medial geniculate bodies,* which relay hearing messages, and the *lateral geniculate bodies,* which relay visual messages, are located in the thalamus adjacent to the midbrain.

The *hypothalamus* occupies only a small area at the floor of the third ventricle below the thalamus, but it is of great importance to the body. It is posterior to the *optic chiasm,* which is where the optic nerves decussate, and it is anterior to the *mammilary bodies,* which are relay centers from limbic system. The hypothalamus, mammilary bodies and limbic system are of paramount importance in memory and emotions, including anger, aggression, fear, pleasure, contentment, sexual desire and orgasm. The hypothalamus has a great deal of influence over sexuality. Several nuclei in the hypothalamus (the suprachiasmatic nucleus and the second and third interstitial nuclei) are two to three times larger in men than in women. These nuclei are significantly smaller in homosexual men than they are in heterosexual men, which points to an anatomic basis for homosexuality. A genetic determinate for homosexuality is suggested by the finding of a high incidence of male and female homosexuality in siblings, especially identical twins. A DNA sequence on one area of the X chromosome has been linked to the development of homosexuality.

The hypothalamus is the major control center of the autonomic nervous system and the endocrine system, and it plays an essential role in homeostatic regulation. It regulates cardiac rate, blood pressure, body temperature, sweating, the constriction of blood vessels in the skin, hunger, satiety, thirst, and the levels of glucose, fatty acids and amino acids in the plasma. Nuclei in the hypothalamus control the circadian rhythm, which is the 24-hour cycle of sleep and alertness. The hypothalamus affects water and electrolyte balance through osmoreceptors, a thirst center, and through the effects of hormones that it secretes. A *portal system* of circulation takes venous blood from the hypothalamus to the pituitary gland.

The *pituitary gland* (also known as the *hypophysis*) is located within the sella turcica just below the hypothalamus. The *infundibulum* is a stalk that attaches the pituitary to the hypothalamus. The pituitary has an anterior lobe and a posterior lobe, each with different functions. The hypothalamus controls hormone secretion by the *anterior lobe* of the pituitary gland by secreting other hormones *(releasing factors)* that stimulate the release of hormones by the anterior pituitary. Releasing factors flood the anterior pituitary by the portal system of circulation from the hypothalamus. The hormones of the anterior pituitary are GH (growth hormone), TSH (thyroid stimulating hormone), FSH (follicle stimulating hormone), ACTH (adrenocorticotropic hormone), and prolactin (stimulates milk production by the mammary glands). Oxytocin and antidiuretic hormone (ADH or vasopressin) are hormones produced by the hypothalamus and stored in the *posterior lobe* of the pituitary. Oxytocin induces labor, and ADH increases water absorption from the renal (kidney) tubules. Too little ADH results in *diabetes insipidus,* a condition in which there is excessive water loss in the urine. Too much ADH production results in water retention and hyponatremia (a low blood sodium concentration).

The ***epithalamus*** is a small area on the roof of the third ventricle. It consists of the habenula and the pineal gland. The ***habenula*** is a relay center from the limbic system to the midbrain. The ***pineal gland*** was once thought to be the center of the soul. A more sophisticated look at the pineal has revealed its importance to be much more modest. The pineal has an endocrine function, and it is active in early childhood, but it rapidly shrinks in size after age seven. It is known to secrete serotonin during the day and melatonin, which induces sleep, at night.

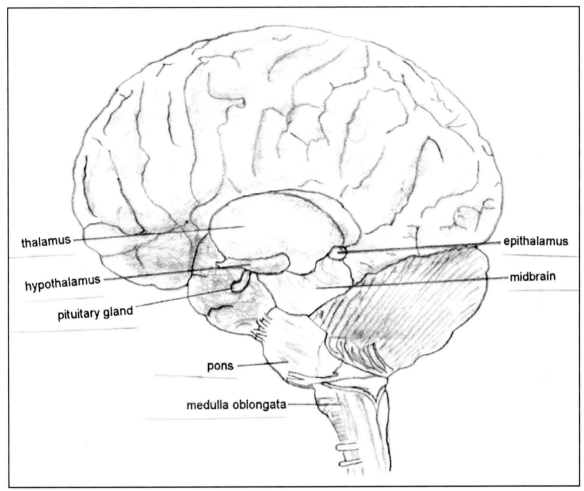

Above: The brainstem is outlined in relief. The temporal lobe would be in front of the brainstem in this drawing, but most of the temporal lobe is not visible so that the position and structure of the brainstem can be shown. The brainstem consists of the diencephalon (thalamus, hypothalamus and epithalamus), mesencephalon (midbrain), pons and medulla oblongata.

Each hemisphere of the ***cerebrum (telencephalon)*** is divided into five lobes, frontal, parietal, occipital, temporal and insula. The ***frontal*** lobes are concerned with intelligence, voluntary motor functions and areas for planning, speech, mood, memory, social judgment, emotion, motivation, foresight and aggression. The frontal lobes are separated from the parietal lobes by the central sulcus. The gyrus rostral to the central sulcus is the ***precentral gyrus*** of the frontal lobe, which is the ***primary motor area*** of the cerebral cortex.

The ***parietal*** lobes contain areas for sensory reception and the integration of stimuli. Immediately behind the central sulcus is the ***postcentral gyrus*** of the parietal lobe, which is the ***primary sensory area*** of the cerebral cortex.

The ***occipital*** lobes are the ***visual centers*** of the brain. They receive input from the retinas of the eyes via the optic nerves and the lateral geniculate bodies of the thalamus.

The ***temporal lobes*** contain areas for the interpretation of hearing, smell, learning, memory, emotional behavior and visual recognition. The temporal lobes integrate sensory input so that it makes sense. The posterior part of the temporal lobe contains ***Wernicke's area***, which is where speech is understood.

The ***insula*** is a small area of cerebral cortex located deep in the lateral sulcus. It plays a part in taste recognition, integration of visual input and understanding spoken language.

The basic function of the ***parietal cortex*** is to perceive stimuli. The ***temporal cortex*** identifies those stimuli, and the ***frontal cortex*** plans what the response will be. Studying people with brain lesions has improved our knowledge of cognition, awareness perception, thinking, knowledge and memory. Studying Individuals with tumors, cerebrovascular accidents and injuries has allowed the identification of several syndromes. **(1)** Patients with the ***contralateral neglect syndrome*** are unaware of one side of their body. This syndrome is caused by an injury to the ***parietal lobe.*** **(2)** ***Agnosia*** is the inability to recognize objects, and ***prosopagnosia*** is the inability to recognize faces. These symptoms may occur with ***temporal lobe*** defects. **(3)** ***Personality and emotional behavioral*** changes with an inability to act appropriately may occur with ***frontal lobe*** defects. **(4)** The visual cortex is located in the occipital lobes, and damage to the occipital lobes may lead to partial or complete ***blindness.***

Cerebral gray matter consists of the ***cerebral cortex*** and the ***basal nuclei (basal ganglia)***. The cortex is only about three mm thick. The mass of the cortex is greatly expanded by folding into gyri and sulci. Gray matter is also present in the cortex of the cerebellum and nuclei throughout the brainstem. From an evolutionary standpoint the cerebral cortex is divided into the ***archicortex***, which in humans exists only in the hippocampus of the limbic system; the ***paleocortex***, which occupies part of the temporal lobe and insula in humans; and the ***neocortex***, which is divided into six layers and accounts for 90% of the cerebral cortex in humans. The neocortex is extensively developed only in primates. Neurons in the cerebral cortex include stellate cells and pyramidal cells. ***Stellate cells*** have dendrites that project in all directions, and these cells receive sensory input and process information on a local level. The ***pyramidal cells*** are largely responsible for voluntary motor movements. They are classified as being either small or large (large pyramidal cells are called Betz cells). Each pyramidal cell has an axon that passes out of the cortex.

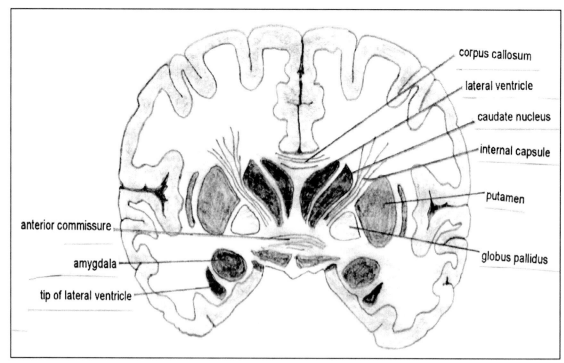

Right: A frontal section through the middle of the brain. This drawing shows the location of the basal ganglia and the internal capsule.

corpus callosum

lateral ventricle

caudate nucleus

internal capsule

putamen

globus pallidus

anterior commissure

amygdala

tip of lateral ventricle

The ***basal nuclei*** (also called the basal ganglia) of the cerebrum are masses of gray matter within white matter.

The basal nuclei are located on each side of the cerebrum lateral to the thalamus. The **_caudate nucleus_**, **_putamen_** and **_globus pallidus,_** are pairs of basal ganglia, and all are involved in motor control. The caudate nucleus and putamen together make up what is known as the corpus striatum. The putamen and globus pallidus together make up the lentiform nucleus. The basal nuclei send signals to and receive signals from the substantia nigra of the midbrain, which is an area rich in inhibitory synapses. Lesions of the basal nuclei make the patient have tremors and move slowly with difficulty initiating movements such as getting out of a chair. Other signs of a lesion in the basal nuclei include chorea, athetosis, dystonia and hemiballismus, which are spasmodic, involuntary, purposeless movements. Pill rolling is an athetotic movement. Hemiballismus is a coarse, sudden, uncontrollable thrashing about or throwing out of the extremities. The changes in muscle tone and posture that result from lesions in the basal ganglia can be similar to those of Parkinson's disease.

The **_cerebral white matter_** includes myelinated tracts that connect the cerebral cortex to the rest of the central nervous system. **_Projection_** tracts are those that extend vertically between the cerebral cortex and the brainstem and spinal cord. Projection tracts form the **_internal capsules and external capsules_**, which are fan-like radiations of white matter from the thalamus and basal nuclei to the cerebral cortex. **_Commissural_** tracts are those that cross from one hemisphere to the other. The **_corpus callosum_** is a wide band of white matter that connects the hemispheres. The anterior and posterior commissures are smaller commissural tracts respectively located rostral and caudal to the corpus callosum. A prefrontal lobotomy is an incision into the rostral portion of the corpus callosum that was performed to quiet patients with schizophrenia in past decades. **_Association_** tracts are those that connect neurons of cortical gray matter in the same hemisphere. Association tracts link perception and memory centers; they enable one to associate and do such things as smell a rose and then be able to name it and picture it.

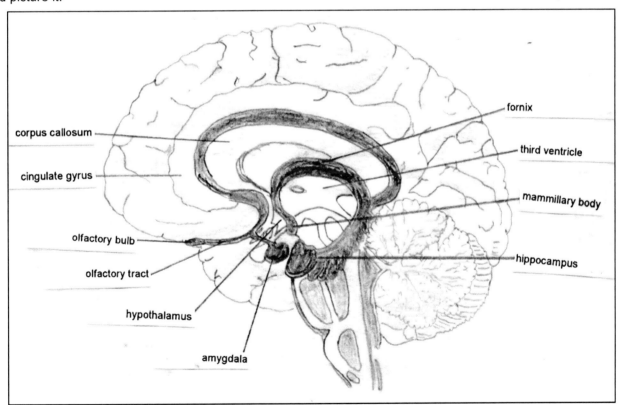

Above: The limbic system (in the darker shade) is a center for emotions and memory. It is closely associated with the sense of smell. The limbic system is made up of the amygdaloid nucleus, hippocampal nucleus, fornix of the hippocampus and the cingulate gyrus of the frontal and parietal lobes.

The **_limbic system_** consists of a loop of cortical structures around the corpus callosum and the thalamus. The four parts of the limbic system are: **(1)** the **_amygdala nucleus_** and the **(2)** the **_hippocampal gyrus,_** both of which are in the medial aspect of the temporal lobe, (3) the _**fornix,**_ which is a white matter tract over the third ventricle, and **(4)** the _**cingulate gyrus**_, which is draped over the corpus callosum. The _**olfactory tracts**_, _**mammilary bodies**_, _**hypothalamus**_ and _**thalamus**_ are closely associated with the limbic system, but they are not part of it. The limbic system is especially involved in _**short term memory**_ and _**emotions.**_ It is well developed in lower animals, which have a keen sense of smell, and it is referred to as the _**rhinencephalon**_ ("nose-brain") in those animals. The _**amygdala**_ is especially important in _**emotion**_ and basic memory, such as remembering what you are doing. The _**hippocampus**_ is responsible for most _**short-term memory**_. The _**fornix**_ extends over the third ventricle to connect the hippocampus to the mammilary bodies. The _**mammilary bodies**_ are in the hypothalamus immediately posterior to the pituitary gland; they relay signals from the limbic system to the thalamus. The _**cingulate gyrus**_ is a gyrus of the cerebral cortex that is draped over the corpus callosum. It is closely associated with smell, and it is connected to the olfactory tracts rostrally and to the hippocampus caudally.

The Cranial Nerves

There are twelve pairs of nerves that exit the brain. Each goes through its specific foramen to emerge outside the cranium and proceed to innervate muscles, glands, sense organs, mucosa and the skin of the head, neck and trunk. Only cranial nerves II and IV decussate; the rest do not.

A mnemonic for remembering the cranial nerves is

<u>O</u>n <u>O</u>ld <u>O</u>lympus' <u>T</u>owering <u>T</u>ops, <u>A</u> <u>F</u>inn <u>A</u>nd <u>G</u>erman <u>V</u>iewed <u>S</u>ome <u>H</u>ops.

The nerves this mnemonic refers to are

<u>O</u>lfactory, <u>O</u>ptic, <u>O</u>culomotor, <u>T</u>rochlear, <u>T</u>rigeminal, <u>A</u>bducens, <u>F</u>acial, <u>A</u>coustic (also known as Vestibulocochlear), <u>G</u>lossopharyngeal, <u>V</u>agus, <u>S</u>pinal accessory (or Accessory), and <u>H</u>ypoglossal.

The cranial nerves are numbered one through twelve, and they are appropriately written by name or Roman numeral. Cranial nerves IX through XII exit the medulla (cranial nerve XI also contains rootlets from the upper five cervical nerves). Cranial nerves V through VIII exit the pons, and cranial nerves III and IV exit the midbrain. The optic tracts enter the lateral geniculate bodies of the thalamus; the optic chiasm is the boundary between the optic nerves (CN II) and the optic tracts. The course of the first cranial nerve is explained below.

The _**olfactory nerve**_ is cranial nerve I. It is the nerve of smell. It is a pure sensory nerve that arises from olfactory cells, which are neurons with non motile _**cilia**_ ("hair cells") in the _**olfactory mucosa**_ at the roof of the nose. This is the only place in the body where neurons are _**exposed**_. Neurons of the olfactory mucosa are also unique in that they are capable of being replaced by stem cells that undergo _**mitosis**_ and differentiate into olfactory neurons. The olfactory nerve is not a single nerve, but a number of small nerve fascicles that penetrate the _**cribiform plate of the ethmoid**_ bone and synapse in the _**olfactory bulb**_, which is located just above the cribiform plate and under the frontal lobes of the cerebrum. From the olfactory bulbs the _**olfactory tracts**_ run in a caudal direction to the _**cingulate gyrus**_ of the cerebrum and other parts of the limbic system.

The _**optic nerve**_ is cranial nerve II. It is the nerve of vision. In embryology the optic nerve and the retina develop as _**part of the forebrain**_. The optic nerve is a pure sensory nerve that receives visual signals from the retinas of the eyes. The right and left optic nerves meet at the _**optic chiasm**_, which is immediately anterior to the pituitary gland. Fifty percent of the fibers of each nerve cross to the other side. From the optic chiasm the _**optic tracts**_ run to the _**lateral geniculate bodies**_ of the thalamus, then to the _**occipital cortex**_.

The _**oculomotor nerve**_ is cranial nerve III. It is primarily a motor nerve that supplies innervation to four of the six small muscles that move each eye. It also innervates the muscle that elevates the upper eyelid (levator palpebrae), the muscle that constricts the pupil, and the muscle that is responsible for accommodation (the ciliary muscle, which allows you to focus on a near object). The muscle that dilates the pupil is innervated by sympathetic nerve fibers that join the oculomotor nerve in the orbit.

The _**trochlear nerve**_ is cranial nerve IV. It is a motor nerve that innervates one muscle that moves the eye (the superior oblique). The trochlear nerve is unique in that it is the only cranial nerve to exit from the dorsal surface of the brain. The trochlear nerve decussates before leaving the midbrain.

The _**trigeminal nerve**_ is cranial nerve V. It is a mixed sensory and motor nerve that has a large ganglion lateral to the cavernous sinus called the Gasserian or semilunar ganglion. Distal to this ganglion the trigeminal nerve divides into ***three divisions***, the ophthalmic, maxillary and mandibular divisions. The trigeminal nerve is the main sensory nerve of the face, and it is responsible for carrying signals of ***pain*** and other somesthetic (widely distributed) senses to the brain. The trigeminal nerve is also the ***motor*** nerve for the powerful ***muscles of mastication*** that close the jaw (temporalis, masseter and medial and lateral pterygoid muscles). Damage to this nerve produces loss of sensation in the face (anesthesia) and impaired chewing. The excruciatingly painful conditions known as trigeminal neuralgia and *tic douloureux* are due to a dysfunction that involves one of the divisions of the trigeminal nerve.

The ***abducens nerve*** is cranial nerve VI. It is a motor nerve that supplies one of the muscles that move the eye (the lateral rectus muscle, which abducts the eye).

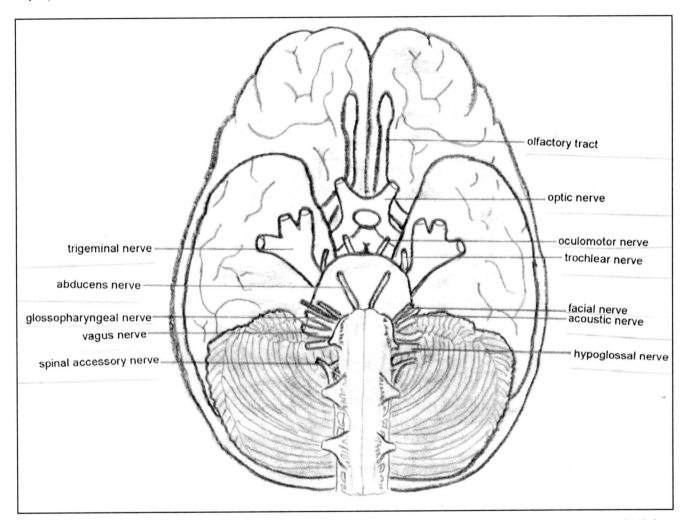

Above: A drawing of the inferior aspect of the brain showing the cranial nerves. Cranial nerves exit the CNS from the cerebrum to the cervical spinal cord. The olfactory tract extends from the lower part of the frontal lobe; the optic tract extends from the lateral geniculate body of the thalamus. Cranial nerves III and IV exit the midbrain. Cranial nerves V, VI, VII and VIII exit the pons, and cranial nerves IX, X, XI and XII exit the medulla. Cranial nerve XI has rootlets from the upper cervical nerves as well as the medulla.

The ***facial nerve*** is cranial nerve VII. It is a mixed nerve that supplies the ***facial muscles***, ***taste buds*** on the anterior 2/3 of the tongue, two pairs of ***salivary glands*** (the sublingual and submandibular), the ***lacrimal gland***, and small glands in the nose, mouth and pharynx. The facial nerve innervates the stapedius muscle, which dampens sound by rotating the stapedius bone in the middle ear. (The tensor tympani muscle, which dampens the effects of sound waves by tightening the eardrum, is innervated by the mandibular division of the trigeminal nerve.) Because both the fifth and the seventh cranial nerves are involved in dampening sound, damage to either nerve can produce undue pain sensations and an increased vulnerability to deafness from loud noises. The facial nerve exits the pons and passes through the ***stylomastoid foramen***, which is a small opening in the temporal bone behind the ear lobe. Swelling around this foramen can paralyze the facial nerve, which results in the disorder known as ***Bell's palsy***. Paralysis of the facial muscles results in sagging of the lower eyelid and corners of the mouth with drooling, tearing and disfigurement. Bell's palsy is usually temporary.

The ***acoustic or vestibulocochlear nerve*** is cranial nerve VIII. It is the nerve of the ***ear***, and it supplies the **cochlea** and the ***vestibular apparatus*** of the ear. It is primarily a sensory nerve for hearing and equilibrium. It exits the pons and travels through the internal auditory meatus to the inner ear.

The ***glossopharyngeal nerve*** is cranial nerve IX. It is a mixed nerve that supplies the ***parotid gland***, ***taste buds*** on the posterior 1/3 of the tongue, skin of the outer ear, and stylopharyngeal muscle, which assists in swallowing. It also innervates the ***carotid sinus***, a barosensitive organ at the junction of the internal and external carotid arteries that detects blood pressure and sends signals to the hypothalamus.

The ***vagus nerve*** is cranial nerve X. "Vagus" means vagabond or wandering, and the vagus got its name from the long, meandering course that it takes to the ***thorax and abdomen***. The vagus is a mixed nerve that supplies motor innervation to smooth muscle, cardiac muscle and glands of the chest and abdomen. It supplies sensation to the internal organs, part of the tongue, part of the pharynx, outer ear, dura mater and epiglottis. It also innervates the ***carotid body***, a small collection of chemoreceptor cells near the carotid sinus. The receptor cells of the carotid body monitor the concentrations of oxygen and carbon dioxide in the blood and the blood pH. This information is sent to the hypothalamus. Life cannot be sustained with the loss of both vagus nerves

The ***spinal accessory (or accessory) nerve*** is cranial nerve XI. It is predominately a motor nerve that supplies muscles of the back and neck including the trapezius, sternocleidomastoid and some small muscles of the pharynx and palate. Rootlets of the accessory nerve exit the CNS between the ***medulla and the fifth cervical nerve;*** the cervical rootlets travel upward through the foramen magnum before exiting the skull through the jugular foramen.

The ***hypoglossal nerve*** is cranial nerve XII. It exits the medulla and joins the ***cervical plexus***. It is primarily a motor nerve that supplies the ***intrinsic and extrinsic muscles of the tongue***. It also supplies the thyrohyoid and geniohyoid muscles, which act on the hyoid bone and the pharynx. If the hypoglossal nerve is damaged on one side, the tongue will deviate toward the injured side.

The Nervous System and Body Regulation

Sleep is a temporary state of unconsciousness from which a person can be fully aroused. ***Stupor*** is the state of arousability to partial cognition. ***Semicoma*** is a minimal ability to arouse, and ***coma*** is the state of unconsciousness with no ability to arouse. The ***reticular formation*** regulates the state of alertness. The suprachiasmatic nucleus of the hypothalamus sets our ***circadian rhythm*** (schedule for being awake and asleep.)

Sleep has ***four stages***. First is a drifting sensation in which the individual often claims he is not asleep. In the second stage, the individual is easily aroused. In the third stage the vital signs change --- the blood pressure, pulse and respiratory rate all drop. The third stage is usually reached after about twenty minutes of sleep. The fourth stage is deep sleep during which arousal is difficult.

The depth of sleep is reflected by movements of the eyes. ***REM sleep*** (rapid eye movement) can take place in stages one, two and three. There are approximately five episodes of REM sleep every night. REM sleep is characterized by an increase in the vital signs, dreaming and penile erections. Despite changes in the metabolic rate, the individual in REM sleep is difficult to arouse. ***Sleep paralysis*** is a feeling of being awake but unable to move. It involves an inhibition of skeletal muscle movements. Both sleep paralysis and ***sleep walking*** occur during REM sleep. REM sleep functions as a time when memories are strengthened and unwanted information is purged from memory. Deprivation of REM sleep does not lead to serious adverse effects. ***NonREM sleep*** is deep, stage four sleep, which has a restorative effect of the brain and is necessary for life. Experimental animals that are deprived of nonREM sleep do not survive long.

An *electroencephalogram (EEG)* is a recording of brain waves as a means of studying the brain. An EEG records rhythmic voltage changes in the cerebral cortex, which occur as a result of synaptic potentials. Electrodes are placed on the scalp, and a series of lines are drawn on a revolving roll of paper. An EEG reflects the state of consciousness from highly alert to deep sleep and coma. Only in death is there a complete absence of brain waves. Brain tumors, epilepsy, degenerative brain disorders and metabolic abnormalities may show EEG abnormalities. Brain waves tend to get faster from infancy to adulthood. The four types of brain waves seen on an EEG are (1) *beta waves*, which occur when the eyes are open and the individual is performing a mental task. Beta waves have a frequency of 14-30 Hertz (Hz or cycles/second). (2) *Alpha waves* occur when the individual is awake and resting with his eyes closed. Alpha waves have a frequency of 8-13 Hz.   (3) *Theta waves* occur during sleep or emotional stress. They are normal in children and sleeping adults, but abnormal in the awake adult. They have a frequency of 4-7 Hz. (4) *Delta waves* occur during deep sleep in adults or in awake infants. They have a frequency of 1-3 Hz. Delta waves are indicative of brain damage if they are seen in an awake adult.

The management of information requires *learning*, *remembering* and the *elimination* of unwanted trivia. Brain injuries can produce an *anterograde amnesia*, which is the inability to store new data, or a *retrograde amnesia*, which is an inability to remember old data. Short-term memory especially involves the *hippocampus*. The hippocampus must send the memory to the cerebral cortex for long-term storage. A lesion involving the hippocampus leads to profound anterograde amnesia. The *amygdala* is involved in basic memory, such as remembering what you are doing, and the *cerebellum* plays a prominent role in remembering motor skills like driving a car, playing the piano or playing basketball.

Although the cortex of the frontal lobe is the seat of judgment, intent and control over our emotions, it is in the *hypothalamus* and the *amygdala* of the limbic system where *emotions* are formed and felt. This includes all sorts of emotions including fear, love, anger and hate. A lesion near the amygdala or hypothalamus can produce either a blunting or an exaggeration of anger, pain, love, aggression, pleasure, etc., as well as abnormalities of learning, memory and motivation.   In some animal study protocols electrodes are implanted into the medial forebrain bundle of the *hypothalamus*, and the animal must press a foot pedal to stimulate this area. Monkeys will continually press this pedal, counted as 17,000 times an hour, and they will neglect food and water in order to do so. Patients have reported a "relief of tension" and "a quiet relaxed feeling" with stimulation of this area.

Nerve signals that arrive at primary sensory areas are processed and interpreted in *association areas*. Visual messages are processed in the occipital lobe. The *primary visual* sensory area is at the rear of the occipital lobe, and it is surrounded by the visual *association area*, which is the area where the brain identifies and makes sense of what the eye is seeing. *Taste* awareness and interpretation occur at the inferolateral end of the postcentral gyrus of the parietal lobe and in the insula. *Smell* appreciation is located on the medial surface of the temporal lobe and in the cingulate gyrus. *Sound* messages from the cochlea of the ear travel to the superior aspect of the temporal lobe and the insula. The auditory association area is in the temporal lobe, which is where the brain identifies the name of a song or the individual speaking. Equilibrium is mainly directed to the cerebellum, but the thalamus and cerebral cortex also receive signals.

The *post central gyrus* of the parietal lobe is the *primary sensory area* for the *somesthetic* (widely distributed) senses, which includes sensations from the skin. The *association* area for somesthetic senses is in the parietal lobe caudal to the post central gyrus. The interpretation of proprioception, touch and pain, and the identification of objects by feel occur in this association area.

The association area for *motor* control is in the frontal lobe anterior to the precentral gyrus. This area is where muscle contractions are planned to carry out an action. The *precentral gyrus* of the frontal lobe is the *primary motor area*, and it processes intent by sending signals to the spinal cord. Pyramidal cells in the precentral gyrus are *upper* motor neurons. These cells send out their signals to connections in the basal ganglia, thalamus, substantia nigra and other areas. Input from the cerebellum further modulates the signals before they reach the corticospinal tracts in the medulla where they decussate. Some of the messages synapse in nuclei of cranial nerves and are sent out from the brain through cranial nerves. Others proceed to synapse with neurons in the spinal cord where they exit the CNS via spinal nerves. Neurons in the cranial nerve nuclei and spinal cord are *lower* motor neurons.

Language

The ability to communicate with language involves reading, writing, speaking and understanding words that are heard. **_Wernicke's area_** is in the temporal lobe at the apex of the lateral fissure and immediately rostral to the angular gyrus of the occipital lobe. This area is responsible for the recognition of spoken and written language. Neurons in Wernicke's area create a plan for speech. Any text that you read is processed into an intelligible format in the angular gyrus adjacent to Wernicke's area. **_Broca's area_** is located immediately rostral to the primary motor cortex in the lateral portion of the frontal lobe. Signals from Wernicke's area to Broca's area are the basis for the initiation of spoken words. Broca's area sends motor signals for speaking to muscles in the larynx, tongue and lips.

    Aphasia is the inability to speak intelligently. A lesion in **_Wernicke's area_** produces **_fluent aphasia_**, which is characterized by babbling nonsense and speaking in jargon with nonsensical, invented words. A lesion near Wernicke's area may also produce **_anomic aphasia_**, which is characterized by an inability to identify pictures or name an object from a picture. Wernicke's area lesions may also produce **_agnosia_** (the inability to recognize objects), or **_prosopagnosia_** (the inability to recognize faces).

    A lesion in **_Broca's area_** produces **_nonfluent aphasia_**, which is characterized by speech that involves few words, which are spoken slowly and with difficulty. Patients with nonfluent aphasia seem to have difficulty choosing words. They know the words they want to use but they cannot articulate them. Their vocabulary for spoken words may be extremely limited. **_Broca's area and Wernicke's area are usually located in the left hemisphere_**. The hemisphere opposite Broca's area (usually the right) contains an area that gives expression to the spoken word. A lesion in this area results in flat, emotionless speech -- a disorder known as **_aprosodia_**. In the hemisphere opposite Wernicke's area is an area that recognizes emotion in the speech of others. A lesion in this area can result in misunderstandings and an inability to understand a joke. **_Remember Wernicke's area as the center for speech interpretation and Broca's area as the center for motor control of speech._**

    The two halves of the cerebrum are not equal. In most people the left temporal lobe is longer than the right. In left handed people the left frontal, left parietal and left occipital lobes are usually wider than those on the right. The hemispheres of most people are specialized for certain types of tasks. In 96% of right handed people and 70% of left handed people the **_left hemisphere_** is the "**_categorical_**" hemisphere and the **_right hemisphere_** is the "**_representational_**" hemisphere."

    Functions of the **_categorical_** hemisphere include the specialization for spoken and written language; sequential and analytical reasoning skills, and the ability to do well in math and science. This is the ability to divide information into fragments and analyze the information in a linear way.

    The **_representational_** hemisphere perceives information in a more holistic way. It is the seat of imagination, insight, musical talent and artistic talent. The perception of patterns and spatial relationships and the comparison of sights, sounds, smells and tastes involve the representational hemisphere.

    You would use your categorical hemisphere to divide data into smaller parts in order to make it easier to learn or work with. You would use your representational hemisphere to lump smaller parts together to give it an association or better meaning. The division of hemispheres into categorical and representational has nothing to do with native ability or the dominance of one hemisphere over another; it is simply the observed fact that some activities and functions primarily involve one or the other hemisphere.

    In half of the people without this particular hemispherical orientation, the hemispheres are reversed, and in the other half there appears to be no hemispherical specialization. Males have larger brains than females, but males have smaller commissures between the hemispheres. As a result, males have more lateralization or specialization of their hemispheres. Smaller commissures and more lateralization mean less communication between the hemispheres, which makes males more susceptible to neurological defects from cerebrovascular accidents and other brain lesions involving one hemisphere.

    The opposite hemisphere of infants frequently can take over the functions of a damaged hemisphere, but that is not true of older children and adults.

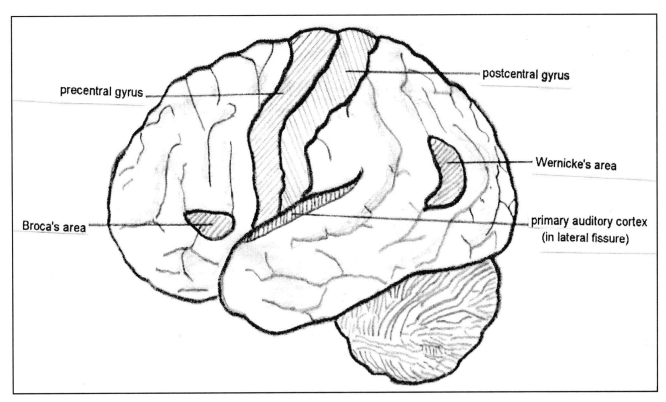

Above: Language centers in the cerebral cortex. Wernicke's area is the center for recognition of speech. Broca's area is responsible for the motor enunciation of speech. Both are in the left cerebral hemisphere in most people, but the opposite hemisphere (usually the right) is involved with understanding nuances of speech and inserting expression into what is spoken.

Brain Landmarks and Terms – A Review

Ectoderm, mesoderm, endoderm.
Neural groove, neural tube.
Rostral, caudal.
Cerebrum, cerebellum, midbrain, pons, medulla oblongata.
Telencephalon, diencephalon, mesencephalon, metencephalon, myelencephalon.
Forebrain, hindbrain.
Gyri (gyrus) and sulci (sulcus) – central sulcus, precentral gyrus, postcentral gyrus, angular gyrus, cingulate gyrus.
Brain stem (diencephalon, mesencephalon, pons and medulla).
Thalamus
Medial and lateral geniculate bodies.
Hypothalamus.
Epithalamus (pineal gland and habenula).
Substantia nigra, cerebral peduncles, superior and inferior colliculi, reticular formation.
Lateral ventricles, third ventricle, fourth ventricle.
Cerebral (mesencephalic) aqueduct.
Choroid plexuses.
Arachnoid villi.
Foramina of Munro.

Foramen of Majendie and foramina of Luschka.
White matter = tracts.
Gray matter = cortex, nuclei.
Fissures: longitudinal, transverse and lateral (Sylvian).
Falx cerebri, tentorium cerebelli, falx cerebelli.
Venous sinuses: superior sagittal sinus, inferior sagittal sinus, transverse sinus, cavernous sinus.
Meninges: dura mater, arachnoid mater, pia mater.
Subdural space, subdural hemorrhage.
Subarachnoid space, subarachnoid hemorrhage.
Medulla landmarks: pyramids, olive nuclei.
Cerebellum: folia, arbor vitae, nuclei, Purkinje cells, ataxia.
Cerebral lobes: <u>Frontal</u> – cognition, planning, memory, primary motor cortex (precentral gyrus).
   <u>Parietal</u> – primary sensory cortex (postcentral gyrus).
   <u>Occipital</u> – vision.
   <u>Temporal</u> – recognition and understanding of sensory stimuli.
   <u>Insula</u> – taste, language and visual understanding.
Basal ganglia: caudate nucleus, putamen, globus pallidus (corpus striatum, lentiform nucleus).
Cerebral cortex: only three mm thick, pyramidal cells, stellate cells.
Internal capsule and external capsule (tracts to and from the cerebral cortex).
Types of cerebral tracts: <u>Projection</u> (connect cerebral cortex with brain stem and spinal cord).
   <u>Association</u> (connect neurons of the same hemisphere).
   <u>Commissural</u> (connect neurons of opposite hemispheres)
Limbic system – cingulate gyrus, hippocampal gyrus, fornix, amygdaloid nucleus.
Rhinencephalon – limbic system plus olfactory connections, hypothalamus, thalamus, mammilary bodies.
Wernicke's area – sensory area of speech interpretation (fluent aphasia).
Broca's area – motor speech control (nonfluent aphasia).
Categorical hemisphere – left, analytical thinking, math and science skills, reasoning.
Representational hemisphere – right, holistic thinking, spatial patterns, imagination, insight, music, art.
Pyramidal cells
Purkinje cells
Cranial Nerves: I. Olfactory, II Optic, III Oculomotor, IV Trochlear, V Trigeminal, VI Abducens, VII Acoustic or Vestibulocochlear, IX Glossopharyngeal, X Vagus, XI Spinal accessory or Accessory, XII Hypoglossal

Study Guide
Know the following:
1. Nuclei within the brain are areas of gray matter containing neurons and synapses.
2. The midbrain (mesencephalon) contains a variety of nuclei including the red nucleus, substantia nigra, tectum, tegmentum, superior and inferior colliculi, central gray matter and a significant part of the reticular system. Cranial nerves III and IV exit the mesencephalon.
3. The substantia nigra contains numerous inhibitory synapses involving the neurotransmitter, dopamine. The substantia nigra is dysfunctional in Parkinson's disease.
4. The reticular formation is involved in maintaining alertness. Dysfunction of the reticular system can result in coma.
5. Visual messages from the retinas of the eyes synapse in the lateral geniculate bodies.
6. Audio messages from the cochlea of the ear synapse in the medial geniculate bodies.
7. The parts of the diencephalon are the thalamus, hypothalamus and epithalamus.
8. Equate the thalamus to a switchboard to and from the cerebral cortex.
9. The epithalamus consists of the pineal gland and the habenula.
10. The pineal gland secretes melatonin and serotonin during childhood.
11. Examine the cerebellum and note that gray matter is on the surface. This gray matter contains Purkinje cells, which make up fifty percent of the total number of neurons in the brain. Know that the cerebellum has prominent connections to the acoustic (vestibulocochlear) nerve, and it is extensively involved in coordination and equilibrium.

Answer the following:

12. Define rostral and caudal.
13. Identify the major anatomical parts of the human brain (cerebrum, diencephalon, midbrain, cerebellum, pons and medulla (medulla oblongata).
14. Understand how brain mass and the number of synapses relate to intelligence.
15. Define gray matter and white matter.
16. The nervous system is derived from which primordial germ cell layer?
17. Compare the embryological development of a human brain with that of a dog. Understand and include the phrase "ontology recapitulates phylogeny."
18. Take a model of a brain and identify the following: gyri, sulci, longitudinal fissure, transverse fissure, lateral fissure, central sulcus, precentral gyrus, postcentral gyrus, frontal lobe, parietal lobe, occipital lobe, insula, temporal lobe, pituitary gland, pineal gland, infundibulum, olfactory tracts, optic nerves, optic chiasm, optic tracts, mesencephalon, pons, cerebellum, pons and medulla.
19. Describe the three meningeal layers (dura mater, arachnoid mater and pia mater), the falx cerebri, tentorium cerebelli and falx cerebelli.
20. Describe the locations of the major venous sinuses (superior sagittal, inferior sagittal, transverse and cavernous).
21. Understand the cause and effect of a subarachnoid hemorrhage and a subdural hemorrhage.
22. Humans are more intelligent and have larger brains than other animals. What are the major disadvantages to a species having a large brain?
23. Describe the ventricles of the brain.
24. Describe where CSF is located and its circulatory route.
25. What are the functions of CSF?
26. Review the blood-brain barrier.
27. Examine the pyramids and olive nuclei in the medulla oblongata. What is contained in these areas? Which cranial nerves exit the medulla?
28. Examine the pons and note its proximity to the cerebellum. Which cranial nerves exit the pons?
29. Which parts of the brain make up the brain stem? (Medulla, pons, midbrain and diencephalon).
30. List the functions of the hypothalamus and the pituitary gland.
31. Name the lobes of the cerebrum, and name a specialized function of each lobe.
32. Which cells of the cerebral cortex are responsible for producing the output of nerve signals from the cerebrum? (Pyramidal cells).
33. What are the names of the basal ganglia? (caudate nuclei, putamen and globus pallidus). Where are they located? (Deep in the cerebrum below and lateral to the lateral ventricles). What is their primary function? (Motor control, with connections to the cerebral cortex and the substantia nigra.)
34. Understand the difference between projection tracts of white matter (those that run between the cerebrum and the spinal cord); commissural tracts of white matter (those that connect the right and left halves of the cerebrum); and association tracts of white matter (those that connect different regions of the same hemisphere).
35. Identify the corpus callosum and the internal capsule on a model or illustration of the brain. Be aware of the structures that each connects.
36. Name the four parts of the limbic system (amygdala, hippocampus, fornix, and cingulate gyrus). Which part is especially involved in emotions? (amygdala). Which part is especially involved in short term memory? (hippocampus).
37. Know the meanings of the terms sleep, stupor, semicoma and coma.
38. Know what REM sleep and nonREM sleep are and their association with dreams, sleep walking and sleep talking.
39. Know that deprivation of nonREM sleep is eventually fatal.
40. What is an EEG? Describe the significance and wavelengths of beta, alpha, theta and delta waves of an EEG.
41. Where do you find the primary motor cortex? (Precentral gyrus of the frontal lobe). Where do you find the primary sensory cortex? (Postcentral gyrus of the parietal lobe).
42. Relate the following syndromes to an injured lobe of the cerebrum: contralateral neglect syndrome (parietal lobe); loss of vision (occipital lobe); inability to recognize objects and/or faces (temporal lobe); and personality and emotional changes (frontal lobe).

43. Understand the meanings of anterograde amnesia and retrograde amnesia.
44. Know the difference between a primary sensory area of the cerebral cortex and an association area. Describe where they are usually located in relation to each other.
45. Where are upper and lower motor neurons located?
46. Describe the location and function of Broca's area. What speech pattern results from an injury to Broca's area?
47. Describe the location and function of Wernicke's area. What speech pattern results from an injury to Wernicke's area?
48. List the differences in specialization between the categorical (usually the left) hemisphere of the cerebral cortex) and the representational (usually the right) hemisphere?
49. List all the cranial nerves by name and Roman numeral and describe the major functions of each.

Chapter Fifteen

The Autonomic Nervous System

Within your nervous system is an inner motor system that controls glandular secretions and contractions of smooth and cardiac muscle. Your consciousness has almost no control over this system. Your blood vessels constrict and dilate; your intestines push food forward; muscles in the iris of your eye change the size of your pupil – all with no input from your consciousness. These activities and many others seem to have a mind of their own as they go about their business. This system is the **_autonomic nervous system_** or **_ANS._**

The autonomic nervous system (ANS) is that part of the **_motor_** system that controls **_involuntary_** contractions of smooth muscle and cardiac muscle and supplies **_efferent_** innervation to glands. It is sometimes called the **_visceral motor system_** to distinguish it from the somatic motor system that controls the skeletal muscles. Autonomic nerve fibers are gray and unmyelinated. They innervate the internal organs, blood vessels, sweat glands and piloerector muscles. It is responses of the ANS that control blood pressure, body temperature, and respiration and maintain homeostasis. "Autonomic" means self-governed, and the ANS acts on its own without the control of our consciousness.

There are two divisions of the ANS, the **_sympathetic_** and the **_parasympathetic_**, which usually have antagonistic effects -- one contracts and the other relaxes. For example, a sympathetic stimulus dilates the pupil and a parasympathetic stimulus constricts the pupil.

The **_sympathetic division_** generally prepares the body for physical activity by increasing the heart rate, increasing blood pressure, dilating bronchioles to increase air flow, and increasing the blood glucose level. The sympathetic system is called the **_"fight or flight"_** system because it revs up in crisis situations when danger and stress are looming.

The **_parasympathetic division_** has a calming effect. Routine functions of the body are stimulated by the parasympathetic system including digestion, defecation and urination. Smooth muscles in the GI tract and urinary tract are stimulated by the parasympathetic system. The pulse, respiratory rate and blood pressure are lowered by the parasympathetic system; for that reason the parasympathetic system is called the **_"rest and digest"_** system.

There is a normal basic level of activity in the two divisions of the ANS which establishes a balance called the **_"autonomic tone."_** Both divisions employ a **_ganglion_** where the neurons synapse. The bodies of the preganglionic neurons are located in the **_brain and spinal cord_**, and the bodies of the postganglionic neurons are located in a **_ganglion_**. The preganglionic neurons of both divisions release **_acetylcholine_** at their synapse in the ganglion. But the postganglionic neurons, which synapse at the end organ, release different neurotransmitters -- the parasympathetic system postganglionic neurons release **_acetylcholine_**, but most sympathetic postganglionic neurons release **_norepinephrine_**.

The ANS employs reflexes in its response to a situation and in maintaining homeostasis. These are called **_visceral reflexes_** to distinguish them from the tendon reflexes of skeletal muscle, which are **_somatic reflexes_**. Visceral reflexes control such things as heart rate, smooth muscle contractions and the secretions of glands in the GI tract and skin. Sensory receptors in the **_carotid sinus, right atrium_**, **_aortic arch_** and **_carotid body_** detect such things as blood pressure, oxygen, carbon dioxide and pH. These visceral sense organs send signals to the hypothalamus, which directs sympathetic and parasympathetic impulses that maintain **_homeostasis_**. This is an example of **_negative feedback_**. You can demonstrate the sensitivity of the carotid sinus by massaging the neck over the bifurcation of the carotid artery. This normally produces a bradycardia, which may be pronounced. This procedure should only be done in the company of a monitor because it potentially could cause unconsciousness.

The fight or flight response of the ***sympathetic nervous system*** is widespread throughout the animal kingdom. The term "sympathetic" came into use because sympathetic preganglionic neurons synapse with multiple postganglionic neurons, and some smooth muscle cells are connected by gap junctions. The impulse is sent to many destinations, and many effector cells react "in sympathy" to a stimulus. There is a great deal of ***neuronal divergence***, which explains why sympathetic responses tend to be widespread. Many organs become involved including the medulla of the adrenal gland, which secretes epinephrine into the blood stream.

The sympathetic system is called the ***thoracolumbar*** system because its preganglionic neurons are located in the lateral horns of the spinal cord between T-1 and L-2. The ganglia of the sympathetic system are in a chain near the vertebrae (***paravertebral ganglia***), which means that the axons of most sympathetic preganglionic neurons are short. There are usually twenty-three pair of paravertebral ganglia lined up along the vertebral column -- three cervical, eleven thoracic, four lumbar, four sacral and one coccygeal. Paravertebral ganglia are linked to spinal nerves by rami. It is apparent that the ganglia must receive fibers from spinal nerves of other levels because only the spinal nerves from T-1 through L-2 contain sympathetic fibers. There are interconnecting fibers between the ganglia, and some nerve fibers pass through ganglia without synapsing. Other nerve fibers do not synapse until they reach a ganglion near the end organ. Ganglia near end organs are called ***collateral ganglia***.

Right: This illustration depicts the paravertebral chain of sympathetic ganglia being fed by spinal nerves T-1 through L-2. Most postganglionic neurons of the sympathetic nervous system are located in the paravertebral ganglion chain and secrete norepinephrine.

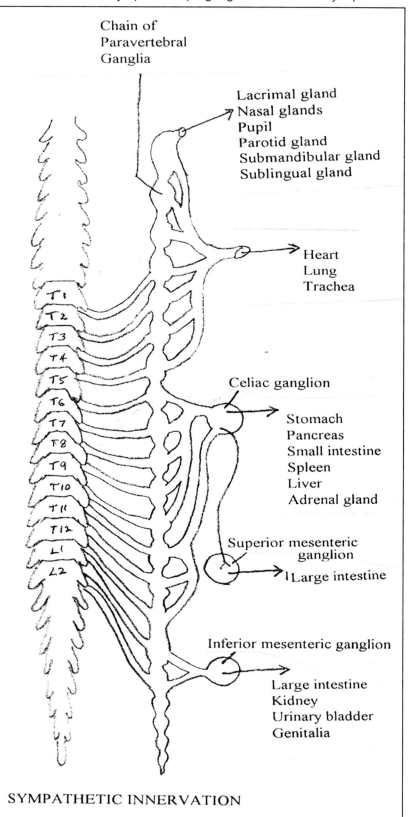

Chain of Paravertebral Ganglia

Lacrimal gland
Nasal glands
Pupil
Parotid gland
Submandibular gland
Sublingual gland

Heart
Lung
Trachea

Celiac ganglion

Stomach
Pancreas
Small intestine
Spleen
Liver
Adrenal gland

Superior mesenteric ganglion
Large intestine

Inferior mesenteric ganglion

Large intestine
Kidney
Urinary bladder
Genitalia

SYMPATHETIC INNERVATION

The **_adrenal glands_** are a pair of endocrine glands that sit above each kidney. Each adrenal gland has a central part (the **_medulla_**) and a peripheral part (the **_cortex_**). The medulla and the cortex are linked by proximity, but they have completely different endocrine functions. The cortex secretes several steroid hormones, and the medulla is part of the sympathetic nervous system. The adrenal medulla is a modified sympathetic ganglion that secretes **_catecholamines_** directly into the blood stream in a crisis, and it acts as part of the fight or flight reaction. 85% of the catecholamines secreted by the medulla is **_epinephrine_** (also known as **_Adrenalin_**), 15% is **_norepinephrine,_** and a trace amount is **_dopamine_**. Norepinephrine acts quickly after being secreted by postganglionic neurons, and its effect is short lived because it is quickly broken down in the synaptic cleft by the enzyme, **_monoamine oxidase_**. Epinephrine secreted by the adrenal medulla does not act quite so quickly, but its effects last much longer because monoamine oxidase is absent from the blood. That is why it takes time for you to calm down after a crisis.

Right: Ganglia of the sympathetic nervous system. The sympathetic system supplies innervation to glands and smooth muscle. That includes the sweat glands, adrenal glands, salivary glands, and the glands of the digestive tract. Smooth muscles in the uterus, male sex organs, heart, and skin (piloerector muscles) are also supplied with innervation from the sympathetic system.

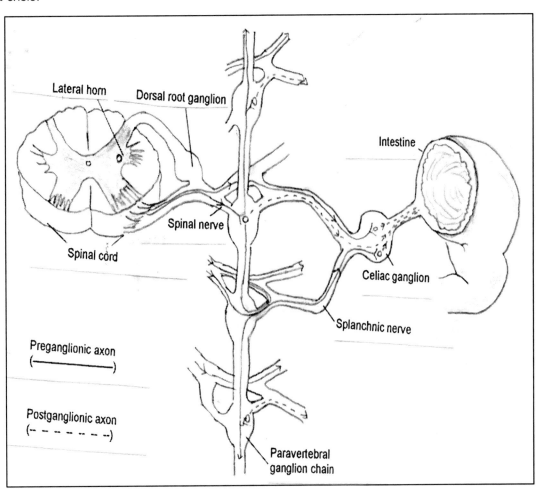

The **_preganglionic neurons_** of the **_parasympathetic_** nervous system are located in cranial nerve nuclei of the midbrain, pons and medulla, and in the lateral horns of the sacral level (S2-S-4) of the spinal cord. Therefore, the parasympathetic system is called the **_craniosacral_** system. Axons from parasympathetic preganglionic neurons travel via cranial nerves and sacral nerves to end organs. The parasympathetic nervous system does not employ paravertebral ganglia; all the ganglia of the parasympathetic system are collateral ganglia located in or near the organs that are being innervated. Examples are the ciliary ganglion behind the eye and the celiac and mesenteric ganglia in the abdomen. Cranial nerves III, V, VII, IX, and X carry parasympathetic fibers; the other cranial nerves do not. **_(1) The oculomotor nerve,_** (CN III), innervates the pupillary constrictor and ciliary muscle of the eye. **_(2) The trigeminal nerve,_** (CN V), innervates the tensor tympani muscle. (**_3) The facial nerve_**, (CN VII), innervates the submandibular and sublingual salivary glands, the lacrimal gland and the stapedius muscle. **_(4) The glossopharyngeal nerve,_** (CN IX), innervates the parotid gland. **_Ninety percent of all parasympathetic fibers_** are carried by the **_vagus nerve,_** (CN X), which innervates the heart, pulmonary tree and most of the GI tract.

Branches of the vagus join sympathetic fibers to form nerve plexuses in the abdomen and thorax. These plexuses include the well known solar plexus in the abdomen.

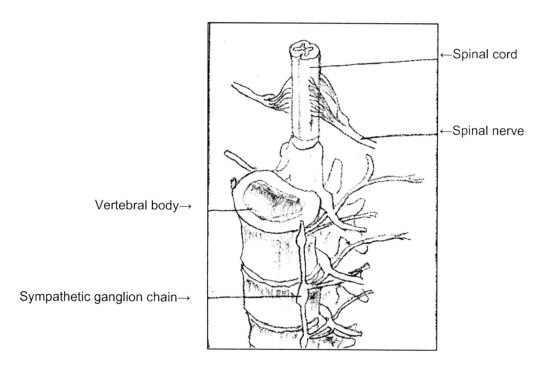

Above: The relationship between vertebrae, spinal nerves and sympathetic chain ganglia is illustrated.

The sacral preganglionic parasympathetic neurons are located in the lateral horns of the spinal cord at the S2-S4 levels. Long preganglionic fibers travel in the **splanchnic nerves** to the inferior **hypogastric plexus** in the abdomen. This plexus sends fibers to the colon, rectum, bladder and sex organs. Preganglionic fibers synapse in **collateral ganglia located in or near the target organs**. Short postganglionic fibers lead to smooth muscle and glands in the target organs. The parasympathetic system shows no neuronal divergence, and the effect of parasympathetic stimulation is not widespread. The usual ratio of preganglionic neurons to postganglionic neurons in the parasympathetic system is 1:1. This contrasts to an average ratio of 1 preganglionic to 17 postganglionic neurons in the sympathetic system.

In addition to the autonomic nervous system there are independent neurons with their own reflex arcs embedded in the walls of the stomach and intestines. Neurons of this system regulate motility and the secretion of acid and enzymes into the gut. The system is called the **"enteric nervous system."** The enteric nervous system does not function well without innervation from the autonomic nervous system.

Nerve fibers of the autonomic nervous system are **cholinergic** if they secrete acetylcholine; they are **adrenergic** if they secrete norepinephrine. Preganglionic and postganglionic fibers of the parasympathetic system are cholinergic, and they secrete acetylcholine. The preganglionic fibers of the sympathetic system are cholinergic, but most of the sympathetic postganglionic fibers are adrenergic and secrete norepinephrine. Ten percent of the neurotransmitters secreted by adrenergic fibers are neurotransmitters other than norepinephrine. These less common neurotransmitters have various effects; some dilate blood vessels, some reduce pain stimuli, some are excitatory and some are inhibitory. **It is the type of receptor in a synapse that determines the response, and not the neurotransmitter.**

Right: This drawing illustrates the parasympathetic nervous system. The nerves of the parasympathetic nervous system include cranial nerves III, V, VII, IX and X, and sacral nerves S-2, S-3 and S-4. Cranial nerve X (the vagus) carries 90% of the total parasympathetic fibers. Cranial nerve V is not included in this illustration, but it carries parasympathetic impulses to the tensor tympani muscle of the ear. Nerve fibers to this muscle are part of the mandibular division of the trigeminal nerve that pass through the otic ganglion before reaching the ear.

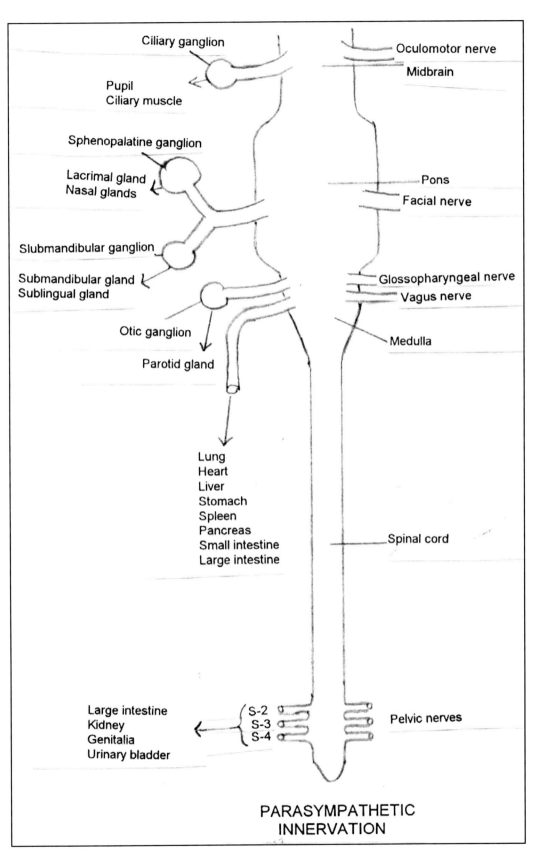

PARASYMPATHETIC
INNERVATION

When acetylcholine is released into the synaptic cleft, it is quickly broken down by the enzyme, **_acetylcholinesterase_**. When norepinephrine is secreted into the synaptic cleft, it is quickly broken down by the enzyme, **_monoamine oxidase_**. **_Pseudocholinesterase_** is an enzyme normally present in the blood that breaks down acetylcholine, but there is no enzyme present in the blood that breaks down catecholamines. Consequently, the epinephrine released into the blood by the adrenal medulla has an effect that lasts about thirty minutes.

Cholinergic and adrenergic synapses can have different types of receptors. Receptors in adrenergic synapses are designated either **_alpha or beta_**. The alpha receptors are usually excitatory, and the beta receptors are usually inhibitory, but exceptions exist. Alpha receptors are further classified as alpha-1 and alpha-2, and beta receptors are further classified as beta-1 and beta-2. **_Alpha_** receptors generally constrict blood vessels and constrict bronchi; **_beta_** receptors increase the heart rate, and they generally dilate blood vessels and dilate bronchi.

There are two types of cholinergic receptors, **_nicotinic and muscarinic,_** and they give different effects. **_Nicotinic_** receptors are present in the neuromuscular junctions of skeletal muscles where they produce a rapid excitatory response. **_Muscarinic_** receptors are in the viscera where they give a slow, tempered response. Muscarinic receptors can be excitatory or inhibitory, and subclasses of muscarinic receptors exist. Most of the viscera receive nerve fibers from both the sympathetic and the parasympathetic systems, and the effect of the two divisions is usually antagonistic; however, some viscera receive unequal innervation from the two divisions of the ANS. For example, sweat glands, piloerector muscles, the adrenal medulla and many blood vessels receive only sympathetic innervation, and the heart receives mostly sympathetic innervation. In these cases it is the antagonistic effects of the alpha and beta receptors that maintain autonomic tone.

Sometimes the effects of stimulation of the two divisions of the ANS are synergistic (cooperative). Thus does parasympathetic stimulation increase the production of saliva of a serous nature from the parotid gland, and sympathetic stimulation increases the production of saliva of a mucous nature from the sublingual gland. The effects of sympathetic stimulation to blood vessels vary with locale. Sympathetic stimulation increases blood flow to the skeletal muscles and the heart by dilating the vessels, but at the same time it decreases blood flow to the skin and GI tract by constricting the vessels there.

To repeat, **_it is the type of receptor in a synapse that determines the response, and not the neurotransmitter._**

There is a myriad of drugs that act on the ANS. Those include **_sympathomimetics_** that stimulate the adrenergic receptors. For example, phenylephrine dilates of the bronchioles, dilates the pupil, and constricts the nasal blood vessels by stimulating alpha-1 receptors. Norepinephrine is primarily an alpha receptor stimulant. Isoproterenol (Isuprel) is primarily a beta receptor stimulant. Epinephrine usually stimulates both alpha and beta receptors. Monoamine oxidase inhibitors prolong the effects of catecholamines, and therefore, they are sympathomimetic drugs.

Sympatholytic drugs suppress sympathetic action either by blocking norepinephrine secretion from the synaptic knob or by binding receptors. For example, Inderal (propranolol) is a beta blocker, and it blocks beta receptors in the heart and blood vessels. The desired effect is usually a slower heart rate.

Parasympathomimetic drugs mimic the effect of acetylcholine. Some parasympathomimetic drugs stimulate parasympathetic receptors (either nicotinic receptors, muscarinic receptors, or both). For example **_pilocarpine_** constricts the ciliary muscle and the pupillary constrictor of the eye. Other parasympathomimetic drugs inhibit acetylcholinesterase, which prolongs the effect of acetylcholine in the synapse. Most **_nerve gases_** and some insecticides are cholinesterase inhibitors. Cholinesterase inhibiting drugs such as **_physostigmine, neostigmine and pyridostigmine_** are used in myasthenia gravis, a disease in which antibodies destroy receptor sites on a postsynaptic cell. These drugs allow the reduced number of receptors present to have an enhanced effect. The **_opioids_** (morphine, heroin, codeine, paregoric and Imodium) have a parasympathomimetic action. They are useful in treating diarrhea because they cause spastic, ineffectual contractions in the intestines.
Parasympatholytic drugs reduce the effects of acetylcholine by either blocking acetylcholine release into the synaptic cleft or by blocking receptor sites. **_Atropine_** blocks muscarinic receptors of the parasympathetic system;

therefore, it inhibits oral secretions, dilates the pupil, causes tachycardia, and it causes fever by blocking vasodilatation in the skin. Atropine is used as an antidote for people who have been exposed to nerve gas. **_Curare_** is a drug used in anesthesia that was first discovered by South American Indians who used it in blowguns. It binds nicotinic receptors and causes paralysis of skeletal muscles. **_Succinyl choline_** is another muscle relaxant that briefly excites nicotinic receptor sites, but it remains bound to the receptors and prevents their stimulation by acetylcholine.   The result is skeletal muscle paralysis.   Succinyl choline is not broken down by acetylcholinesterase in the synapse, but it is broken down by pseudocholinesterase in the blood. Some people lack the enzyme pseudocholinesterase. The paralytic effect of succinyl choline is prolonged in these people, and assisted ventilation must be continued for hours after an injection of succinyl choline. Both curare and succinyl choline have proved useful in anesthesia because the muscle relaxation they produce greatly facilitates the insertion of a tube into the airway. Neither drug affects consciousness so they are given after a short acting barbiturate or other sedative has induced sleep. Both have been used without sedation in wartime as a form of torture used in the interrogation of prisoners. The paragraph that follows is an actual description of the sensation of muscle paralysis induced by curare.

"When an appropriate dose of curare is injected intravenously in man, the onset of effects is very rapid. The progress of events has been vividly described by a nonpremedicated trained observer who was injected with two and one-half times the dose of d-tubocurarine required for complete respiratory paralysis, pulmonary exchange being maintained by artificial means. Slight dizziness and a sensation of warmth are first experienced. Difficulty in focusing and weakness in the jaw muscles are then observed, and difficulty in speech and in keeping the eyelids open soon follows. Ptosis, strabismus, diplopia, dysarthria, and dysphagia are indicative of the early involvement of the small muscles of the head and neck. Relaxation of the small muscles of the middle ear improves acuity of hearing for low tones. The limbs feel heavy and are difficult to move. Respiratory movements become more diaphragmatic as the intercostal muscles are involved. Despite adequate artificially controlled respiration, "shortness of breath" is experienced. The accumulation of unswallowed saliva in the pharynx may prove most annoying and causes the sensation of choking. Head movement soon becomes impossible, and ultimately the ability to move the limbs and trunk is lost. Throughout the stage of complete muscular paralysis, consciousness and sensorium remain entirely undisturbed. The experience is definitely unpleasant. Facial and diaphragmatic muscles are the first to recover, followed in order by those of the legs, arms, shoulder girdle, trunk, larynx, hands, feet, and pharynx." (Goodman and Gilman)

Other agents that affect the ANS include several drugs that have recently become popular for treating clinical depression. **_Prozac_** and **_Zoloft_** block the reuptake of the mood elevating neurotransmitter, **_serotonin_**, by the synaptic knob, which prolongs the presence of serotonin in the synaptic cleft. **_Monoamine oxidase (MAO) inhibitors_** interfere with the breakdown of catecholamines (epinephrine, norepinephrine and dopamine). **_Adenosine_** consists of adenine plus ribose, and it is a breakdown product of ATP. Adenosine acts as an inhibitory neurotransmitter that causes sleepiness, and it builds up toward evening and after activity. **_Caffeine_** reverses the effect of adenosine by competing with adenosine receptors. **_Cocaine_** prolongs the effects of dopamine by decreasing dopamine reuptake by the synaptic knob. The prolonged existence of dopamine in the synaptic cleft leads to the diffusion of dopamine out of the synaptic cleft and the subsequent degradation of dopamine stores. Cocaine addiction results from the depletion of dopamine. Amphetamines stimulate the release of dopamine and norepinephrine from the synaptic bulb, and they also prevent their reuptake. A result of chronic use is low dopamine levels and symptoms mimicking Parkinson's disease and Alzheimer's disease. The eventual destruction of dopamine synapses leads to permanent tremors, lack of coordination, memory defects and loss of cognitive learning. Methamphetamine is the most potent, the most addictive and the most toxic amphetamine.

Here are some points to remember about the autonomic nervous system or ANS (the visceral motor system):
The ANS is an involuntary motor system with two divisions, the sympathetic and the parasympathetic.
The **_hypothalamus_** is the major control site for the visceral motor system. Fight or flight originates here, as does hunger, thirst, thermoregulation, emotion and sexual desire.
 The hypothalamus has strong connections to the **_limbic system_**, which has a major effect on **_emotions._**
The **_cerebral cortex_** has control over the actions we take as a result of our emotions or a fight or flight situation.
Biofeedback is a process by which an individual is made aware of his ANS to an extent. It has been successful in lowering the blood pressure of some people.

Nuclei of the ***reticular formation*** are strung out from the thalamus to the medulla. These nuclei regulate responses to visceral stimuli, usually by increasing the excitatory responses. Reticular formation nuclei maintain alertness. Damage to nuclei in the reticular formation can result in an irreversible coma.

Spinal cord reflexes can control defecation and micturition (urination), but the cerebral cortex can consciously overcome these reflexes. Exceptions to this are infants and paraplegics.

In stress or a crisis the sympathetic nervous system kicks in with sympathetic stimulation of organs and vessels and the secretion of catecholamines by the ***adrenal medulla***. The result is a faster heart rate, increased blood flow to the skeletal muscles, and increased glucose production from proteins and fats (gluconeogenesis). Chronic stress leads to exhaustion of the adrenal glands and ANS dysfunction.

Study Guide

1. Define the autonomic nervous system (ANS). Note that it is an involuntary motor system consisting of gray, unmyelinated nerve fibers.
2. Associate the sympathetic division of the ANS with "fight or flight," and the parasympathetic division with "rest and digest."
3. Which neurotransmitter is usually employed by postganglionic fibers of the sympathetic division?
4. Which neurotransmitter is employed by the postganglionic fibers of the parasympathetic division?
5. The ANS controls ***visceral*** reflexes that maintain homeostasis by negative feedback. Name some of these reflexes.
6. How do neuronal divergence and the adrenal medulla relate to the naming of the sympathetic system?
7. What hormones does the adrenal medulla secrete?
8. Which division of the ANS is the craniosacral division?
9. Which division of the ANS is the thoracolumbar division?
10. Describe the paravertebral chain of ganglia and its relation to the ANS.
11. Review the terms cholinergic, adrenergic, preganglionic neuron, and postganglionic neuron.
12. Recognize that alpha and beta receptors are part of the sympathetic division of the ANS.
13. Recognize that muscarinic and nicotinic receptors are part of the parasympathetic division of the ANS.
14. Recognize that nicotinic receptors are in skeletal muscle and muscarinic receptors are in smooth muscle and glands.
15. Define the following terms as they relate to effects on the ANS: sympathomimetic, sympatholytic, parasympathomimetic and parasympatholytic.
16. Understand how caffeine, opioids, cocaine, methamphetamine, Prozac and acetylcholinesterase inhibitors affect the nervous system.

Chapter Sixteen

The Sense Organs

The Eye

The eye is the organ of vision. The ***occipital lobe*** of the brain is almost entirely occupied with the interpretation of visual impulses sent to it from the retina of the eye. The ***retina*** perceives ***light***. Light is a form of energy that is emitted from excited atoms. Light may be looked upon as particles known as ***"photons,"*** which are quanta of ***light waves***. Heat and other forms of energy can cause atoms to release photons. Photons (light waves) are surrounded by an electric field and a magnetic field, and they make up part of the ***electromagnetic spectrum***. Energy from the waves of the electromagnetic spectrum is called "radiant energy."

Other parts of the electromagnetic spectrum besides visible light include ***radio waves, infrared rays, ultraviolet rays and gamma rays***. The shorter the wavelength, the more energy a radiant wave possesses. ***Gamma rays (X-rays)*** have the shortest wavelengths and the greatest amount of energy. Ultraviolet waves have wavelengths below 400 nanometers (nm). Infrared rays have wavelengths greater than 700 nm. Ultraviolet and infrared rays are not visible. ***Visible light has wavelengths between 400 and 700 nm***. Short wave radio waves are longer still; microwaves are short radio waves with a wavelength between one mm and thirty cm. Long wave radio waves have the longest wavelengths and the least amount of energy. Some radio waves are more than 10,000 km (6000 miles) long.

Visible light waves are between 400 and 700 nm in length. The violet waves are the shortest, then the blue, green, yellow, orange and the red waves, which are the longest. Physicists regard light as a wave and as a particle (photon) in quantum mechanics because it behaves as both. Energy from uv rays possesses ***ionizing radiation***, which ionizes organic molecules and produces free radicals. Free radicals cause rapid, indiscriminate movement of electrons from one molecule to another, which damages DNA and other organic molecules and kills cells. Infrared rays (wave length over 700 nm) are less energetic than ultraviolet rays or visible light rays, and they do not cause chemical reactions. Infrared rays can warm tissues, however.

Vision is the perception of objects in the environment according to the light they emit or reflect in the visible spectrum (wave length 400-700 nm).

Adnexa are the tissues surrounding an organ. The adnexa of the eye include the ***eyebrow***s and ***eyelids***, which are part of the external anatomy of the eyes. The eyebrows give some protection from glare and a perspiring forehead. The eyelids and their lashes (called cilia) protect the eye from desiccation and foreign objects. The medial and lateral margins (corners) of the eyelids are the ***commissures***. ***Canthal ligaments*** are fibrous structures in the commissures that give structural support to the corners of the eyes. The upper and lower eyelids contain fibrous plates of dense connective tissue called ***tarsal plates,*** which provide stiffness to the lids. ***Meibomian*** glands are sebaceous glands within the tarsal plates; these glands open to the surface at the lid margins. They secrete oils that keep the tear film from evaporating. The follicles of eyelashes contain modified sebaceous glands (glands of Zeiss) and modified sweat glands (glands of Moll). The ***levator palpebrae*** muscle elevates the upper eyelid. It inserts into the tarsal plate and skin of the upper lid by a broad aponeurosis. The levator palpebrae is innervated by the oculomotor nerve. The levator and four of the six extrinsic muscles that move the eye originate at the annulus of Zinn, a circular band surrounding the optic foramen. The ***orbicularis oculi*** muscle is a facial muscle innervated by the facial nerve. Its insertion and origin are at the canthal ligaments. It acts as a sphincter to forcibly close the eye.

The ***cornea*** is a translucent window in the eyeball through which the iris and pupil can be seen. The cornea is about one mm thick. Starting on the outside, the layers of the cornea are **(1)** the epithelium -- a thin layer of nonkeratinized stratified squamous cells; **(2)** the basement membrane, which is known as Bowman's membrane; **(3)** the stroma, which is a relatively thick layer of regular collagen fibers and modified fibroblasts called keratocytes; **(4)** Descemet's membrane layer, and **(5)** and a layer of simple squamous endothelium on the inner surface. The cornea is continuous with the ***sclera,*** which is the tough covering of dense irregular connective tissue that is the white of the eye. The ***limbus*** is the circular area where the cornea meets the sclera.

The **conjunctiva** is a thin mucous membrane that contains blood vessels. Conjunctiva covers the inner surface of the eyelids and the anterior surface of the sclera; it is anchored to the limbus. An infection of the conjunctiva is known as conjunctivitis, which is popularly known as "pink eye."

Tears are produced by the **lacrimal gland**, which is located under the upper orbital rim laterally. The **glands of Krause and Wolfring** are small accessory lacrimal glands located throughout the conjunctiva. Tears are a watery liquid containing **lysozyme**, a bactericidal enzyme that helps prevent infections. Tears are collected in two tiny **puncta**, which are openings to **canaliculi.** Canaliculi are tubules in the upper and lower lids near the medial commissure. The canaliculi drain into the **lacrimal sac**, which is located in the lacrimal fossa at the lateral side of the nose. Tears drain from the lacrimal sac through the **nasolacrimal duct** into the nose under the inferior turbinate. A blockage in the nasolacrimal duct produces tearing and frequent infections in the lacrimal sac. Baseline tears are produced primarily by the glands of Krause and Wolfring. The lacrimal gland is innervated by CN VII, and it is responsible for the excessive tear production brought about by irritation or emotion.

Right: The lacrimal apparatus. Tears are produced by the lacrimal glands and accessory lacrimal glands in the conjunctiva. They drain into the nose via the canaliculi, lacrimal sac and the naso-lacrimal duct.

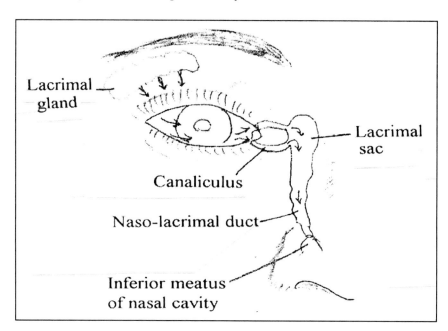

There are six **extrinsic muscles** that move the eyeball in different directions. The **lateral rectus** is innervated by the abducens nerve; the **superior oblique** is innervated by the trochlear nerve. The **medial rectus, inferior rectus, superior rectus and inferior oblique** muscles are innervated by the oculomotor nerve. Contraction of one muscle will move the eye in the direction of the muscle tendon. The same muscles of the two eyes do not act as a pair in moving the eyes. Thus the medial rectus of the right eye is paired with the lateral rectus of the left eye to move the eyes to the left. The oblique muscles rotate the eyes, and they also serve to elevate or depress the eyes. **Strabismus** is any disorder in which the eyes are not aligned. **Esotropia** refers to a crossed eye; **exotropia** refers to a wall eye (turned outward). **Hypertropia** and **hypotropia** refer to vertical misalignment.

The **anterior chamber** is the small space behind the cornea and in front of the **iris**. It is filled with a watery fluid called **aqueous humor**. The **lens** is behind the iris. The **posterior chamber** is the narrow space between the lens and the iris; it is filled with aqueous humor. The **iris** contains melanocytes, which give it color, and two muscles, which change the size of the pupil. The constrictor muscle of the pupil (parasympathetic) makes the pupil smaller; the dilator muscle (sympathetic) makes the pupil larger. A cloudy or opaque area in the lens is called a **cataract.** The lens is acted on by the **ciliary muscle**, which is attached to the lens through suspensory ligaments called **zonules.** When the ciliary muscle constricts, the zonules relax. That allows the lens to change shape to a rounder form, which is the way your eye bends light rays by different amounts so that near objects can be brought into focus. That process is called **accommodation**. The **near reflex** includes constriction of the pupil and contraction of the ciliary muscle. The near reflex is accompanied by **convergence**, or the contraction of both medial rectus muscles so that the eyes cross slightly to align with a near target. If too much convergence occurs when accommodation is stimulated, the eyes will cross excessively when looking at a near object. The ciliary muscle and the constrictor of the pupil are innervated by parasympathetic fibers in the oculomotor nerve. The dilator muscle of the pupil is innervated by sympathetic fibers that join the oculomotor nerve in the orbit.

Right: The extrinsic muscles of the eye. This is a lateral view of the left eye.

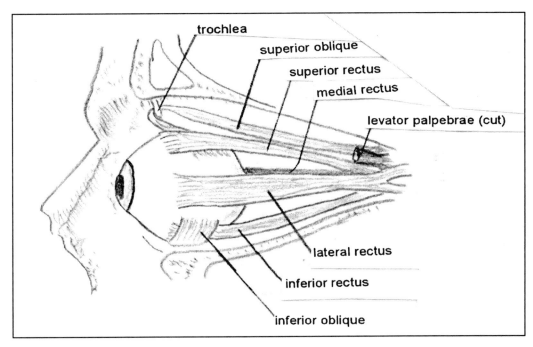

The **_cornea_** and the **_lens_** provide the refractive powers of the eye. They do this by bending light rays that enter the eye so that light comes to a point focus on the retina. Light rays will focus behind the eye if the eyeball is too short or the refractive powers of the lens and cornea are too weak. This condition is known as **_hyperopia_** or farsightedness; it is corrected by convex spectacle lenses. If the eyeball is too long, or the refractive powers of the lens and cornea are too great, light rays will focus in front of the retina, a condition known as **_myopia_**, or nearsightedness. Myopia is corrected by concave spectacle lenses. If light rays focus on the retina without spectacle correction, it is called **_emmetropia._** **_Astigmatism_** is an asphericity of the refractive powers of the eye (more convexity in one plane than the other.)

The **_trabecular meshwork_** is in the limbus at the anterior root of the iris. It is a sponge-like tissue where aqueous humor leaves the anterior chamber and enters the blood stream. The **_angle_** is the cleft between the cornea and the iris that points to the trabecular meshwork. The angle can be visualized, and the degree to which it is open can be gauged by placing a lens called a gonioscope on the cornea. Aqueous humor is secreted into the posterior chamber by cells of the **_ciliary body_**, an area of folded tissue interior to the ciliary muscle. The zonules are anchored to the ciliary body. Normally a pressure of 10 and 20 mm of Hg (mercury) exists in the eye, and the ciliary body must secrete aqueous humor against a gradient. **_Glaucoma_** is the condition of having too much pressure in the eye, which causes damage to fibers of the optic nerve at the back of the eye. There are different types of glaucoma. The common types are open angle glaucoma and narrow or closed angle glaucoma. In **_open angle glaucoma_** there is a microscopic block of aqueous outflow through the trabecular meshwork. Open angle glaucoma is typically a chronic disorder that is treated medically or by burning the trabecular meshwork with a laser. Surgery is limited to intractable cases. However, in **_closed angle glaucoma_** the block is initially at the pupil; the space between the iris and the lens disappears at the margins of the pupil, and aqueous cannot flow from the posterior chamber to the anterior chamber. This comes about because the front of the eye is too small, the structures of the eye are crowded, and the angle is narrow. Nearly all eyes with narrow angles are hyperopic. American Indians and Eskimos have a high incidence of narrow angles. The block of aqueous flow through the pupil leads to higher pressure in the posterior chamber than the anterior chamber. As a result of this pressure differential, the iris bulges forward and closes the narrow angle, which covers the trabecular meshwork. Aqueous humor no longer can reach the trabecular meshwork; the intraocular pressure continues to build until the ciliary body shuts down and no more aqueous is secreted. Sudden closure of an angle is an emergency. The treatment consists of making an opening in the iris called an iridectomy, which reestablishes the flow of aqueous from the posterior chamber to the anterior chamber. The iris falls back, and that opens the angle. An iridectomy will not be effective if treatment is delayed because permanent adhesions will form over the angle. Most iridectomies are done with a laser.

The large cavity behind the lens is the ***vitreous cavity***. It is filled with a jelly-like substance called ***vitreous humor***, which is rich in GAG compounds, especially hyaluronic acid.

The covering of the posterior 2/3 of the eye consists of three layers: the outer layer is the ***sclera,*** the middle layer is the ***choroid*** and the inner layer is the ***retina***. The ***choroid*** is a layer rich in ***blood vessels and melanocytes.*** Blood vessels in the choroid provide cells in the outer portion of the retina with nutrients, and pigment in the choroid enhances the capacity of the retina to capture light waves.

The outer layer of the ***retina*** is the ***retinal pigment epithelium*** (RPE). The basement membrane of the RPE is known as ***Bruch's membrane***. The inner layer of the retina is the ***sensory retina***. There is a potential space between the RPE and the sensory retina that a ***retinal detachment*** forces open. The precursor of a detached retina is an opening in the sensory retina that allows fluid in the vitreous to dissect into the potential space between the RPE and the sensory retina. When fluid seeps into this space, it peels the sensory retina into the vitreous cavity where it cannot survive because it is removed from the blood supply of the choroid.

Right: A sagittal section of an eye.
 (1) Vitreous cavity
 (2) Lens
 (3) Retina
 (4) Choroid
 (5) Sclera
 (6) Optic nerve
 (7) Iris
 (8) Cornea
 (9) Posterior chamber
 (10) Anterior chamber
 (11) Ciliary body

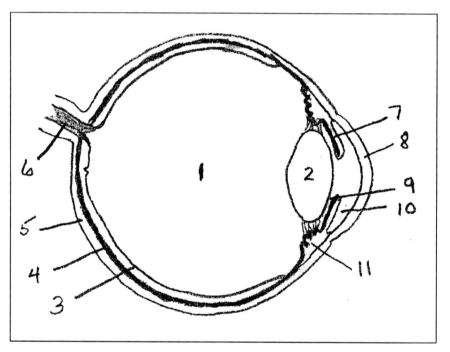

There are two types of ***photoreceptors*** (light sensitive cells) in the retina, the ***rods*** and the ***cones***. These cells are located in the sensory retina just inside the RPE. Light coming into the eye must pass through the full thickness of the sensory retina to reach the photoreceptors. The ***rods*** are highly sensitive in dim light (***scotopic vision***), and the total number of rods outnumbers the total number of cones in the retina by 130 million rods to 6.5 million cones. The ***rods*** are predominant in the ***peripheral*** retina, and the ***cones*** are predominant in the ***central*** retina, where visual acuity is greatest. There is an average ratio of 114 rods to each optic nerve fiber. This reflects a great deal of neuronal ***convergence,*** which leads to inability of the rods to provide a clear image to pyramidal cells of the occipital lobe.

Cone cells have little or no neuronal convergence, and they provide a clear image to the visual cortex. Cones are most sensitive when light is abundant (***photopic vision***). There are three types of cone cells, each with a different sensitivity peak in the visible light spectrum. Cones are named according to the color that corresponds to the wavelength to which they are most sensitive. The types of cones are **_blue_** cones (peak sensitivity of 420 nm), **_green_** cones (peak sensitivity 531 nm), and **_red_** cones (peak sensitivity 558 nm). The brain interprets color according to the prevalence of the signals it receives from each type of cone cell. Inherited color vision defects are due to the absence or dysfunction of one of the cone cell types, usually the red or green. **_Color blindness_** is inherited as a **_sex linked recessive_** trait. The gene is located on the X chromosome, which means that the disorder is seen much more commonly in males. If both the red and green cones are defective, the patient is said to be a **_blue cone monochromat_**. Blue cone monochromats are not only color blind; they also have poor central visual acuity.

The light reaction is the chemical reaction that occurs when photons in the visible spectrum enter the eye and strike a photoreceptor. Energy from photons bends a molecule in the photoreceptor cells known as **_retinal_** from the *cis* isomer to the *trans* isomer. This elicits an action potential, which travels to the optic nerve, optic tract, lateral geniculate body of the thalamus, and eventually to the occipital lobe of the cerebrum. A combination of the protein, opsin, and retinal makes up **_rhodopsin_** in the rods. Rhodopsin containing *cis*-retinal is purple in color, and it is called "visual purple." Rhodopsin with *trans*-retinal is colorless. *Cis*-retinal and a slightly different variation of opsin make up **_photopsin_** in the cones. *Trans*-retinal is transformed back to cis-retinal in the RPE. Retinal is a vitamin A derivative.

Above: **Retinol** is vitamin A. **Retinal** is the aldehyde form of vitamin A that is present in the eye. Retinal exists in two forms, *cis* and *trans*. The change of retinal from the *cis* form to the *trans* form is what elicits nerve impulses that are responsible for vision. The change from *cis*-retinal to *trans*-retinal is caused by energy in light rays striking the rods and cones

The nuclei of rod and cone cells are in the **_outer nuclear layer_** of the retina. Bipolar cells synapse with rods and cones and are the first order neurons of the visual pathway. The nuclei of **_bipolar cells_** are in the **_inner nuclear layer_**. **_Horizontal cells_** and **_amacrine cells_** are retina cells that form horizontal connections, which enhance contrast and perception; they are spread about in the retina. **_Ganglion cells_** are in the ganglion cell layer; they are the second order neurons. Axons of the ganglion cells lie on the inner surface of the retina; they collect at the **_optic disc_** to form the optic nerve. A few ganglion cell axons go to the oculomotor nuclei in the midbrain where they synapse with fibers that innervate the pupillary constrictor muscle. Shining a light in one eye will constrict both pupils because each oculomotor nucleus is innervated by ganglion cell fibers from both eyes. This is the pathway of the **_pupillary light reflex_** (photopupillary reflex). Any disorder of the retina, optic nerve, optic tract, oculomotor nuclei of the midbrain, or the oculomotor nerve could affect the photopupillary reflex. By contrast a lesion in the occiput can produce blindness, but it would not affect the photopupillary reflex.

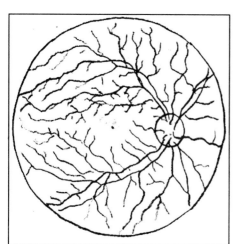

Above: A view of the retina with a direct ophthalmoscope. The circle is the optic disc (optic nerve head). The radiating lines are retinal arteries and retinal veins. The central dot is the fovea centralis.

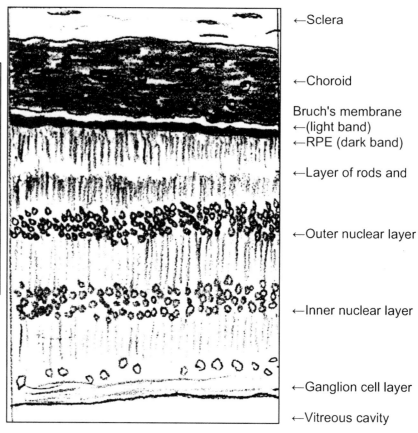

←Sclera

←Choroid

Bruch's membrane
←(light band)
←RPE (dark band)

←Layer of rods and

←Outer nuclear layer

←Inner nuclear layer

←Ganglion cell layer

←Vitreous cavity

Above: The histology of the retina, choroid and sclera.

Photoreceptors are absent in the **_optic disc_**, which is a blind spot (**_scotoma_**) known as the **_physiologic blind spot._** An ophthalmologic examination of the eye includes visualizing the optic disc, blood vessels and retina. The **_macula lutea_** is a slightly darker area lateral to the optic disc. Nerve fibers bypass the macula making the retina thinner there. The **_fovea centralis_** is a tiny pit in the middle of the macula. The fovea contains only cone cells; it is the most highly sensitive area of the retina for vision. There is no neuronal convergence of cone cells in the macula, but cone cells in the peripheral retina have a small amount of neuronal convergence.

Optic nerve fibers are axons of ganglion cells in the retina. The optic nerves partially decussate at the **_optic chiasm_**. Nasal retinal fibers from each eye cross to the other side at the chiasm. This pattern of decussation leads to interesting findings in the **_fields of vision_** of the eyes, which can direct an observer to determine the site of a neurological lesion. A lesion in an optic nerve will create a **_field defect_** in only one eye. A lesion at the chiasm, such as a pituitary gland tumor, can lead to loss of the nasal fibers from both eyes. Since the nasal fibers provide lateral (temporal field) vision, loss of lateral vision in both eyes is indicative of a chiasmal lesion. When the complete temporal field of both eyes is lost, it is called bitemporal hemianopsia. An occipital lobe lesion produces field defects that are congruous (similar) in the two eyes. For example, a left lower quadrant defect in each eye would suggest a right occipital lobe lesion. Complete destruction of one occipital lobe involves both eyes and leads to blindness to the opposite side of the occipital damage. An occipital lobe lesion would not affect the pupillary light reflex because fibers from the eyes to the oculomotor nuclei would not be affected.

The Ear

The ear is two sense organs in one; it is the organ of *hearing,* and it is the organ of *equilibrium,* both of which are contained within the *temporal* bone. The ear consists of the outer ear, the middle ear and the inner ear. The *outer ear* is called the *auricle*. It is composed of elastic cartilage covered with skin. It is structured like a funnel, which makes it effective in catching sound waves. The *middle ear* is an *air filled cavity* where sound is transmitted through the ossicle bones to the inner ear. The *inner ear* contains the sense organs of hearing and equilibrium.

The acoustic (vestibulocochlear, or cranial nerve VIII) nerve innervates the sense organs of the ear. It is primarily a sensory nerve, but it also carries motor fibers to the outer hair cells of the cochlea.

Sound waves are pressure waves that can be transmitted through air, liquid, or by vibrations of a solid. Sound waves do not exist in the vacuum of outer space. The loud engine and motion noises of spaceships in science fiction movies cannot exist outside the pressurized cabin of the spaceship. Consider sound waves to be similar to waves on a body of water. They have *frequency,* which is measured in *cycles/second or Hertz*. The frequency of a sound wave is perceived by our ear as the *pitch* of a sound. Healthy human ears are able to hear sound between *20 and 20,000 Hertz.* Low frequency sounds are low-pitched sounds; high frequency sounds are high-pitched sounds. Dogs can hear sounds well above 20,000 Hertz. Sound waves below 20 Hz are inaudible by the human ear, but bones of the skull can sense them. Sound waves over 20,000 Hz are called ultrasonic. The human ear is most sensitive to sound waves in the 1500-4000 Hz range.

The *loudness or amplitude* of a sound is measured in *decibels (dB),* which is a measure of the height of the sound wave. Using waves on water as an analogy, ripples on a pond have a low amplitude; a tsunami has a high amplitude. The loudness of a sound is its *intensity,* and it is a measure of the *energy* a sound wave has. The threshold of a healthy human ear is close to zero decibels in the 1500 to 4000 Hz range. The measurement of sound in decibels is exponential like the measurement of earthquakes, so that any increase of loudness by ten decibels is an increase of 10 x 10 in energy. Normal conversation emits about 60 dB; 120 dB is painful. Prolonged exposure to noise over 90 dB is capable of causing *noise induced deafness*. Louder sounds produce deafness in a shorter period of time. Two small muscles, the tensor tympani and the stapedius, act to dampen sound as it crosses the ossicles. The *tensor tympani* muscle tightens the ear drum, and the *stapedius* muscle rotates the stapes. These muscles respond to loud sounds by a reflex with a latency period of only 40 milliseconds. Unfortunately that is not fast enough to protect the ear from the noise of gunshots and sudden explosions. The tensor tympani is innervated by the trigeminal nerve and the stapedius by the facial nerve.

Sound waves collected by the outer ear (auricle) are directed into the *external auditory canal* (ear canal). The external auditory canal contains sebaceous glands and *ceruminous glands,* which are modified sudoriferous (sweat) glands. The secretions of these glands make up *cerumen,* or ear wax, which keeps the eardrum pliable, waterproofs the ear canal and has a bactericidal effect. The ear canal is curved as it penetrates the temporal bone. In order to visualize the *tympanic membrane* (ear drum), you must pull the outer ear upward and backward to straighten the ear canal. This gives you visual access to the tympanic membrane and the underlying malleus. The ear canal ends at the tympanic membrane. The tympanic membrane is a semitransparent membrane with a layer of skin on the outside, a mucous membrane on the inside, and a tightly stretched fibrous layer in the middle that vibrates like a drum when struck by sound waves. Behind the eardrum is the air filled middle ear.

Behind the ear drum in the *middle ear* are the three small bones called the *ossicles* (the *malleus, incus and stapes*). The ossicles were named for their shapes. In English the malleus is hammer, the incus is anvil, and the stapes is stirrup. These three tiny, slightly moveable bones are linked in a series and stretched across the middle ear cavity to the *oval window*, which is a hole in the temporal bone covered by a membrane that separates the middle ear from the inner ear. The manubrium is the rounded end of the malleus that is in contact with the tympanic membrane, and the footplate of the stapes is in contact with the oval window. The incus lies between the two other ossicles. The ossicles convey vibrations from the tympanic membrane to the oval window. The middle ear is also called the *tympanic cavity*. It is connected to the posterior nasopharynx by the *Eustachian tube.* A flap of nasal mucosa usually covers the Eustachian tube in the nasopharynx, but when you raise your palate as happens when you swallow, the orifice of the tube will open, thus allowing an equilibration of air pressure between the middle ear and the outside atmosphere. Viral infections of the nasal mucosa may close the opening of the Eustachian tube, which can lead to **_otitis media_** (a middle ear infection), or **_serous otitis_** (fluid in the middle ear). Excessive redness of the tympanic membrane is present in otitis media. Because a normal eardrum is semitransparent, fluid can often be seen in the middle ear in serous otitis. Fluid in the middle ear may be visible as bubbles or a fluid level behind the eardrum. The pain of an ear infection is due to the build up of pressure in the middle ear that accompanies infection. The air cavity of the middle ear is connected to air cells in the mastoid process of the temporal bone; thus an infection in the middle ear can cause **_mastoiditis._** Mastoiditis can be a chronic and serious infection that can lead to breakdown of the temporal bone, an abscess and meningitis.

Right: A view of the ear.
 (1) Temporal bone
 (2) Malleus
 (3) Incus
 (4) Stapes
 (5) Semicircular canals
 (6) Vestibular nerve
 (7) Cochlear nerve
 (8) Cochlea
 (9) Tensor tympani muscle
(10) Eustachian tube
(11) Temporal bone
(12) Round window
(13) Tympanic cavity
     (middle ear)
(14) Tympanic membrane
(15) External auditory
     canal

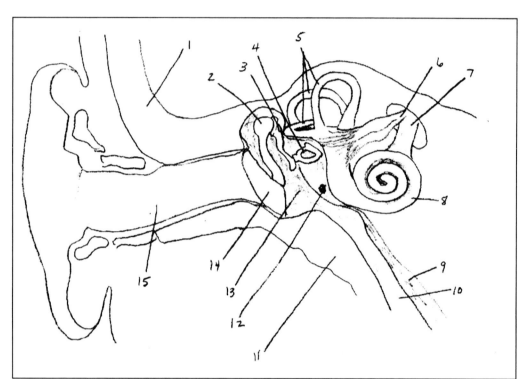

The temporal bone contains the organ of hearing (the **_cochlea_**) and equilibrium (the **_vestibular apparatus_**). These organs are located in tiny tubular passageways called the **_bony labyrinth_**. The bony labyrinth contains chambers filled with two different fluids, **_perilymph_** and **_endolymph._** **_Perilymph_** is continuous with cerebrospinal fluid through an opening in the temporal bone, and it resembles CSF. The oval window has air of the middle ear on its outer side and perilymph on its inner side. **_Endolymph_** is formed in the **_endolymphatic sac_**, a small tuft that intrudes into CSF in the subarachnoid space, but endolymph does not have a direct connection to CSF. Endolymph resembles intracellular fluid somewhat.

The eardrum (tympanic membrane) has a surface area eighteen times greater than the oval window, which means that the oval window receives a considerably greater force per unit area than the tympanic membrane. Sound vibrations are carried by perilymph to the cochlea. The cochlea is a small spiral that is shaped like a snail. It has three parallel fluid chambers that extend the length of the spiral. Those are: **(1)** the **_scala vestibuli_**, which is filled with perilymph and abuts the oval window. **(2)** The middle chamber is the **_cochlear duct_** or **_scala media._** It is filled with endolymph, and it contains the **_organ of Corti_**, which is the organ of hearing. **(3)** The **_scala tympani_** is filled with perilymph; it leads to the **_round window_**, a membrane with perilymph on its inner surface and air of the middle ear on its outer surface. The round window serves to eliminate pressure vibrations that have traveled through the cochlea. Sound vibrations are transmitted through the tympanic membrane to the ossicles, oval window, scala vestibuli, cochlear duct, scala tympani, and end at the round window. The scala vestibuli and the scala tympani are continuous at the apex of the cochlea, which is called the helicotrema.

The ***organ of Corti*** responds to the pressure of vibrations carried from the scala vestibuli to the cochlear duct. These vibrations move the basilar membrane up and down, which causes stereocilia on the inner hair cells of the organ of Corti to rub against the overlying tectorial membrane. The louder the sound, the more vigorously the basilar membrane vibrates. Stimulation of the hair cells creates an action potential; the impulse is carried to the ***spiral ganglion*** of the cochlea where the neurons synapse. The impulse then goes to the pons, midbrain, and eventually to the temporal lobe of the cerebrum. There are two varieties of hair cells in the organ of Corti, the ***inner hair cells*** and the ***outer hair cells.*** The ***outer hair cells*** receive motor nerve fibers that cause them to contract, which dampens vibrations in select areas of the basilar membrane. This allows the ***inner hair cells*** to respond more precisely to pitch, and it gives one the ability to hear sounds that would otherwise be below threshold.

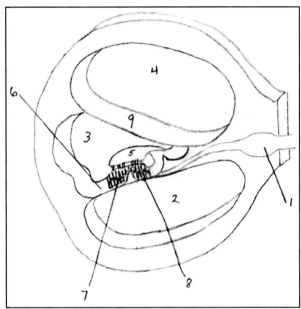

Left: The cochlea. Sound is transmitted from the **scala vestibuli** (4) to the **vestibular membrane** (9). Vibrations of the vestibular membrane affect the endolymph in the **cochlear duct** (3) and cause the **basilar membrane** (6) to vibrate. Cilia on the **inner hair cells** (8) and the **outer hair cells** (7) are stimulated by the overlying **tectorial membrane** (5) and a nerve impulse is initiated. The nerve impulse is carried to the **spiral ganglion** (1) and to the brain via the cochlear nerve, a branch of the eighth cranial nerve. The pressure waves of sound are dissipated through the **scala tympani** (2) to the round window.

The two types of deafness are conduction deafness and nerve deafness. ***Conduction deafness*** results from a defect in the transmission of sound from the outer ear to the cochlea. Some things that cause conduction deafness are a damaged eardrum, otitis media, a blocked external auditory canal, and otosclerosis (fibrosis of the ligaments connecting the ossicles).

Nerve deafness or sensorineural deafness is due to damage to the cochlea or the acoustic nerve. It includes noise induced deafness, which is characterized by destruction of the stereocilia of hair cells and the subsequent death of hair cells. ***Tinnitus*** (ringing in the ears) is a symptom of damage to these cells. Lower pitched sounds are heard at the apex, or helicotrema, of the cochlea; higher pitched sounds are heard at the base of the cochlea. ***The higher pitched sounds are lost first in noise induced deafness.*** Individuals with moderate noise induced deafness may have no trouble detecting vowel sounds in normal speech, but some consonants, such as "c", "g", "s", "t" and "x" have higher frequencies that would be inaudible. This leads to an inability to understand many words, even with loud speech. Hearing aids may be useless to these people. Other things that can cause nerve deafness include certain antibiotics and other drugs, toxins, infections and a genetic susceptibility.

The ***vestibular apparatus*** is the sensory organ of equilibrium. It is located in the inner ear adjacent to the cochlea, and it is part of the bony labyrinth that includes the cochlea. Its tiny chambers are lined by a thin membrane called the ***membranous labyrinth***. ***Endolymph*** fills the membranous labyrinth, and ***perilymph*** surrounds the membranous labyrinth. The ***vestibule*** is a space containing perilymph that is juxtaposed to the oval window.

The sensory parts of the vestibular apparatus are the saccule, the utricle and the three semicircular canals. The ***saccule and the utricle*** are endolymph filled chambers in the vestibule. The saccule and the utricle each contain a *macula,* which is a patch of ciliated *hair cells,* and a gelatinous membrane (the *otolithic membrane*) that floats over the hair cells. Tiny particles called *otoliths* are suspended in the otolithic membrane. The saccule and the utricle sense acceleration by the bombardment of cilia on the hair cells by otoliths. Hair cells of the saccule and utricle are oriented so that the saccule senses vertical acceleration, and the utricle senses horizontal acceleration.

The *three semicircular canals* (ducts) are oriented in different planes, and so they are able to sense rotary acceleration in three planes. The anterior and posterior semicircular canals are in vertical planes ninety degrees apart. The lateral canal is 30 degrees off the horizontal plane. Each canal has a dilated end called the *ampulla*, which contains a mound of hair cells. A gelatinous membrane called the *cupula* overlies these hair cells. When the head turns, endolymph in the canal of the proper plane lags behind and pushes the cupula, which stimulates the hair cells.

The saccule, utricle and semicircular canals do not sense continuous motion; they sense *acceleration* and *deceleration.* When you are spinning and suddenly stop, vertigo is initiated by stimulation of the semicircular canals by deceleration.

Nerve fibers from the hair cells of the vestibular apparatus synapse in the nearby *vestibular ganglion*; then they travel to the pons through the vestibular portion of the eighth cranial nerve. Most of these fibers synapse in the vestibular nucleus of the pons; others go directly to the cerebellum. Nerve tracts from the pons and cerebellum carry vestibular information to the superior colliculi of the midbrain, which connects to the nuclei of cranial nerves III, IV, and VI and allows our eyes to track while acceleration is occurring. This allows us to focus on a page and read even while our head is moving.

Whereas cochlear dysfunction causes deafness, vestibular dysfunction causes *vertigo*. Vertigo differs from dizziness in that *dizziness* is a spinning sensation in the upright position, and vertigo is a spinning sensation unrelated to positioning. Vertigo can result from cerebral, cerebellar or brain stem lesions as well as a vestibular disorder. *Meniere's disease* (endolymphatic hydrops) is a vestibular disorder characterized by distension of the membranous labyrinth. The cause is unknown, but it is thought to be due to either an overproduction of endolymph or a failure of adequate reabsorption of endolymph. Symptoms include vertigo, deafness and tinnitus. Only one ear is involved in most cases. Treatment is largely symptomatic, but ablative surgical procedures are available.

The Sense of Smell

There is a patch of epithelium in the top of the nose that has specialized neuroepithelial cells called *olfactory cells*. Olfactory cells are the only *exposed* neurons in the body. Epithelial cells called supporting cells and basal cells are also seen in this patch of epithelium. Unlike other neurons the basal cells are *capable of mitosis and differentiating* into olfactory neurons. An olfactory cell has a lifespan of about sixty days. Each olfactory cell has about twenty cilia that are called *olfactory hairs*. These cilia are immobile. They have binding sites for molecules that have an odor. In order to have an odor, a molecule must be *volatile* and be able to elicit an action potential in an olfactory cell. Olfactory cilia are tangled in a thin layer of mucus. In a nasal infection or nasal allergy, the mucus layer may become so thick that the binding sites of the olfactory cells are buried, and odor molecules cannot reach them.

The basal end of an olfactory cell forms an axon. Multiple axons from these cells collect in fascicles, which perforate the *cribiform plate of the ethmoid bone*. The multiple fascicles of all olfactory axons make up cranial nerve I, the olfactory nerve. The axons synapse in the *olfactory bulb*, which is just above the cribiform plate and immediately below the frontal lobe of the cerebrum. Postganglionic fibers from the olfactory bulb form the *olfactory tracts*, which go to the cingulate gyrus, temporal lobe, hypothalamus and amygdala.

Impulses from the cerebral cortex to the olfactory bulbs are capable of reducing sensitivity to an odor. Connections between the olfactory system and the limbic system can influence emotions.

The olfactory sense is ancient in evolution, and lower animals have a much keener sense of smell than do humans. Dogs are used in the detection of illegal drugs and dead bodies because of their keen sense of smell. The olfactory epithelium of a human is about 5 square centimeters in size, and it contains 10-20 million olfactory cells. The olfactory epithelium of a bloodhound occupies a space of about 380 square centimeters and contains four billion olfactory cells. The sense of smell in lower animals is closely connected to their behavior. This includes their search for food, revulsion to some odors, and their sexual behavior. Smell is such an important sense to many animals that their brain has a large area called the ***rhinencephalon*** (literally the "nose-brain"). Vestiges of the rhinencephalon in humans are the olfactory bulbs, olfactory tracts and the limbic system. Humans retain some associations between the old rhinencephalon and behavior. ***Pheromones*** are human body odors that can affect sexual behavior. For example, ovulation in women is affected by the presence of men. Women secrete chemicals called copulines at the time of ovulation, which increase men's testosterone levels and make their beards grow faster. These effects are wired through the limbic system and the hypothalamus.

The Sense of Taste

Special sense organs called ***taste buds*** are located on the tongue. There are also a few taste buds on the soft palate, pharynx, buccal mucosa and epiglottis. Each of us has about 4000 taste buds total.

Lingual taste buds occur at special places on the tongue called ***papillae.*** There are four types of papillae on the tongue: **(1)** vallate (circumvallate), **(2)** fungiform, **(3)** foliate, and **(4)** filiform.
Vallate papillae are 7-12 in number. They are the largest of the papillae, and they are located at the rear of the tongue in a "V" configuration. Although they are few in number, they contain about half of all the taste buds -- about 250 per papilla. Each vallate papilla is surrounded by a trench, which contains the taste buds.
Fungiform papillae are widely distributed over the tongue. Each is shaped like a mushroom, and each has three taste buds.
Foliate papillae are not well developed in humans. They are located mostly on the sides of the tongue, about 2/3 of the way back from the tip. In humans most of their taste buds have degenerated by the age of two or three years.
Filiform papillae are the most abundant papillae on the tongue, but they do not contain taste buds. They are shaped like tiny spikes that are used to detect texture.

Taste buds are located in a pit in the epithelium, and they are shaped like a lemon. All taste buds look alike without regard to the taste sensation they elicit or the type of papilla where they reside. A taste bud has basal cells and supporting cells in addition to taste cells. Taste cells are ***epithelial cells*** with a sensory nerve fiber at their base. Taste cells are located at the external surface of the taste bud. "Hairs," which are actually ***microvilli***, extend from the taste cells through a pore (***the taste pore***) to the surface.
To be tasted, molecules must be in solution, and the solution must enter the taste pore. A dry tongue tastes nothing. Humans are able to detect five primary taste sensations, **(1)** salty, **(2)** sweet, **(3)** sour, **(4)** bitter, and **(5)** umami. All the primary tastes can be detected throughout the tongue, but they tend to be concentrated in certain regions. Sweet tastes are best appreciated at the tip of the tongue, salty and sour on the lateral margins, and bitter at the rear.

Metallic ions are perceived as ***salty***, especially ions of sodium, potassium and calcium. ***Sweet*** tastes come from sugars and some other compounds such as aspartame and saccharin. Sucralose (Splenda), is a molecule created from sucrose by replacing three hydroxyl groups with three chlorine atoms. Sucralose is 600 times sweeter than sucrose. ***Sour*** tastes are created by acids. The taste of vinegar is due to acetic acid, and the taste of lemons and grapefruit is due to citric acid, which is used extensively as a food additive. ***Bitter*** tastes are received from alkaloids, which are nitrogen containing alkaline compounds that are found in many plants. Spoiled food and toxins contain alkaloids. Nicotine and caffeine are alkaloids with a bitter taste. Taste buds are most sensitive to bitter tastes and least sensitive to sweet and salty tastes.
Umami (pronounced "Ooo-mommy") is a Japanese word meaning savory. The taste of meats and their amino acids, especially aspartic acid and glutamic acid, are umami tastes. Both aspartic acid and glutamic acid are neurotransmitters, and they are usually of the excitatory type. The sweetener aspartame is derived from aspartic

acid. MSG (monosodium glutamate) is a "flavor enhancer" that is used extensively in Chinese food. It is a derivative of glutamic acid, an amino acid that also functions as an excitatory neurotransmitter. Large doses of MSG cause seizures in susceptible people.

Foods such as jalapeño peppers stimulate pain receptors and give a "hot" sensation. Texture, temperature, appearance, and especially **_smell_** influence our sensation of taste for foods. We have only five primary taste sensations, but our sense of smell can detect ten thousand different odors. Without smell, coffee and peppermint are bitter and taste alike.

Once stimulated, a taste cell releases a neurotransmitter that creates an impulse on the dendrites of a nerve fiber. Taste buds on the anterior 2/3 of the tongue send sensory impulses to the brain via the facial nerve (CN VII), and those on the posterior 1/3 of the tongue via the glossopharyngeal nerve (CN IX). Taste buds on the palate, pharynx and epiglottis send impulses to the brain via the vagus nerve (CN X), and pain receptors in the mouth via the trigeminal nerve (CN V). Sensory impulses from taste buds synapse in the **_medulla_**; the fibers then proceed to the **_hypothalamus and amygdala_**, where they connect with reflex arcs that cause salivation, gagging and vomiting. You become aware of the sense of taste in the **_postcentral gyrus of the parietal lobe_**, which is the primary sensory area of the cerebral cortex.

Right: Two taste buds. Taste buds are embedded in the epithelium of the tongue. Hairs on gustatory cells (taste cells) sense salts of metallic ions, sugars, amino acids, other acids and alkaloids. Those substances must be in an aqueous solution, and the solution must enter the taste pore in order for a substance to be tasted. The hairs of taste cells are microvilli that elicit a nerve impulse.

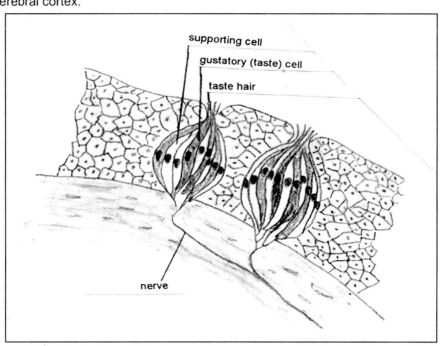

Somesthetic Senses

Somesthetic senses are those that are widely distributed throughout the body. Examples include receptors in the skin and internal organs that sense pain, heat, cold, light touch, pressure, stretch and tension. **_Bare dendritic nerve endings_** in the skin can sense pain, heat and cold; they are bare dendrites that branch from the afferent axon of a unipolar neuron in a dorsal root ganglion. Bare dendritic nerve endings are present in both epithelial and connective tissue, including the epidermis and the dermis. They are especially prominent around the base of hair follicles.

Merkel discs are small unencapsulated nerve endings in the epidermis that distinguish light touch.

Encapsulated nerve endings include: **(1) _Meissner corpuscles_**, which are located in the dermal papillae. They are especially common in the fingers, sensitive areas of the face and the genitalia. They detect light touch. **(2) _Krause end bulbs_** are similar to Meissner corpuscles, but Krause end bulbs are located in mucous membranes. **(3) _Pacinian corpuscles_** are lamellated corpuscles that sense deep pressure, stretching, tickling sensations and vibrations. They are seen in the dermis, especially the hands, feet, breasts, and genitalia, and they are seen in the viscera. **(4) _Ruffini corpuscles_** are present in the dermis, hypodermis, tendons, ligaments and joint capsules. They detect heavy touch, pressure, joint movements and stretching.

Right: Illustrations of sensory nerve endings.

Bare (free) nerve endings are widespread in the skin, mucous membranes and connective tissues. They detect pain, cold and heat.

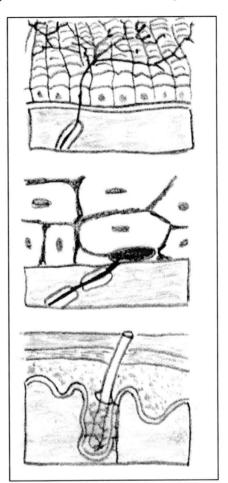

Merkel discs are present in the epidermis. They respond to light touch, and they detect texture, edges and shapes.

Hair receptors are nerve endings around hair follicles. They detect movement and pain.

Right: **Ruffini corpuscles** are found in the dermis, subcutaneous tissue and joint capsules. subcutaneous tissue and joint capsules. They respond to heavy touch, pressure, stretching and movement.

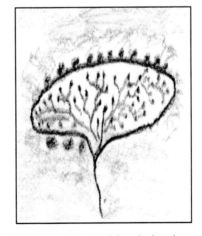

   Proprioception is detected by **_muscle spindles_**, which are located in skeletal muscles near their tendons. Muscle spindles are special organs within muscles. They contain specialized contractile muscle cells called **_intrafusal fibers_**, which have motor end plates and are innervated by gamma efferent motor nerves. Muscle spindles contain **_annulospiral nerve endings_**, which are sensory nerve endings that are coiled around the intrafusal fibers. They detect the amount of contracture of the intrafusal fibers, and the CNS interprets that information as the sense of **_proprioception._**

Golgi tendon organs are located in tendons; they sense tension and stretching. They function to balance contractions in a muscle and to prevent excessive tension from developing in the tendon.

Right: A muscle spindle, a sense organ for proprioception.

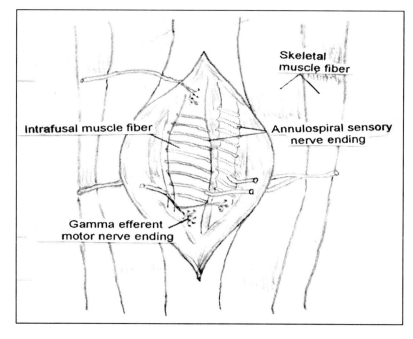

Below: Golgi tendon organs are seen in this drawing as branched nerve endings on the tendon. They detect stretching.

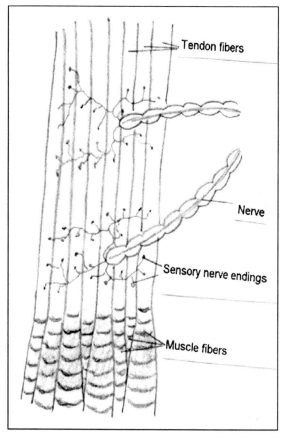

Right: **Tactile corpuscles** are also known as **Meissner corpuscles.** They are located in dermal papillae of the fingertips, tongue, nipples and genitalia. They respond to light touch.

Right: **Krause end bulbs** are found in mucous membranes. They detect touch.

Right: **Lamellated corpuscles** are also known as **pacinian corpuscles.** They are located in the dermis, joint capsules, breasts, genitals and some of the viscera. They respond to deep pressure, stretch, tickle, and vibration.

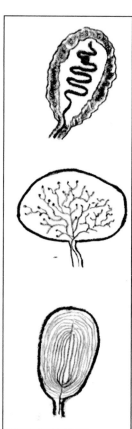

Right: The brain showing the primary motor area and the primary sensory area.

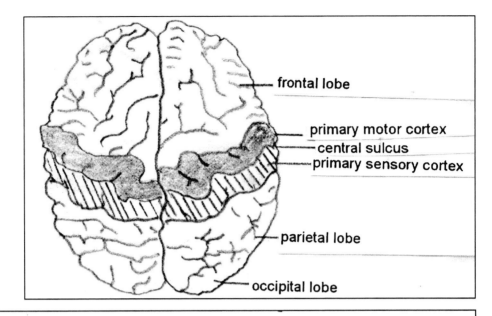

Right: A sensory homunculus showing where sensation from different areas of the body is represented in the cerebral cortex.

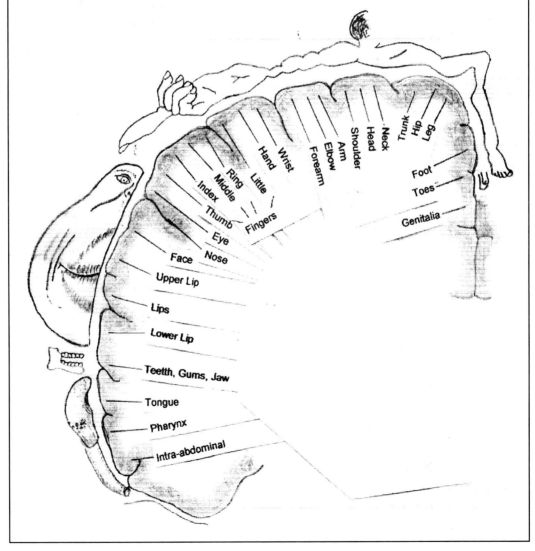

Pain receptors are called *nociceptors*. They are ubiquitous in the body except for the brain. Headaches do not originate in the nervous tissue of the brain. Headaches can be caused by the stimulation of pain receptors in the meninges, eyes, sinuses, face, blood vessels of the head, or in muscles, tendons and ligaments of the neck. Nociceptors are most densely located in the skin. Pain fibers may be myelinated, in which case they travel quickly and produce a sharp, stabbing localized pain, or they may be unmyelinated, in which case they travel slowly and produce a longer lasting, dull, diffuse, aching or burning pain.

Pain arising from skin, muscles and joints is *somatic pain.* If pain is from the skin, it is sharp and stabbing, and the sensory nerve fibers are myelinated. If the pain is from deeper tissues it is aching or burning, and the sensory nerve fibers are unmyelinated.
Visceral pain can arise from stretching, ischemia (loss of blood supply) or from chemical irritants. It is poorly localized and often associated with nausea.

Injured tissues release chemicals that stimulate pain fibers. The most potent pain stimulus known is *bradykinin,* which is found in basophiles in tissues and in blood. Bradykinin is released following an injury; it causes vasodilatation as well as intense pain. Bradykinin is an *eicosenoid,* which is a *prostaglandin,* a group of compounds derived from fatty acids. Prostaglandins were first discovered in the prostate gland, but they are found in all tissues. Histamine, serotonin, potassium ions and ATP are also capable of eliciting pain when they are released into the tissues from ruptured cells following an injury. Possibly the most painful experience is caused by a dissecting aneurysm, which is a rent or tear in the aorta. A dissecting aneurysm ruptures the aorta longitudinally, and blood creates a new channel through the wall of the aorta.

Pain sensations below the head synapse in dorsal root ganglia or the dorsal horn of the spinal cord. They form the *spinothalamic tracts*, which decussate and ascend to the thalamus. From the thalamus they proceed to the *postcentral gyrus* of the parietal lobe, which is the primary sensory cortex. Pain fibers from the viscera connect with the hypothalamus and the limbic system as well as the parietal lobe.
Facial pain travels to the pons via the *trigeminal* nerve (CN V), where it joins the spinothalamic tracts going to the thalamus and parietal lobe.

Referred pain is pain that is interpreted as coming from a site other than where it actually arises. Thus cardiac pain can be felt in the left shoulder and on the inside surface of the left arm, and gall bladder pain can be felt in the right shoulder. The mix-up involving cardiac pain sensation occurs because spinal nerves that innervate the heart are from the same level as those that innervate the shoulder area (T-1 to T-5).

The CNS has mechanisms for modulating severe pain. Receptors on neurons called *enkephalins,* *endorphins* and *dynorphins* are peptides that bind to receptors. They act as neuromodulators, neurotransmitters and hormones that are secreted in times of pain and during exercise. They inhibit pain sensations, and they cause feelings of euphoria and well being. Receptors that respond to these neuromodulators are the same as those that bind to opium compounds (heroin, morphine, codeine, etc.). Endorphins, enkephalins and dynorphins are naturally secreted by the midbrain, pituitary gland, and other organs.
Another mechanism of pain modulation is created by stimulation of mechanoreceptors (touch and pressure sensors) in the skin and tissues, which inhibits interneurons in the spinal cord from transmitting pain stimuli. Thus does rubbing the scalp after bumping your head help decrease the sensation of pain.

Study Guide
1. Trace a visual impulse from the retina to the optic nerve, optic chiasm, optic tract, lateral geniculate body to the occipital lobe.
2. List wavelengths for the various energetic waves in the electromagnetic spectrum from the short, highly energetic gamma waves to the long radio waves. Know the wavelengths in nanometers of visible light (400-700 nm), ultraviolet light (< 400 nm), and infrared light (> 700 nm).
3. How does the energy of a wave relate to its wavelength?
4. Relate the color spectrum to wavelength.
5. Familiarize yourself with the following structures: meibomian glands, glands of Zeiss and Moll, tarsal plates (tarsus), levator palpebrae muscle, orbicularis oculi muscle, glands of Krause and Wolfring, lacrimal gland, canaliculi of the lacrimal system, lacrimal sac, nasolacrimal duct, commissures and canthi.

6. Be able to identify the following: sclera, cornea, iris, pupil, ciliary body, ciliary muscle, zonules (suspensory ligament of the lens), choroid, retinal pigment epithelium, and sensory retina.
7. Where is the vitreous humor located, and what is its consistency?
8. Where is the aqueous humor located, and what is its consistency?
9. Locate the following in a model or illustration of the eye: physiologic blind spot, optic disc, macula lutea, fovea centralis, limbus, trabecular meshwork, and ciliary body.
10. Name the two types of photoreceptor cells.
11. Take note of the following differences between rods and cones:
    Cones specialize in photopic (daytime) vision; there are fewer cones than rods in the retina; cones fill up the fovea centralis; foveal cones have no neuronal convergence; peripheral cones have only a small amount of neuronal convergence; cones are responsible for color vision; there are three types of cones: red, green and blue, each being named according to the portion of the color spectrum to which it is most sensitive.
    Rods are more plentiful in the retina than are cones; rods are responsible for scotopic (night) vision; there is only one type of rod; rods are absent in the fovea; rods have a considerable amount of neuronal convergence; consequently they can provide only a blurred image to the occipital lobe.
12. Locate and describe the conjunctiva.
13. Name the extrinsic and the intrinsic muscles of the eye, and give the innervation of each.
14. Understand convergence, adduction and abduction as they relate to ocular movements.
15. Define strabismus. Define astigmatism.
16. Note that light rays are refracted by the cornea and the lens. This results in focusing light onto the retina.
17. Know that visual purple is the photochemical of rods that is modified when it is struck by light. The photochemical of cones has a slightly different protein component. Each photochemical consists of a protein and retinal, which is a vitamin A derivative.
18. Recognize that the ear is two sense organs in one — hearing and equilibrium.
19. Know the three anatomical parts of the ear (outer, middle and inner).
20. Where is air found in the ear and how does it get there?
21. Understand the vocabulary for the parameters of sound waves -- amplitude, loudness, frequency, pitch, Hertz, cycles per second and decibels.
22. Know the effects of contraction of the tensor tympani muscle and the stapedius muscle.
23. Know the significance and location of the following: tympanic membrane (ear drum), ossicles (malleus, incus and stapes), oval window, mastoid air cells, vestibule, perilymph, endolymph, vestibule, saccule, utricle, semicircular canals, macula of the saccule and utricle, ampulla of the semicircular canals, cochlea, inner and outer hair cells, basilar membrane, tectorial membrane, organ of Corti and round window.
24. Follow a sound wave from the auricle to the external auditory canal, tympanic membrane, ossicles, oval window, perilymph, scala vestibuli, scala media, and scala tympani to the round window.
25. What is the significance of the Eustachian tube? How does this tube relate to otitis media (infection in the middle ear)?
26. Understand the difference between conduction deafness and sensorineural or nerve deafness. Give examples of each type.
27. What is tinnitus? What causes it?
28. To what does each of the following respond -- utricle, saccule, and semicircular canals? (The utricle responds to horizontal acceleration and deceleration, the saccule to vertical acceleration and deceleration, and the semicircular canals to rotary acceleration and deceleration).
29. Where are olfactory cells located? Are they neurons or epithelial cells? Where is the olfactory nerve? Where do olfactory neurons synapse? Trace the axons of secondary neurons from the olfactory bulb to various parts of the limbic system.
30. How do the volatility of a chemical and the presence of increased nasal mucus affect the sense of smell?
31. Which lingual papillae contain taste buds and which do not? (Vallate and fungiform do; others do not.)
32. Are taste cells epithelial cells or neurons?
33. Name the five sensations of taste.
34. Which two cranial nerves carry sensory impulses from taste buds in the tongue to the brain?
35. What are somesthetic senses? Give examples.
36. Name the specialized receptors for touch that are located in the skin. (Merkel discs, pacinian corpuscles, Meissner corpuscles, Ruffini corpuscles)
37. Name the specialized receptors for proprioception and stretch that are located in muscles or tendons.

38.   Name the chemical that produces the most excruciating pain when injected into the tissues.   Note that bradykinin is a prostaglandin.
39.   Define referred pain.
40. Note that endogenous opioids are naturally occurring peptides that decrease pain. They are secreted by the CNS in times of stress and during exercise.

Chapter Seventeen

The Endocrine System

The glands of the body consist of **_(1) exocrine glands_**, which secrete their product into a duct, **_(2) endocrine glands_**, which secrete **_hormones_** directly into the blood stream, and **_(3) paracrine glands_**, which secrete their product into surrounding tissues. Exocrine secretions and paracrine secretions have only local effects, but endocrine secretions are carried by the blood to all parts of the body, and they will affect any organ with the proper receptors.

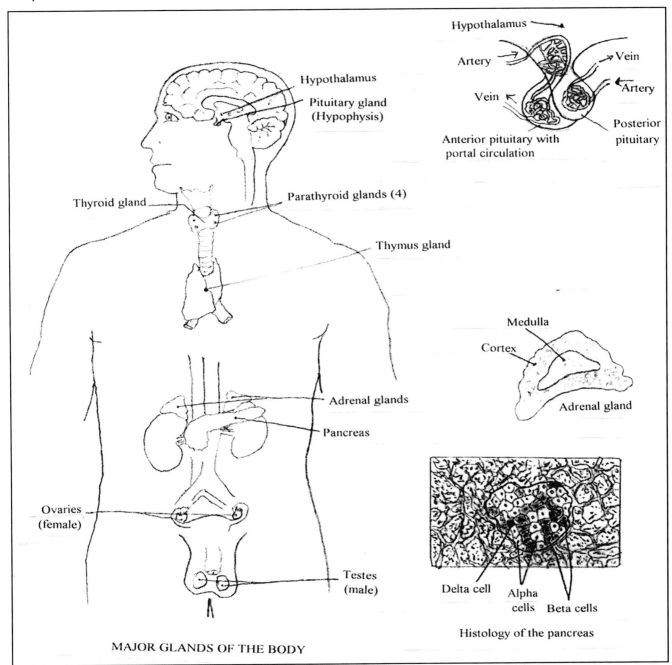

Above: The endocrine glands of the body.

A *__hormone__* is a chemical secreted by an endocrine gland into the blood stream. Hormones exert their effect on a target organ that is distant from the gland of their origin. Hormones are effective in low concentrations, and they exert their effect by binding with specific receptors on specific target cells.

Hormones are classified into three groups according to their chemical structure. Those groups are: (1) *__peptides and proteins__*; (2) *__amines__* (including the monoamines), and (3) *__steroids.__*

Hormones that are *__peptides or proteins__* are chains of amino acids. Included in this group are *__insulin, glucagon, growth hormone, calcitonin, ACTH, parathyroid hormone, prolactin, oxytocin and ADH__* (antidiuretic hormone).

Some of the peptides secreted by the anterior pituitary also have a carbohydrate moiety and are classified as *__glycoproteins.__* They include *__FSH, LH (ICSH) and TSH__*.

Hormones with an *__amine__* structure are synthesized from the amino acids *__tyrosine__* or *__tryptophan__*. The *__catecholamines__* (epinephrine, norepinephrine and dopamine) and *__thyroid hormone__* (thyroxin, or T-4 and triiodothyronine, or T-3) are derived from *__tyrosine.__* *__Serotonin__* and *__melatonin__*, which is sometimes classified as a hormone, are derived from *__tryptophan__*.

__Steroid__ hormones are a group of compounds derived from cholesterol, and they have the basic four-ring sterol structure of cholesterol. Unlike proteins, peptides and amines, steroids are lipophilic, and they are classified as lipids. Hormones that are classified as steroids include *__aldosterone__*, *__cortisol__* (*__hydrocortisone__*), the *__estrogens, progesterone__*, and the *__androgens__* (including *__testosterone__*).

Above: Steroid hormones, showing the pathways of their synthesis.

The secretion of most hormones is by _**negative feedback loops**_. Secretion is increased when more hormone is called for; secretion is decreased when less is needed. There are different triggering mechanisms for hormone release. For example, the amount of glucose in the blood determines insulin secretion. Thyroid hormone, cortisol and the sex hormones are released in response to the presence of a stimulatory _**trophic**_ hormone from the pituitary gland.

**Oxytocin** triggers uterine contractions; it differs from other hormones in that it is released through a positive feedback mechanism during childbirth. Oxytocin release by the _**posterior pituitary**_ is triggered by the stretching of uterine smooth muscle. Once childbirth begins, the infant's head stretches smooth muscle in the lower uterus (cervix), which triggers more oxytocin release by the pituitary. The _**positive feedback**_ release mechanism continues until the infant is delivered.

Most of the glands of the body are ectodermal or endodermal in origin. A tumor arising from a gland is called an adenoma if it is benign. A malignant tumor of glandular origin is an adenocarcinoma.

The pituitary gland (_**hypophysis)**_ is called the _**master gland**_ because many of its hormones are trophic (tropic) hormones that stimulate and control the release of hormones from other glands. The pituitary gland is located in the _**sella turcica of the sphenoid bone**_ immediately posterior to the optic chiasm. It is connected to the hypothalamus by a short stalk called the _**infundibulum**_. The adult pituitary is divided into two sections: (1) the _**anterior pituitary**_ or adenohypophysis, and (2) the _**posterior pituitary**_ or neurohypophysis.

The different hormones of the _**anterior hypophysis**_ are produced by different types of cells. Those hormones include:

(1) _**Growth hormone**_, which is also called _**GH or somatotropin**_. GH is a peptide that stimulates bone growth and protein synthesis. Its secretion is regulated by two hormones from the _**hypothalamus,**_ GH releasing factor, which increases GH secretion, and _**somatostatin,**_ which inhibits GH and TSH secretion. Somatostatin is a peptide that is also secreted by the pancreas and monocytes of the immune system.

(2) _**Thyroid stimulating hormone**_ (_**TSH**_) is a glycoprotein. It stimulates the release of thyroid hormone by the thyroid gland. TSH release is controlled by thyrotropin releasing hormone from the hypothalamus.

(3) _**Adrenocorticotropic hormone**_ (_**ACTH**_) is a peptide that stimulates the release of _**cortiso**_l and similar _**glucocorticoid**_ steroid hormones from the adrenal cortex. ACTH release is controlled by corticotropin releasing factor from the hypothalamus.

(4) _**Prolactin**_ is a peptide that stimulates the mammary glands to produce milk. Prolactin release is controlled by two hormones from the hypothalamus.

(5) _**Follicle stimulating hormone**_ (_**FSH**_) is a glycoprotein that stimulates development of the germ cells, which are the egg cells in females and sperm cells in males.

(6) In females _**luteinizing hormone**_ (_**LH**_), a glycoprotein, is responsible for ovulation and the development of the corpus luteum in the ovaries, which produces progesterone. In males LH is known as _**interstitial cell stimulating hormone**_ (_**ICSH**_); it stimulates the interstitial cells to produce testosterone. The secretion of FSH and LH (ICSH) is regulated by releasing hormones from the hypothalamus. FSH and LH (ICSH) are collectively called _**gonadotropins**_ due to their effects on the gonads (ovaries and testes).

Tumors of the anterior pituitary may produce an abnormally high secretion of a specific hormone. A tumor of the cells that produce _**GH**_ may produce an excess of GH, which may result in gigantism and _**acromegaly.**_ Acromegaly is characterized not only by excessive height, weight and bone size, but also by coarse features and diabetes mellitus.

An overproduction of _**ACTH**_ will cause the adrenal cortex to produce an excessive amount of _**cortisol**_, which leads to _**Cushing's syndrome**_, a disorder characterized by central obesity, easy bruisability, hypertension, muscle weakness and diabetes mellitus.

The hormones of the posterior pituitary are _**oxytocin and antidiuretic hormone (ADH)**_. Both are peptides. _**Oxytocin**_ is released when uterine smooth muscle is stretched. In males oxytocin stimulates smooth muscle contractions in the spermatic ducts and prostate gland, which produces the emission of semen. _**ADH**_ (also called _**vasopressin**_) increases the reabsorption of water in the kidney tubules, which decreases urinary volume and increases blood volume. Osmoreceptors in the hypothalamus measure the tonicity of the blood, and they control the secretion of ADH. An overproduction of ADH results in water retention and dilution of the blood, which leads to hyponatremia and mental confusion. This syndrome is called an *"inappropriate" secretion of ADH*. One cause of inappropriate ADH secretion is overzealous use of respiratory therapy. Respiratory therapy increases the intrathoracic pressure, which decreases the return of blood to the heart and lowers the cardiac output. Sensors in the carotid sinus and the aortic arch alert the hypothalamus that the blood volume is low, which stimulates the hypothalamus to secrete ADH. A lack of ADH is called *diabetes insipidus*, a situation that is characterized by excessive urine production. *"Diabetes insipidus"* means excessive urine production without taste (no sugar), which differentiates this disease from diabetes mellitus.

The *hypothalamus* controls the secretion of hormones by the anterior pituitary and the *posterior pituitary*. The hormones of the posterior pituitary (oxytocin and ADH) are *produced in the hypothalamus and stored in the posterior pituitary.*

The hypothalamus produces *releasing hormones* that are secreted into a capillary network. Venous blood from this network is then shunted by *hypophyseal portal veins* to another capillary network that surrounds the *anterior pituitary*. The cells of the anterior pituitary are exposed to high concentrations of hypothalamic releasing hormones by this special portal circulatory system. By that means the hypothalamic releasing hormones control secretions by the anterior pituitary.

The *thyroid gland* is located in the neck, anterior to the trachea and below the larynx. *Thyroxin (T-4) and triiodothyronine (T-3)* are thyroid hormones that are secreted in response to TSH from the pituitary. Both T-3 and T-4 are active, and both contain *iodine*. T-3 is somewhat more active than T-4, but the thyroid secretes more T-4 than it secretes T-3. Thyroxin and triiodothyronine are amines that are derived from tyrosine. They *increase the metabolic rate* and heat production. They stimulate protein synthesis, growth and maturation. A lack of thyroid hormone produces *cretinism* in an infant and *myxedema* in an adult. Cretins are dwarfish and mentally dull. Myxedema is characterized by lethargy, weakness, generalized edema, dry skin and hair loss. *Grave's disease* is caused an overproduction of TSH and other hormones, which leads to an overactive thyroid. Exophthalmos (bulging eyes), tachycardia (fast heart rate), and hyperactive reflexes are symptoms of Grave's disease.

The thyroid is susceptible to tumors and hypertrophy. A *goiter* is a benign enlargement of the thyroid gland. A lack of iodine in the diet may produce a goiter.

The thyroid also produces *calcitonin*, a hormone that encourages bone growth by inhibiting the activity of osteoclasts. Calcitonin thereby lowers the blood levels of calcium and phosphate. Calcitonin has measurable effects in children, but it has little or no effect in controlling calcium blood levels in adults.

The *parathyroid glands* are four small glands embedded within the posterior surface of the thyroid gland. These glands produce *parathyroid hormone* (*PTH*), a polypeptide, in response to low blood calcium levels. Parathyroid hormone stimulates bone reabsorption by the osteoclasts, and it raises the calcium level in the blood. Therefore, parathyroid hormone and calcitonin have opposite effects on bone and blood calcium levels.

A lack of parathyroid hormone results in *hypocalcemia,* which leads to *tetany*. Thyroid surgery has resulted in the inadvertent removal of all four parathyroid glands, which results in a total lack of parathyroid hormone. Fatal tetany can occur as soon as four days following surgical excision of all parathyroid glands. A parathyroid tumor may result in *hypercalcemia* due to an excess production of parathyroid hormone. High blood calcium levels lead to sluggish reflexes and possible cardiac arrest.

The *pancreas* is located in the left upper quadrant of the abdomen, behind the intestines and behind the peritoneum (retroperitoneal). The hormones of the pancreas include *insulin and glucagon.* Both are polypeptides. *Insulin* lowers the amount of glucose in the blood by facilitating the transport of glucose across the plasma membranes of muscle cells and adipose cells. *Glucagon* raises the blood glucose by stimulating the liver to break down glycogen into glucose (glycogenolysis). The glucose is then released into the blood.

Somatostatin is a *paracrine* secretion of the pancreas that helps to control blood sugar levels by inhibiting the secretion of insulin and glucagon, and by inhibiting some digestive functions. Insulin, glucagon and somatostatin are produced in isolated cellular clusters in the pancreas called *"islets of Langerhans."* Each hormone is produced by a specific type of cell in the islets - *insulin* by *beta* cells, *glucagon* by *alpha* cells, and *somatostatin* by *delta* cells.

Destruction of the beta cells of the Islets of Langerhans causes insulin-dependent diabetes mellitus (type I diabetes). There are other physiologic causes for diabetes mellitus, including destruction of insulin receptor sites and the presence of insulin antibodies. Insulin is necessary for the entry of glucose into muscle tissue and adipose tissue. Insulin is not required for glucose uptake by the brain, liver, kidneys and red blood cells.

The pancreas is also an **_exocrine_** gland that secretes digestive **_enzymes_** into the pancreatic duct, which leads into the duodenum (upper small intestine).

The **_adrenal glands_** are situated like a cap over each kidney. The adrenal medulla and the adrenal cortex have completely different endocrine functions. The **_adrenal medulla_** secretes catecholamines, and the **_adrenal cortex_** secretes steroid hormones.

Catecholamines are secreted into the blood by the **_adrenal medulla_** in response to stimuli from the sympathetic division of the autonomic nervous system. 85% of the adrenal medulla secretions is epinephrine, 15% is norepinephrine and a trace amount is dopamine. The adrenal medulla secretes catecholamines in situations of crisis. Catecholamines increase the blood pressure and pulse rate, and they increase blood flow to skeletal muscles.

The steroid hormones secreted by the **_adrenal cortex_** are classified as: **_(1) glucocorticoids_** (chiefly **_cortisol_**), **_(2) mineralocorticoids_** (chiefly **_aldosterone_**) and **_(3) sex steroids_** (androgens [male hormones] and estrogens [female hormones]). Glucocorticoids are secreted as a response to ACTH from the pituitary. Mineralocorticoids are secreted as a response to low blood volume or low blood pressure.

The effects of **_cortisol_** and other **_glucocorticoids_** on the body include anti-inflammation, protein and fat catabolism, and an elevation of the blood glucose. Glucocorticoids promote the formation of glucose from proteins and fats, a process that is known as **_gluconeogenesis._** Cortisol and hydrocortisone are two names for the same compound. Cortisone and corticosterone are glucocorticoids that are similar to cortisol in structure and effect. **_Cushing's syndrome_** occurs when glucocorticoid production by the adrenal cortex is excessive. Symptoms of Cushing's syndrome include truncal obesity, muscle wasting, weakness, easy bruisability, hypertension and diabetes mellitus. The overproduction of glucocorticoids by the adrenal cortex in Cushing's syndrome could be secondary to a pituitary tumor that produces an excessive amount of ACTH, or it could be due to an adrenal tumor that secretes glucocorticoids independent of ACTH.

Aldosterone is the primary mineralocorticoid secreted by the adrenal cortex. Its primary effect is on the kidneys, where it enhances sodium reabsorption and potassium excretion. The sodium preserving effect of aldosterone results in water retention, an increase in blood volume, and an increase in blood pressure. A total lack of aldosterone would be fatal.

The adrenals produce more **_androgens_** (male hormones) than **_estrogens_** (female hormones). Adrenal androgen production in males is greatly overshadowed by androgens from the testicles. However, in females adrenal androgens in females are responsible for the growth of axillary and groin hair, and for sexual libido. Adrenal estrogens have little effect in either sex.

When the cortices of both adrenal glands are nonfunctional, it results in a lack of glucocorticoid, mineralocorticoid, androgen and estrogen secretion by the adrenals. This condition is known as **_Addison's disease_**. The patient suffering from Addison's disease exhibits sodium wasting in the urine and a reduction in blood volume, which results in low blood pressure, hyponatremia, hyperkalemia and dehydration. ACTH production by the pituitary rises due to the lack of negative feedback from adrenal steroids. Melanocyte stimulating hormone (MSH), a derivative of ACTH, is also produced in excess by the pituitary in Addison's disease, and it results in darkening of the skin. Severe Addison's disease is fatal without aldosterone replacement therapy. Glucocorticoid replacement therapy is desirable, but not necessary for life.

The **_gonads_** are the **_ovaries and the testes_**. The development of ova (eggs) in the ovaries is stimulated by **_FSH_** (follicle stimulating hormone) from the anterior pituitary. **_LH_** (luteinizing hormone) stimulates ovulation and the development of the **_corpus luteum_**. The **_follicle cells_** of the **_ovaries_** secrete estrogen, and estrogen promotes the maturation of egg cells (ova). Estrogen also stimulates the secondary sex characteristics of the female including breast development and uterine growth. The **_corpus luteum_** of the ovaries produces **_estrogen and progesterone,_** which stimulate growth and development of the endometrium of the uterus and secretory cells of the mammary glands.

Sperm production in the testes is stimulated by **FSH** from the anterior pituitary. **ICSH** (interstitial cell stimulating hormone) from the anterior pituitary stimulates the **interstitial cells** of the **testes** to produce **testosterone**. (**ICSH is identical to LH**.) Testosterone promotes the secondary sex characteristics of the male, including growth of the penis, larynx, skeletal muscle, and the development of facial and body hair.

Inhibin is a hormone secreted by the ovaries and the testes. Inhibin decreases the production of **FSH** by the pituitary. It functions to regulate the timing of ovulation in the female and the rate of spermatogenesis in the male.

The **thymus** gland is located in the mediastinum, above the heart and between the right and left lungs. It secretes thymopoietin and thymosins, which are hormones that **regulate T lymphocytes**, a type of blood leukocyte. The thymus gland is relatively large in infants, but it involutes after puberty, and it is almost entirely replaced by fibrous and adipose tissue in the elderly. **Myasthenia gravis**, an autoimmune disease of the neuromuscular junction, is sometimes associated with hypertrophy of the thymus or a thymic tumor.

The **pineal gland** is part of the epithalamus, which is part of the diencephalon. The pineal gland is active in young children, but it begins to involute after the age of seven years. It secretes **serotonin** by day and **melatonin** by night. Both serotonin and melatonin are monoamines. The pineal may have a function in regulating the timing of puberty.

The placenta, heart, liver, skin, kidneys, stomach and small intestines also secrete hormones.

(1) The **placenta** secretes large amounts of estrogen and progesterone during pregnancy.

(2) The **heart** (specifically the right atrium) produces **atrial natriuretic peptide**, a peptide that lowers blood pressure by promoting sodium excretion by the kidney and by blocking the effects of angoitensin II (see below).

(3) Keratinocytes in the **epidermis** of the **skin** produce vitamin D-3 when exposed to ultraviolet light. Vitamin D-3 is a precursor of vitamin D. Vitamin D-3 is converted to calcidiol in the **liver**, and the **kidneys** convert calcidiol into **calcitriol**, the most active form of vitamin D. Vitamin D is classified as a vitamin, but it acts like a hormone.

(4) **Erythropoietin** (EPO) is a hormone produced by the **kidneys** (85%) and the **liver** (15%). EPO stimulates blood cell production in the bone marrow. Individuals with chronic renal disease are typically anemic due to the lack of erythropoietin.

(5) The **kidneys, liver and lungs** have a role in the **angiotensin-renin** mechanism to elevate blood pressure. **Angiotensinogen** is a polypeptide produced by the liver. **Renin** is an enzyme produced in the kidneys that converts angiotensinogen to **angiotensin I**. Angiotensin I is converted to **angiotensin II** by the effect of **angiotensin converting enzyme (ACE)** in the lungs and the kidneys. **Angiotensin II raises blood pressure** by several mechanisms: **(1)** it is a powerful vasoconstrictor; **(2)** it stimulates ADH secretion by the posterior pituitary; **(3)** it stimulates aldosterone secretion by the adrenal cortex, and **(4)** it increases sodium reabsorption by the kidneys.

(6) The **stomach and intestines** secrete at least ten different hormones. In general these hormones coordinate the functions of the digestive system. **Gastrin** is one of the most important of these hormones. Gastrin stimulates the secretion of hydrochloric acid, enzymes and intrinsic factor into the stomach.

(7) **Prostaglandins** are produced by nearly all cells of the body. They usually behave as **paracrine** secretions and not endocrine secretions. Functions of prostaglandins are many and varied. Some of their effects include inflammation, pain stimulation, blood clotting, vasoconstriction, constriction of the bronchioles, vasodilatation, uterine contraction and digestive gland secretion. Prostaglandins are synthesized from **arachidonic acid**, an essential fatty acid found in phospholipids. Most of the body's phospholipids are in the cell membrane. Aspirin acts to alleviate inflammation and pain and to inhibit blood clotting by its effects on prostaglandins and prostaglandin synthesis.

Study Guide

1. Know the three types of hormones according to chemical structure (peptides and proteins, amines and steroids).
2. Know into which of the above types individual hormones fall.
3. Know what regulates the secretion of individual hormones.
4. Recognize the hormones produced by the hypothalamus.
5. Recognize the hormones produced by the anterior pituitary.
6. Recognize the hormones produced by the posterior pituitary.
7. Study the pituitary hormones according to their function.

8. Be familiar with the hormones produced by the adrenal medulla, adrenal cortex, thyroid, parathyroid, ovary, testicle and pancreas.
9. Understand what is meant by corticotropin, glucocorticoid, mineralocorticoid, and gonadotropin.
10. Recognize that the thymus and the pineal are endocrine glands only in the young.
11. Be familiar with the steps involved in the synthesis of calcitriol.
12. Be acquainted with hormones produced by the liver and kidneys and the angiotensin-renin system.
13. Recognize the terms acromegaly, diabetes mellitus, diabetes insipidus, Cushing's syndrome, Addison's disease, myxedema and cretinism.

Chapter Eighteen

Blood

Hematology is the study of blood, its components and its associated abnormalities. A hematologist is one who studies blood and blood abnormalities.

The ability of the blood to circulate causes it to be involved in all bodily systems and functions including respiration, nutrition, waste elimination, thermoregulation, immune defense, acid-base balance, hydration and internal communication.

Blood is a connective tissue. Plasma is a clear extracellular fluid that makes up the matrix of blood. The formed elements of blood are the red and white blood cells and the platelets.

Ionized metallic salts (especially sodium and chloride ions) constitute most of the osmolarity of blood. The millions of erythrocytes (red blood cells or *RBCs*) in blood are responsible for most of the viscosity of blood. *Plasma proteins*, especially *albumin*, significantly add to the osmolarity and viscosity of blood. Centrifugation of the blood separates the red cells and white cells (*WBCs)* from the plasma. The RBCs are heaviest and are at the bottom after centrifugation. Above the red cells is a thin layer of white cells called the buffy coat. RBCs normally constitute 37-52% of the volume of the blood. The percentage of the blood that is RBCs is called the *hematocrit* or *packed cell volume* (PCV). A hematocrit below 37% is termed *anemia*.

Serum is the clear fluid left behind after blood has clotted. In effect serum is *plasma* that has had its clotting proteins removed.

Albumin, various *globulins* and *fibrinogen* are the most numerous proteins in plasma. *Albumin* is the smallest and most abundant plasma protein, and therefore, it contributes more to osmolarity and viscosity than other plasma proteins.

There are three classes of *globulins*: alpha, beta and gamma. The globulins of each class have markedly different functions.

Fibrin is the protein that forms the framework of a clot. *Fibrinogen* is the precursor of fibrin that is in plasma (fibrinogen is absent in serum). Most of the blood proteins, including albumin, fibrinogen and many of the globulins, are *produced by the liver.*

Any time proteins, peptides or amino acids are broken down, nitrogenous wastes are produced. Those wastes include ammonia, which is transformed into urea by the liver. Urea is transported by the blood to the kidneys, where it is excreted in the urine.

Erythrocytes

Hematopoiesis, or hemopoiesis, is the process by which the blood cells are created. The *red bone marrow* is the primary hematopoietic tissue in the body. Red blood cells, platelets and most white blood cells are produced in red marrow. The liver, spleen and thymus gland are capable of hematopoiesis in the fetus.

Erythropoiesis is the production of erythrocytes (RBCs); *myeloid hematopoiesis* is the production of *leukocytes* (WBCs) in the marrow. *Lymphocytes* (a type of WBC) are produced in the marrow and also in lymphoid tissues throughout the body including lymph nodes, tonsils, adenoids, thymus gland, spleen and lymphoid tissue in the intestines known as Peyer's patches.

Your red marrow generates about two and one-half million RBCs per second!

Erythrocytes and leukocytes evolve from precursor cells called *hemocytoblasts.* Hemocytoblasts that are destined to become erythrocytes are first transformed into *erythroblasts* and then into *reticulocytes* before they become mature erythrocytes. Erythroblasts, reticulocytes and immature erythrocytes are normally found in the marrow but *not the blood*. The nucleus of the precursor cells is gradually lost, and mature erythrocytes lack a nucleus. Other cellular changes that occur in erythrocyte maturation include a reduction in cell size and the synthesis of hemoglobin.

During the process of maturation, an RBC loses not only its nucleus but other organelles as well. It becomes essentially an enclosed packet of hemoglobin, which functions to transport oxygen. Normal erythrocytes are shaped like a disc with a thinner, indented central area. The discoid shape helps expose intracellular hemoglobin molecules to the plasma, and it thereby helps to transport oxygen. Erythrocytes also help transport carbon dioxide (CO_2), and they contain the enzyme **carbonic anhydrase**, which catalyzes the production of carbonic acid (H_2CO_3) from water and carbon dioxide. Carbonic acid is a buffer, and its presence helps maintain the pH of the blood at a constant 7.4. Carbonic acid aids in the transport of carbon dioxide and hydrogen ions so they can be eliminated by the lungs and kidneys.

Erythropoietin (EPO) is a hormone secreted by the kidneys and the liver by a negative feedback mechanism. Erythropoietin is secreted in hypoxic (low tissue levels of oxygen) and anemic states; it stimulates the production of mature erythrocytes from precursor cells. Individuals with renal (kidney) failure typically have low levels of erythropoietin, and they are anemic.

Red blood cells are essentially tiny packets of **hemoglobin (Hb)**, and hemoglobin accounts for over 95% of the intracellular proteins of a red cell. Hemoglobin is capable of binding with oxygen, and oxygen is distributed throughout the body by the hemoglobin in RBCs. Hemoglobin that has bound with oxygen has a bright red color. Non oxygenated hemoglobin has a much darker maroon to burgundy color. Thus arterial blood is bright red and venous blood is a dark purplish red.

Cyanosis is a blue tint imparted to the skin by the presence of hemoglobin lacking oxygen. **Erythema** is a red or pink flushing of the skin that is caused by the dilation of skin capillaries containing oxygenated hemoglobin. Generalized erythema occurs during fever and after exercise, and it occurs locally with inflammation due to trauma or infection.

Hemoglobin is a large molecule consisting of **four long protein** chains called **globins** and **four smaller moieties called heme**, each of which contains a ferrous iron (Fe++) ion in its center. Each heme moiety has the ability to weakly bind an oxygen molecule (O_2). It is **the ferrous ion in heme that binds with oxygen**. **CO_2 binds with the globin** moieties of hemoglobin. When **oxygen** is bound to the heme moiety in hemoglobin, it is called **oxyhemoglobin.** When **carbon dioxide** (CO_2) bound to the globin moieties in hemoglobin, it is called **carbaminohemoglobin**. **Carbon dioxide does not compete with oxygen binding**, and hemoglobin may transport both gases simultaneously. However, **carbon monoxide** (CO) is highly toxic because it competes with oxygen for binding sites on the heme moiety. Carbon monoxide not only competes with oxygen for the same binding sites, but it is 250 times more tightly bound to those sites than is oxygen. Therefore, CO will interfere with hemoglobin's oxygen carrying ability for hours or days. Hemoglobin bound to carbon monoxide (**carboxyhemoglobin or HbCO**) normally constitutes less than 1.5% of our total hemoglobin. Atmospheric CO levels will build up inside an enclosed garage with a gasoline motor running. An atmospheric concentration of CO of only 0.01% produces symptoms, and a concentration of 0.1% will bind half of your hemoglobin. A concentration of 0.2% is quickly fatal.

Anemia is the state of having too few erythrocytes in the blood. Anemia is a sign of another disorder, and there are many causes including blood loss, iron deficiency and renal disease. Symptoms include pale skin, lethargy and breathlessness.

The normal PCV (packed cell volume or hematocrit) is between 37-52%, with males averaging about 5% higher than females. A hematocrit below 37 denotes anemia.

The red blood cell count (RBC count) is a count of the number of erythrocytes in a microliter of blood. The normal level for the RBC count is between 4.2 and 6.2 million.

The hemoglobin content in 100 cc of blood can also be measured. The normal hemoglobin level is between 12-18 g/dL (grams per 100 cc). The average size of RBCs and their average hemoglobin content can be determined by comparing the RBC count, hematocrit and hemoglobin. Erythrocytes in iron deficiency states are typically small and contain lower levels of hemoglobin; this is termed a **microcytic, hypochromic anemia**. Pernicious anemia results from a vitamin B12 deficiency; a similar anemia is produced by a deficiency of folic acid, another B vitamin. The red blood cells are large (**macrocytic**) in patients with either of these deficiencies. RBCs in patients with hereditary spherocytosis are round rather than discoid, and they contain more hemoglobin than normal.

The normal hematocrit, hemoglobin and RBC count values are all higher in males.   Androgens (male hormones) stimulate erythropoiesis. Blood tends to clot more quickly in males than in females.

**Polycythemia** is the condition of having too many erythrocytes in the blood. Polycythemia can be secondary to a respiratory disorder such as emphysema, or it can be due to a primary disorder such as polycythemia vera. People with polycythemia have a dark, dusky red complexion with prominent subcutaneous veins, and they are described as _**plethoric**_. Patients with polycythemia may require intermittent removal of some of their blood. The intentional removal of blood for therapeutic purposes or for donation is called a _**phlebotomy.**_

Anemia, lung disorders, cardiac disorders and high altitudes can result in a low oxygen content, which is called _**hypoxemia**_ (low blood oxygen) and _**hypoxia**_ (low tissue oxygen).   The earth's atmosphere at altitudes over 10,000 feet does not have enough oxygen for normal body functions. People who live above 10,000 feet develop a compensatory physiologic polycythemia to adapt to the low amount of oxygen in the atmosphere; they will typically have 40-50% more erythrocytes in their blood than people living at sea level.   Athletes trained for endurance will also have higher levels of RBCs in their blood than normal.   "Blood doping" is transfusion of an athlete's own RBCs that were collected previously.   It increases the number of RBCs in circulation, and it increases endurance.

Right: The structure of **heme**. There are four heme moieties in each hemoglobin molecule. Oxygen binds to the ferrous ions in the center of the porphyrin rings.

Hemolysis is the premature and uncontrolled disruption of erythrocytes, which results in the release of hemoglobin into the plasma. Heme is converted into **bilirubin** by the liver.

Heme moiety in hemoglobin

Oxidation of the ferrous ion (Fe++) of heme to the ferric ion (Fe+++) cancels the ability of hemoglobin to bind with oxygen. _**Methemoglobin**_ is the oxidized (ferric) form of hemoglobin. Normally less than 1.7% of hemoglobin is methemoglobin. A higher level of methemoglobin in the blood is called _**methemoglobinemia**_; it can result from exposure to a number of drugs and chemicals including Sulfa drugs, phenacetin and nitrites. Cyanosis, hypoxia and lactic acidosis are signs of methemoglobinemia. Reducing agents in the blood such as ascorbic acid (vitamin C) can reduce methemoglobin to the ferrous form. Hereditary forms of methemoglobinemia exist. These people have an enzyme defect that leads to constantly elevated levels of methemoglobin in their blood, and they are strikingly cyanotic.

In the 120 day cycle of an erythrocyte, glucose slowly and irreversibly binds with hemoglobin forming _**glycosylated (glycated) hemoglobin or hemoglobin A1c**_. The amount of hemoglobin A1c in the blood reflects the average blood sugar levels for the previous month or two. Therefore, measurement of the hemoglobin A1c level in the blood is an indicator of blood sugar control in diabetics. The normal level of hemoglobin A1c in the blood is 4-6%.

The four chains of **_globins_** in a hemoglobin molecule can vary among individuals. In most adults there are two alpha chains and two beta chains. This genetic allele results in what is called hemoglobin A. But in a small number of adults the globin moieties are made up of two alpha chains and two delta chains. In the fetus two alpha chains and two gamma chains are present, which is called **_fetal hemoglobin_**. Fetal hemoglobin binds oxygen more tightly than does hemoglobin A. (The difference between beta, delta and gamma chains is due to a substitution of one or two amino acids in the protein). There are over a dozen alleles for different forms of hemoglobin, some of which produce disease.

Sickle-cell hemoglobin (HbS) is a common allele found in people of sub-Saharan African descent. The homozygous state of HbS (SS) results in sickle cell disease. The heterozygous state (SA, or hemoglobin S plus hemoglobin A) usually does not cause problems and is called sickle cell trait. When individuals with sickle cell disease exercise, the resulting hypoxemia leads to a change in the shape of the erythrocytes; they become elongated, curved and pointed. The misshapen RBCs clump together (agglutinate), and they can block small vessels, which may result in tissue damage, organ failure and premature death. The accepted theory of how the allele for sickle hemoglobin became common in Africa is intriguing. Malaria is a tropical disease caused by a parasite that invades erythrocytes, and it has been found that erythrocytes with sickle hemoglobin are relatively resistant to malaria. The persistence and frequency of HbS in the African genome is thought to be due to a greater resistance to the malaria parasite.

Two other genetic disorders involving hemoglobin are **_thalassemia_** and **_hemoglobin C disease._** Globin is defective, and globin production is deficient in thalassemia, resulting in slow erythropoiesis and fragile, short-lived erythrocytes. The heterozygous state for thalassemia is diagnosed as thalassemia minor; the homozygous condition is called thalassemia major because the symptoms are more severe. An individual with the combination of HbC and HbS (called S-C disease) has a disorder similar to those with the SS genotype, except SC sufferers have an especially poor prognosis with pregnancy.

The incidence of hemoglobinopathies differs among the races. Thalassemia is widespread, but it is most common among Mediterranean peoples. The alleles for hemoglobin S and C are exclusively of African origin.

Iron is not easily absorbed by the digestive system; the ferrous (Fe^{++}) valence is much easier to absorb than the more oxidized ferric (Fe^{+++}) valence. To be absorbed, iron ions must be bound to a protein in the stomach (gastroferritin) and then transported by transferritin, a protein in the blood. Iron is stored by binding with the protein, ferritin. Iron in tissue sections is identifiable as **_hemosiderin,_** which consists of clumps of iron and ferritin. Iron deficiency is most often caused by chronic blood loss, but a dietary deficiency can also be the etiology (cause). Iron absorption normally slows nearly to a stop in individuals with saturated iron stores, but patients with **_hemochromatosis_**, a genetic disorder, acquire an excessive amount of stored iron in their tissues, which can lead to organ failure. The heart, liver and pancreas are particularly susceptible to damage in hemochromatosis. People with familial hemochromatosis are treated by phlebotomy (intentional blood removal), which reduces their iron stores.

Erythrocytes survive in the blood for about four months; by that age the RBCs have become rigid and less functional. The **_spleen_** is the primary organ where RBCs are broken down and removed from circulation. Red cells can also be broken down in the liver and in the bone marrow. RBCs programmed for destruction are engulfed by phagocytes. The globins are broken down into amino acids, which are reutilized in protein production or burned as fuel. Iron is stripped from the heme moieties and reutilized. The heme moiety (a porphyrin) is converted into **_biliverdin,_** which has a green color and accounts for the greenish tint of severe bruises. Biliverdin is converted into **_bilirubin_**, a yellow-orange compound, which the liver secretes into the bile. Bile travels through the bile duct from the liver to the small intestine. Bilirubin is further broken down into urobilinogens, urobilins and stercobilins; these compounds are responsible for the color of the stool and urine. When bilirubin is present in excessive amounts in the blood and the tissues, it imparts a yellow tint that can be seen in the skin and the sclera of the eyes. This condition is called **_jaundice_**. Jaundice can be caused by liver disease, obstruction of the bile duct or excessive **_hemolysis_** (RBC breakdown).

Heme belongs to a class of compounds called **_porphyrins_**. Porphyrins consist of four **_pyrrole_** moieties (a pyrrole is a five ring structure containing nitrogen and methyl groups [CH_3]). The **_porphyrias_** are a group of inherited diseases characterized by excessive porphyrin production and excretion. Attacks of abdominal colic, skin lesions, hemolytic anemia, jaundice, psychoses and neurological disorders are symptoms of porphyria. The porphyrins are bright yellow, red and burgundy compounds, and some porphyrics will have red or brown urine, skin and teeth. Individuals with some forms of porphyria must avoid sun exposure because porphyrin deposits in their skin create an extreme sensitivity to sunlight.

Clotting

Platelets are tiny cellular fragments released from red marrow into the blood. They consist of fragments of cytoplasm surrounded by a membrane. They are created by a pinching-off process from the plasma membranes of large marrow cells known as *megakaryocytes.* Megakaryocytes evolve from hemocytoblasts, the same cells that are the precursors of RBCs and WBCs. Platelets are also known as *thrombocytes*. This term implies that they are true cells, but platelets are cellular fragments. They are not true cells, and they do not contain a nucleus, although they may contain lysosomes, endoplasmic reticulum, mitochondria and Golgi bodies. Platelets of some mammalian species do contain a nucleus and are true cells. The concentration of platelets can be measured from a blood sample. The normal count is >100,000 per microliter, but unless a platelet count is specifically requested, most technicians will simply survey a blood smear and call the number of platelets "adequate" if scattered platelets are seen and appear to be of sufficient number. *Thrombocytopenia* is the term for the condition when too few platelets are present in the blood.

Platelets have the ability to clump together to form a *platelet* plug, which is the first step in the clotting process. They also promote vasoconstriction, which helps stop bleeding. A *thrombus* is a blood clot within a blood vessel; thrombi form as a result of platelets sticking to the wall of the vessel. An *embolus* is any material that abnormally and briefly circulates in the blood stream. A thrombus may become an embolus if it becomes dislodged from the wall of a blood vessel. Emboli travel through the circulation, and they may occlude small vessels in the lungs or any other organ or tissue.

The clotting of blood is necessary for *hemostasis*, which literally means "cessation of bleeding." Platelets secrete five of the factors necessary for clotting, but those are not the only factors involved in clotting. *Calcium ions* in the blood and *numerous clotting factors* are necessary for normal clotting to occur. The liver synthesizes a majority of the clotting factors and releases them into the blood stream. The liver requires *vitamin K* to synthesize four of the factors it produces, and large doses of vitamin K are given to counteract some anticoagulants (the warfarin drugs) and to promote prenatal clotting. There are over thirty chemical reactions going on during clot formation, and there are two separate pathways by which clots form, depending upon whether tissue has been cut or not. If tissue has been cut, *tissue thromboplastin* is released, which sets up a cascade leading to *thrombin* production. Thrombin is an enzyme that catalyzes the conversion of *fibrinogen* to fibrin, and fibrin forms the framework for a blood clot. Once a clot has formed and bleeding has stopped, *clot retraction* begins, which pulls the edges of the ruptured blood vessel closer together and helps seal the vascular wound. After the wound has been sealed, the clot begins to dissolve by a process known as *fibrinolysis.*

If bleeding occurs in a tissue due to blunt trauma, and there has been no incision into tissue, a series of reactions involving several clotting factors eventually leads to thrombin formation. *Factor VIII* is one of those factors. A genetic defect in factor VIII production is the cause of *classic hemophilia*, or *hemophilia A*. This *sex-linked recessive* inherited disease affects one in five thousand males, and it is the cause of 83% of all hemophilia. Contrary to popular belief, classic hemophiliacs have little to fear from minor skin cuts or incisions because tissue thromboplastin is released by the cut, and clot formation would not require factor VIII. However, classic hemophiliacs are susceptible to bleeding from blunt trauma, which does not release tissue thromboplastin. Hemophiliacs often find that they will bleed into joints following minor blunt trauma, and repeated bleeding into joints can result in joint destruction.

There are other types of hemophilia in which clot formation is defective including *von Willebrand's disease* and *factor IX deficiency*. In von Willebrand's disease a factor is missing that binds and stabilizes factor VIII. Factor IX deficiency is called *hemophilia B;* it is a *recessive sex-linked* inherited disorder that affects one in thirty thousand males and accounts for 15% of all hemophilia. Factor II deficiency is called *hemophilia C*. Hemophilia C is a rare *autosomal recessive* disorder that affects males and females equally.

Anticoagulants are substances that prevent clot formation. They act in various ways to block one of the steps in the clotting process. Warfarin drugs like coumadin and dicumerol interfere with the action of vitamin K, which is necessary for the liver to produce ***prothrombin***, a precursor of thrombin. Warfarin anticoagulants are found in red clover. Cattle that graze on red clover are subject to hemorrhagic conditions. Warfarin anticoagulants are the prime ingredient in rat poisons. Large doses of vitamin K are given to counteract the anticoagulant effect of warfarin.

TPA, or tissue plasminogen activator, is capable of dissolving recently formed clots by stimulating ***plasmin*** production. (Plasmin is an enzyme that breaks down fibrin). Unwanted and uncontrollable bleeding can be an undesirable side effect of TPA.

Streptokinase and urokinase are enzymes that lead to the creation of plasmin.

Heparin is an anticoagulant that activates antithrombin-III, which blocks thrombin formation. Protamine is a drug that blocks the anticoagulant effect of heparin.

Aspirin (acetylsalicylic acid or ASA) and many other drugs inhibit platelet agglutination and platelet enzymes.

EDTA (ethylenediaminotetroacetic acid) is used in the laboratory to prevent blood samples from clotting. It is also used as a preservative in solutions, foods and medications. EDTA prevents clotting by binding with calcium ions.

CDP (citratephosphate dextrose) is used in blood banks to keep blood from clotting so it can be stored for long periods of time. CDP acts by binding with calcium ions.

There are several laboratory tests that determine the ability of blood to clot. Some are seldom used today. The ***clotting time*** is done by simply putting blood into a tube and determining how long it takes to form a clot. The ***bleeding time*** is determined by placing a blood pressure cuff on the arm, and then making a small shallow cut into the skin of the forearm. The length of time it takes for the cut to stop bleeding is the bleeding time. A bleeding time of one to nine minutes is normal. The ***prothrombin time*** measures the amount of prothrombin in the blood by measuring the time required to form thrombin. This test is frequently used to check the proper dose of warfarin anticoagulants. The ***partial thromboplastin time*** (PTT) is a good screening test for clotting disorders because a deficiency of most factors will produce a prolonged PTT. ***Heparin*** is an anticoagulant that is used frequently to prevent clotting. The correct dose of heparin is monitored by the PTT.

Leukocytes

Whereas there are between 4.2 and 6.2 million RBCs per 100 cc of blood, there normally are only 5-10 thousand white blood cells (***leukocytes*** or WBCs) per 100 cc of blood normally. Leukocytes are considerably larger than erythrocytes, and there are several types of leukocytes. The process of leukocyte production involves the differentiation of hemocytoblasts into three types: ***(1)*** the granulocyte-monocyte-megakaryocyte precursors, ***(2)*** the B lymphocyte and NK (natural killer) lymphocyte precursors, and ***(3)*** the T lymphocyte precursors.

Neutrophiles, eosinophiles and basophiles are classified as ***granulocytes*** because they contain large granules in their cytoplasm. The granules of neutrophiles do not take up ***hematoxylin and eosin*** (H&E) stain well, but the granules of eosinophiles stain red, and the granules of basophiles stain dark blue with an H&E stain. (Hematoxylin and eosin are two stains that are combined for tissue staining. The hematoxylin stain is blue; the eosin stain is red). Granulocytes have amoeboid movement, and they are capable of migrating out of the blood and into the tissues. Neutrophiles and eosinophiles are capable of phagocytizing debris, viruses and bacteria (pathogens). Neutrophiles are the first WBCs to arrive at an injury site, and they contain numerous ***lysosomes*** whose enzymes attack invaders. The number of neutrophiles in the blood increases dramatically in most bacterial infections.

Eosinophiles become numerous in the blood in allergic conditions and in helminthic (worm) infestations.

Basophiles are much less common than neutrophiles or eosinophiles. Their granules contain ***histamine and heparin***, and these compounds are released into areas of injury. Histamine dilates blood vessels and makes them more permeable, and heparin prevents clotting. Tissue basophiles are called ***mast cells***. Mast cells also release histamine and heparin, but they are distinct from blood basophiles, and they have a different origin.

Monocytes are large cells that are derived from the same precursor cells as granulocytes (hemocytoblasts). Although monocytes contain fine granules in their cytoplasm, they are not considered to be granulocytes, and they are classified as ***agranulocytes***. Many monocytes leave the blood stream and enter the tissues where they are known as ***macrophages***.

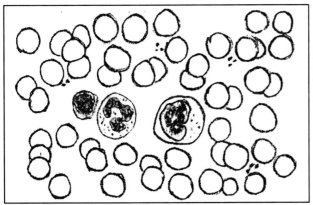

Left: This drawing shows, from left to right, a small lymphocyte, a neutrophile and a monocyte. There are numerous erythrocytes visible. The small dark bodies scattered about are platelets.

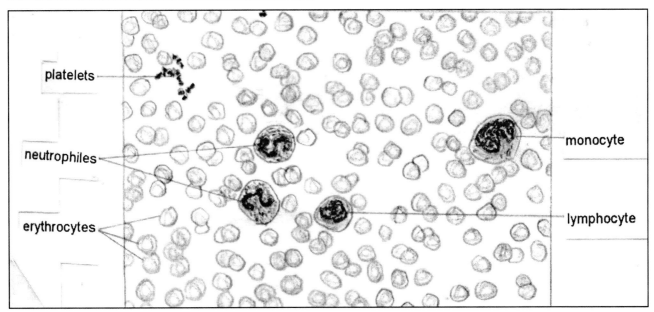

Above: A typical blood smear. Platelets and numerous erythrocytes are visible. Four leukocytes are seen in this drawing. Neutrophiles are usually the most common leukocyte, followed by lymphocytes.

There are three main categories of _**lymphocytes:**_ (1) _**T cells**_ (thymus-dependant), (2) _**B cells**_ (bone marrow-derived), and (3) _**NK**_ (natural killer) cells. Most lymphocyte production takes place in the bone marrow, but one group of lymphocyte stem cells travels to the thymus gland of young individuals where thymic hormones transform them into _**T cells**_. These cells then leave the thymus and travel to the bone marrow and lymphoid organs such as the spleen.

85% of the circulating lymphocytes are _**T cells.**_ There are three types of T cells, _**helper**_ T cells, _**suppressor**_ T cells and _**cytotoxic**_ T cells. _**Helper T cells**_ stimulate the activation of both T cells and B cells. _**Suppressor T cells**_ inhibit the activation and function of T cells and B cells. _**Cytotoxic T cells**_ attack foreign cells and cells infected by viruses. The attack by cytotoxic cells commonly involves direct contact. T cells are the primary cells involved in _**cell-mediated immunity**_. An infection by the human immunodeficiency virus is the cause of AIDS (acquired immunodeficiency syndrome). This virus suppresses immunity by preferentially attacking helper T cells.

**B cells** account for 10-15% of circulating lymphocytes. When stimulated (by a helper T cell), B cells are activated to differentiate into _**plasma cells**_. Plasma cells and B lymphocytes produce _**antibodies,**_ which are proteins that bind to _**antigens**_. Antigens are chemical substances often associated with _**pathogens**_ (disease causing microorganisms). _**B cells and plasma cells are responsible for**_ _**antibody-mediated immunity**_, which is also known as _**humoral**_ (liquid, or blood) _**immunity**_.

Plasma cells develop from activated B lymphocytes. They are tissue cells that produce ***gamma globulin*** (antibodies). Plasma cells are not usually seen in the blood except in a few neoplastic states such as plasma cell leukemia and multiple myeloma. Atypical monocytes are seen in the blood in large numbers in infectious mononucleosis ("mono"), and these cells may somewhat resemble plasma cells.

5-10% of all circulating lymphocytes are ***natural killer cells (NK cells).*** **NK cells** attack foreign cells and virus infected cells. They are a natural defense against cancer, and they are capable of killing cancer cells. The continuous policing of body tissues by the NK cells has been called immunological surveillance.

A ***differential count*** involves identifying 100 WBCs in a smear of blood, which establishes the percentage of each type of leukocytes in the blood. Normal proportions for leukocytes in the blood are
neutrophiles – 50-70%
eosinophiles – 2-4%
basophiles – less than 1%
lymphocytes – 20-30%
monocytes – 2-8%

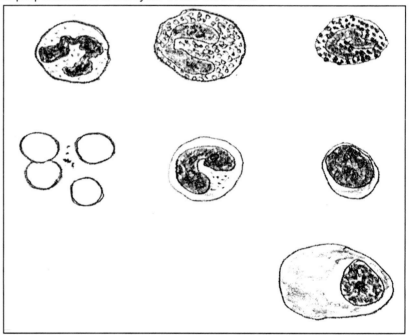

Right: A drawing of leukocyte types.
(Reading left to right)
Top row: Granulocytes. Specifically, neutrophile; eosinophile; basophile. The granules of eosinophiles stain red with eosin; the granules of basophiles stain blue with hematoxylin. The granules of neutrophiles and monocytes do not stain well with either eosin or hematoxylin.

Second row: Erythrocytes and platelets; monocyte; lymphocyte

Third row: Plasma cell (normally absent in a blood smear.)

When the number of leukocytes in the blood is lower than normal, it is called ***leukopenia***. Leukopenia may be seen in radiation sickness, heavy metal toxicity (Pb, Hg, As), and in some viral infections including AIDS.

When the normal leukocyte count of 5-10,000 is exceeded, it is called ***leukocytosis.*** Leukocytosis secondary to an excessive number of neutrophiles is seen in most bacterial infections. Viral infections frequently tend to cause a small increase in ***agranulocytes*** (lymphocytes and monocytes). ***Leukemia*** includes a group of neoplastic disorders with greatly increased numbers of leukocytes in the blood. Myelogenous leukemia is characterized by an increased number of granulocytes; lymphocytic leukemia is characterized by an increased number of lymphocytes. The leukemias are classified as acute or chronic. Acute leukemia appears suddenly and progresses rapidly. Chronic leukemia progresses slowly and may not result in mortality for many years or decades.

Blood typing
Blood typing involves identifying genetic markers on the surface of red cells. Many types of antigens exist as carbohydrates that make up the glycocalyx of our red cells. The best known and most important markers are those in the ***ABO system***. There are two specific antigens (called A and B) on erythrocytes in this system. The A and B antigens are inherited as autosomal dominant traits. The presence or absence of these antigens determines the ABO blood type. The O antigen is the absence of either the A or B antigen.

Six different genetic inheritance patterns are possible in this system. They are (1) homozygous AA, (2) homozygous BB, (3) heterozygous AO, (4) heterozygous BO, (5) homozygous OO, and (6) heterozygous codominant AB.

Individuals with the genotype AA or AO would have type A blood, since the A antigen would be present in both genotypes. Individuals with the BB or BO genotype would have type B blood, and individuals with the OO genotype would have type O blood. Individuals with the genotype AB would have both A and B antigens present, and they would have type AB blood.

The antigen on type A erythrocytes is a four sugar branched moiety with the structure
Cell membrane—glucose—galactose--fucose
                                                |
                              N-acetylgalactosamine

The antigen in type B erythrocytes is similar to type A, but with a galactose moiety in place of the N-acetylgalactosamine. Its structure is
Cell membrane---glucose---galactose---fucose
                                      |
                            galactose

In type O individuals, the glycocalyx is a nonantigenic trisaccharide with the structure
Cell membrane—glucose—galactose—fucose.

All RBCs, no matter the blood type, contain the O trisaccharide, which is the basis for both the A and the B antigen; consequently the O trisaccharide is not antigenic. All type AB erythrocytes have both the type A antigen and the type B antigen on their cell membranes. Individuals with the genotype AA or AO lack the B antigen on their erythrocytes. Individuals who have the genotype BB or BO lack the A antigen on their erythrocytes.

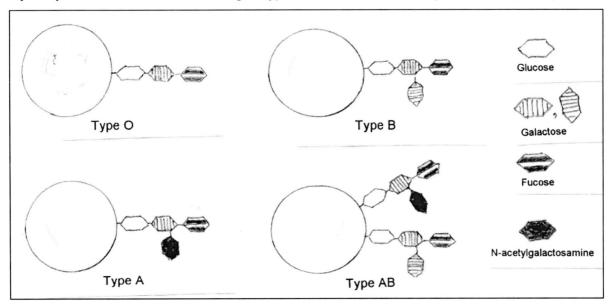

Above: This drawing depicts the glycocalyces of type O, type A, type B and type AB blood.

Blood typing in the laboratory is determined by mixing an individual's blood with antisera (serum containing a specific antibody) to the A or B antigens. When blood containing type A antigen is mixed with antiserum with type A antibodies, a visible agglutination occurs. The same is true if blood with type B antigen is mixed with antiserum with type B antibodies. Type AB blood would agglutinate when mixed with either anti A or anti B antisera, and type O blood would agglutinate with neither.

When transfusing a patient, care must be taken that the donor's blood cells do not agglutinate. If the recipient has blood type O, he will have antibodies to both A and B antigens, and therefore, he can receive only type O blood. Someone with type A blood could receive either type A or type O blood, and someone with type B blood could receive either type B or type O. A patient with type AB blood could receive either type A, type B, type AB or type O because the patient with type AB blood would have no antibodies to any of the antigens. Thus type AB is called the **_"universal recipient,"_** and type O is called the **_"universal donor."_** However, it is usually best to transfuse blood of the same type as the recipient. Although a type AB recipient can usually receive type O blood without a reaction, the presence of anti A and anti B antibodies in the donor blood can cause mild agglutination of the recipient's type AB red cells.

If blood is transfused incorrectly, the agglutination process results in **_hemolysis_** (RBC disruption). Hemolysis releases hemoglobin into the plasma. If the transfusion reaction is significant, the free hemoglobin can block tubules in the kidneys and be fatal.

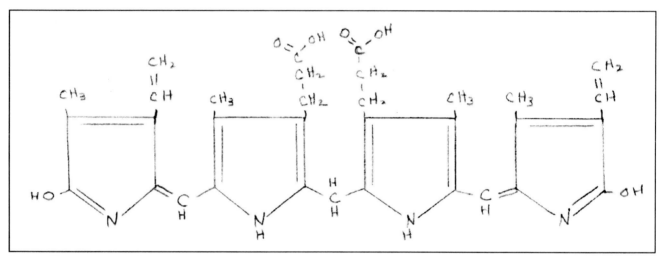

Above: The structure of bilirubin. In the formation of bilirubin the porphyrin ring of heme is broken into a chain with four pyrroles. Each pyrrrole is a five ringed structure containing nitrogen and methyl groups.

Blood typing also involves the determination of other antigens, the next most important being the **_Rh factor_**. Those with the Rh antigen on their RBCs are called Rh positive (Rh+), and those lacking this antigen are called Rh negative (Rh-). Only Rh- individuals who have been exposed to Rh+ blood will have antibodies to the Rh factor. This is especially important during pregnancy because Rh antibodies can cross the placenta, unlike antibodies to the A and B antigens. Mothers who are Rh- are often sensitized to the Rh factor during the birth of an Rh+ infant because mixing of maternal and fetal blood occurs during the birth process. This causes no problem with the first Rh+ child because maternal antibodies have not had time to form. But any subsequent Rh+ babies conceived by this mother are exposed to maternal Rh antibodies. Hemolysis may occur from any antigenic incompatibility, but an Rh incompatibility between Rh+ infants and sensitized Rh- mothers tends to cause an exceptionally severe hemolysis in the infant. Hemolysis in these infants may occur before birth or soon after birth, and it can lead to a severe hemolytic anemia and jaundice.   The anemia may be mild, but severe cases are diagnosed as **_erythroblastosis fetalis_**, or **_hemolytic disease of the newborn_**. Bilirubin levels may reach such high levels that brain damage occurs due to the precipitation of bilirubin in the brain – a condition known as **_kernicterus_**. Also the kidneys and other organs may fail due to the precipitation of bilirubin and hemoglobin. Treatment for these infants includes complete exchange transfusions to replace the infant's Rh+ erythrocytes with Rh- erythrocytes, which would not be destroyed by the mother's antibodies. The mother's antibodies remain in the infant for one to two months, and without a complete exchange transfusion these antibodies would hemolyze any new RBCs produced by the baby. In the worst cases it may even be necessary to induce a premature delivery so that the fetus can undergo an exchange transfusion immediately after birth.   Ultraviolet light breaks down bilirubin as it passes through capillaries in the skin, and uv lamps are frequently used to treat hemolytic conditions in the newborn.

Sensitization of an Rh- mother who has delivered an Rh+ baby can usually be prevented if anti Rh antibodies are given to her in late gestation, during delivery and immediately after delivery. This is carried out using the product **_RhoGam_**, which consists of anti Rh antibodies. RhoGam destroys the infant's Rh+ cells that have reached the mother's circulation before those cells can stimulate an immune response in the mother. Despite the availability of RhoGam, there is a twenty percent incidence of sensitization to the Rh factor in an Rh- mother who has delivered an Rh+ infant.

The prevalence of A and B antigens differs among races. The A antigen exists in about 40% of Caucasian Americans and 27% of Black Americans. The B antigen is present in 11% of Caucasian Americans and 20% of Black Americans. Type O is the most common blood type in the U.S.; 47% of White Americans and 45% of all Americans have type O blood.

Type B is uncommon in Caucasians, but it frequently is present in the Chinese and the people of India. American Indians have no B antigens and a very low incidence of A antigens. Over 97% of American Indians are type O.

The presence of the Rh factor also differs among the races. Eighty-six percent of all Americans are Rh+. The highest incidence of Rh negativity is 29% in the Basques of Spain and France. Other Caucasian groups have significant numbers of Rh- people. Rh negativity is less common in African Blacks, and it is rare in the Chinese. All American Indians and Australian Aborigines who have been tested have been found to be Rh+.

In the process of matching blood for transfusion, many other antigens are checked in order to get the best possible match.

Study Guide

1. Know the meaning of hematology and the following laboratory tests: packed cell volume (PCV), hematocrit, and red blood cell count (RBC count) and hemoglobin.
2. What are the proteins of blood, and where are most of them produced?
3. What is hematopoiesis? What is erythropoiesis?
4. Where does erythropoiesis take place in the adult? -- In the fetus?
5. What is erythropoietin and where is it produced?
6. What is cyanosis and what are its causes?
7. What is the difference between oxyhemoglobin, carbaminohemoglobin and carboxyhemoglobin?
8. What moieties are in hemoglobin? Which moiety contains Fe?
9. Which part of the hemoglobin molecule combines with oxygen? Which combines with carbon dioxide? Which combines with carbon monoxide?
10. Define anemia, microcytic anemia and macrocytic anemia.
11. Define polycythemia.
12. What reaction is catalyzed by the enzyme, carbonic anhydrase?
13. Know that hemoglobin S, hemoglobin C and thalassemia are abnormalities of the globin part of hemoglobin.
14. Recognize that the spleen is the major organ for removing old, worn out erythrocytes from the circulation.
15. Understand the metabolism of the porphyrins, hemoglobin and bilirubin.
16. Where are platelets produced, and what is their function?
17. What is a thrombus?
18. What is an embolus?
19. Understand the clotting reactions taking place following an incision into the skin and following blunt trauma.
20. What are the different classes of lymphocytes?
21. Know where helper T cells, suppressor T cells, cytotoxic T cells, B cells, plasma cells and natural killer (NK) cells are produced and how they function.
22. Define leukocytosis, leukopenia and leukemia.
23. Understand blood typing and its relation to the glycocalyx.
24. What is erythroblastosis fetalis? What is kernicterus?
25. Why are infants with erythroblastosis fetalis and kernicterus jaundiced?

Chapter Nineteen

Blood Vessels

In 1628 William Harvey, an English anatomist, became the first to discover and describe the flow of blood through the body. No one before Harvey had a correct understanding of how blood circulates through the heart and blood vessels.

The blood vessels include the *arteries, capillaries and veins*. Small arteries are called *arterioles*. Small veins are called *venules*. *Sinusoids* are dilated capillaries. The heart pumps blood into the arteries, which lead to a network of capillaries. Blood returns to the heart through the veins.

Blood flows from the heart into two separate circuits, the *systemic circuit* and the *pulmonary circuit.*
In the *systemic circuit* oxygen-rich blood is pumped from the left ventricle of the heart into the aorta, which is the largest artery in the body and the trunk of the arterial tree. Blood then flows into smaller arteries and arterioles to a capillary network where blood gives up oxygen and nutrients to the tissue cells and receives carbon dioxide and wastes from the tissues. Veins then carry oxygen-poor blood back to the superior and inferior vena cava, which empty into the right atrium of the heart.

In the *pulmonary circuit* oxygen-poor blood is pumped from the right ventricle of the heart into the pulmonary artery trunk, which divides into a right and a left branch that go to the right and left lungs respectively. Smaller arterial branches lead to capillary beds in the lungs where the blood picks up oxygen and releases carbon dioxide. The pulmonary veins then carry the oxygen-rich blood to the left atrium of the heart.

Arteries

An *artery* is a three-layered tube. The inner layer, or tunica interna, is a simple squamous epithelial layer called the *endothelium*. The endothelium has a smooth surface so that blood will not clot. The middle layer, or *tunica media*, contains smooth muscle and elastic connective tissue. This layer controls the diameter of the arterial lumen, and therefore, it controls blood pressure. Smooth muscle of the tunica media receives input from the sympathetic division of the autonomic nervous system. Larger arteries have a *tunica adventitia*, which is an outer layer of strong, fibrous connective tissue that helps prevent rupture of the artery. Only the endothelium and smooth muscle layer continue into the smaller arteries and arterioles.

Right: An artery and a vein. The layers are
(1) Endothelium
(2) Basement membrane
(3) Layer of smooth muscle
(4) Elastic layer
(5) Connective tissue
The tunica intima is the endothelium with its basement membrane.
The tunica media is the smooth muscle and elastic tissue layer.
The tunica adventitia is fibrous connective tissue around an artery or vein. Veins lack the elastic layer, and the layer of smooth muscle around a vein is considerably less developed than that around arteries.

Right: Capillaries are tiny thin walled tubes consisting only of an endothelial cell and its basement membrane.

The ***aorta*** is a continuous vessel from the heart to the pelvis, where it bifurcates into the right and left common iliac arteries. The aorta is given various descriptions according to its regional location. Those include the ascending aorta, the aortic arch, the descending aorta, the thoracic aorta and the abdominal aorta. The ascending aorta is a short, one inch long, trunk extending from the heart to the aortic arch. The aortic arch is a curve in the aorta that ends in the descending aorta. The descending aorta includes the abdominal aorta and part of the thoracic aorta.

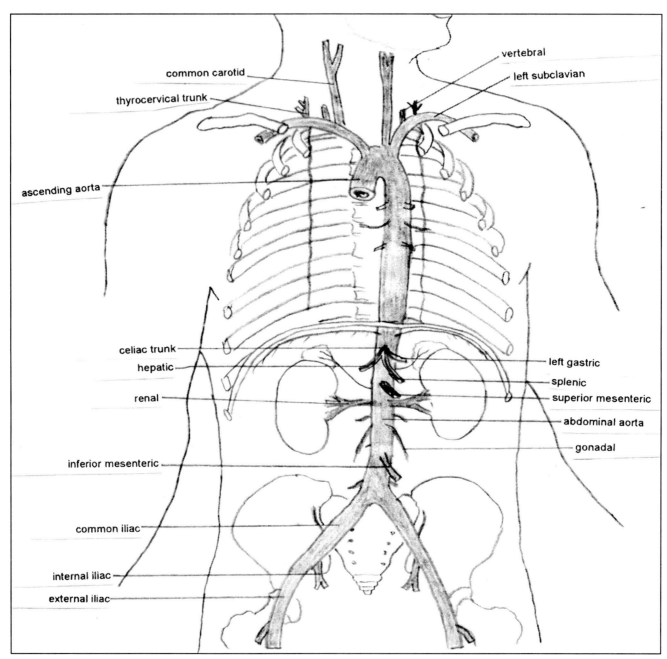

Above: The arteries of the trunk.

The right and left ***coronary arteries*** supply the heart muscle with blood; they are the only branches of the ***ascending aorta.*** Arteries that branch off the ***aortic arch*** go to the head, neck and upper extremities; they are the ***right brachiocephalic*** artery (to the right side of the head and right arm), the ***left common carotid*** (to the left side of the head), and the ***left subclavian arteries*** (to the left arm).

The descending aorta gives off vessels that supply tissues and organs in the thorax, abdomen and pelvis, including branches to the liver, kidneys, spleen, digestive organs, reproductive organs, and muscles. The aorta divides into two **_common iliac arteries_** at the L-2 level, and each of these arteries divides into an internal and an external iliac artery.   The **_femoral arteries_** are branches of the external iliac arteries that supply the lower extremities with blood.

Superficially located arteries have pulsations that can be felt through the skin. Such arteries are designated as **_palpable_**. They include the superficial temporal artery in front of the ear, the carotids in the neck, and the radial artery at the lateral flexor surface of the wrist. In the lower extremity the femoral artery is palpable in the groin, the posterior tibial artery is palpable behind the medial malleolus, and the dorsalis pedis artery is palpable on the dorsum of the foot and ankle.

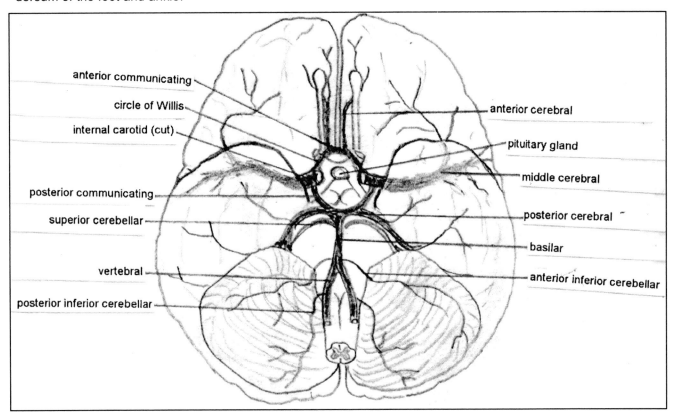

Above: The arteries of the brain. The circle of Willis is an anastomotic circle of cerebral arteries around the pituitary gland.

An **_anastomosis_** is a short cut connection between vessels; it can be an artery to an artery, an artery to a vein, or a vein to a vein. Anastomoses exist in branches of the coronary arteries, and these anastomoses can shunt oxygenated blood where needed. Venous anastomoses are ubiquitous in the body; they serve to bypass obstructed channels.

Arterio-venous anastomoses can be created surgically. This is occasionally done in patients who require repeated transfusions or hemodialysis because their veins become scarred and fibrotic due to repeated venapunctures. Transfusing blood and the administration of venous fluids become increasingly difficult in these patients. A surgically created A-V anastomosis is called a shunt. It dilates the proximal veins, which greatly facilitates the placement of an IV needle.

Not all anastomoses are beneficial. The **_circle of Willis_** is made up of artery to artery anastomoses between the anterior cerebral, middle cerebral and posterior cerebral arteries and three communicating arteries (the anterior communicating artery and the right and left posterior communicating arteries). Blood to the circle of Willis comes from the right and left carotid arteries and the basilar artery. The circle of Willis is a common site for arterial

aneurysms (bubble-like bulges of an arterial wall).   Rupture of an aneurysm in the circle of Willis, if not immediately fatal, can create an arterio-venous (A-V) anastomosis that empties into the surrounding cavernous sinus. The flow of shunted blood through such an anastomosis is often audible to the patient and the physician.

Blockage of the left subclavian artery can lead eventually to the dilation of arterial vessels that are collateral channels between the left carotid artery and the left subclavian artery beyond the block. Blood moving through these vessels is shunted from the left side of the head to the left arm. Arterial insufficiency to the brain may result, which is a condition known as the "***subclavian steal syndrome***."

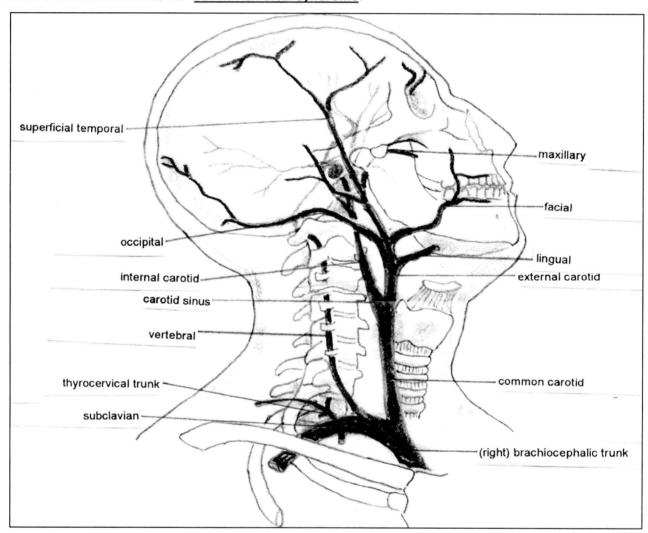

Above: The arteries of the head and neck.

There are interesting peculiarities in the position of some arteries. The gonadal arteries supply the ovaries and testes. The right gonadal artery is a branch of the aorta, but the left gonadal is a branch of the left renal artery, which is an important anatomical discrepancy when an operation such as a nephrectomy (kidney removal) is done. The intercostal arteries are branches of the descending aorta in the thorax. The intercostal arteries and veins are located adjacent to the lower margins of the ribs. Knowledge of the position of the intercostal vessels is necessary to prevent unnecessary bleeding when doing a perforating incision into the chest cavity.

Veins

Arteries are under considerable pressure due to the pumping action of the heart and the contraction of smooth muscle and elastic tissue in their ***tunica media***. Arterial blood is pumped by the heart and squeezed by the smooth muscle and the elastic tissue in the tunica media. This is what produces the ***blood pressure***. In contrast the walls of ***veins*** are much thinner that that of arteries, and consequently blood in the veins is under little pressure. However, veins have a layer of smooth muscle, and they can constrict, which is important in controlling a hemorrhage. ***Venules*** are small veins that carry blood into larger veins.

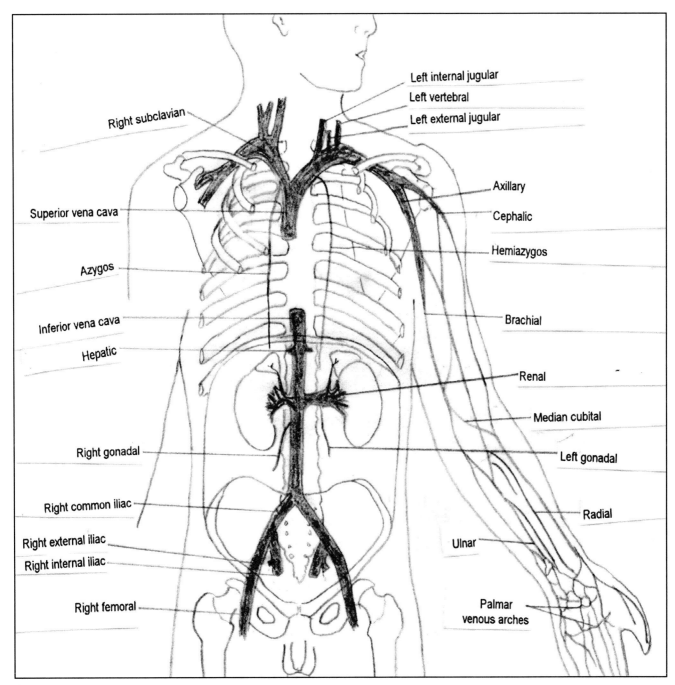

Above: Veins of the trunk and upper extremity. The inferior and superior venae cava drain into the right atrium of the heart. The heart is not shown in this illustration. Note that the right gonadal vein empties into the vena cava, but the left gonadal vein empties into the left renal vein.

When one is standing, blood in the legs has difficulty returning against gravity to the heart because venous blood is under little pressure. ***Valves*** in the veins of the legs help accomplish venous return to the heart. Walking requires intermittent contraction of the leg muscles, which helps propel the blood in the veins upward. Prolonged standing leads to stasis of blood flow in the legs, venous distension, insufficiency of the valves of the leg veins, and the formation of dilated venous sacs called ***varicose veins***. A ***varix*** is a single out-pouching or bulge in a vein.

Right: The veins of the head and neck.

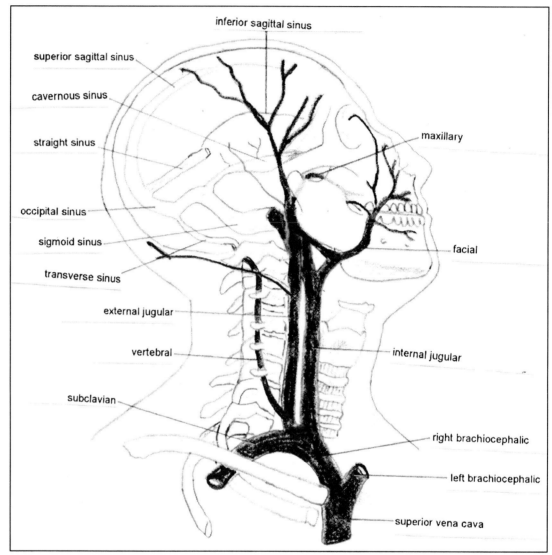

Veins in the extremities are classified as deep or superficial. Venous arches in the foot send blood to the deep and superficial vessels of the leg. The deep veins of the leg unite to form the ***popliteal vein*** near the knee. The ***femoral vein*** of the thigh receives blood from the popliteal vein and other veins. Superficial veins of the lower extremity include the ***great saphenous*** medially and the ***small saphenous*** laterally. The great saphenous is the longest vein in the body. It empties into the femoral vein near the hip. The small saphenous vein empties into the popliteal vein.

The veins of the forearm receive blood from a deep and a superficial ***palmar venous arch*** in the hand. The deep palmar veins drain into the ***radial vein*** and the ***ulnar vein***. These two veins fuse above the elbow to form the ***brachial vein***, which becomes the ***axillary vein*** in the axilla.

The superficial palmar arch empties into the ***cephalic vein*** laterally, the median antebrachial vein, and the ***basilic vein*** medially. The median antebrachial vein joins the basilic vein below the elbow. The cephalic vein sends a branch to the basilic vein near the elbow (the ***median cubital vein***). This branch is the site from which most blood samples are taken. The basilic vein joins the brachial vein in the upper arm. The cephalic vein drains into the axillary vein to form the subclavian vein.

Intravenous fluids are most often given through catheters in the superficial veins of the hand or forearm. Other preferred sites for entry into the venous system for cardiac procedures and long term catheters include the femoral veins, subclavian veins and cephalic veins. The great saphenous vein is the preferred donor vessel for arterial bypass procedures.

Right: The veins of the brain.

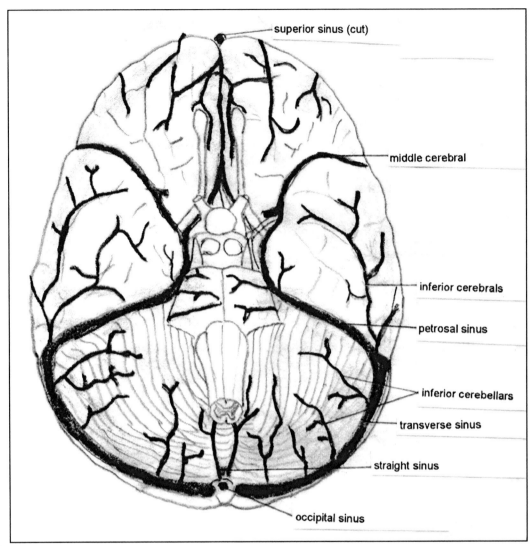

Capillaries

Arteries branch into smaller efferent vessels called **_arterioles._** Arterioles lead into **_capillaries,_** which are tiny blood vessels that make up a vascular network between arterioles and venules. The capillary network is where oxygen and nutrients diffuse from the blood to the tissues, and carbon dioxide and wastes enter the blood. The wall of a capillary consists only of a thin layer of simple squamous epithelium called the **_endothelium_** and its basement membrane. The thinness of capillary walls assures that diffusion of materials can occur to and from the capillaries and the tissues.

Most tissues have an extensive capillary network; however, capillaries are absent from the epidermis, cartilage, and from the lens and cornea of the eye.

Precapillary sphincters are rings of smooth muscle at the arterial end of capillary networks. They regulate the amount of blood flow to an area.

Sinusoids are large dilated capillaries. Sinusoids are more permeable than other capillaries, and they allow the passage of large substances such as proteins and erythrocytes. Sinusoids are found in the liver, spleen, bone marrow and pituitary gland.

The Hepatic Portal Circulation

The **_hepatic portal circulation_** is a special system of venous circulation within the systemic circulation. The mesenteric and splenic arteries supply the stomach, intestines, pancreas and spleen with blood. Venous blood from these organs drains into the **_portal vein_**, which leads to a sinusoidal capillary bed in the **_liver._** The liver absorbs much of the **_chyle_** (digested food material) that is carried by the portal vein. Blood flows from the liver to hepatic veins, which drain into the inferior vena cava. The inferior vena cava empties into the right atrium of the heart. Two **_capillary networks_** are present in the hepatic portal system. The first capillary network is in the spleen and the organs and glands of the digestive tract. The second capillary network is in the liver; it consists of dilated, porous, sinusoidal capillaries. Digested material from the intestines is transported to the liver via the portal vein. These substances are acted upon in the liver, where glucose is turned into glycogen, amino acids are turned into proteins, and cholesterol and lipoproteins are synthesized. The liver absorbs and detoxifies ethyl alcohol, ammonia and other toxins that it receives from the digestive tract. The liver receives oxygen rich blood from the **_hepatic artery_**, a branch of the celiac trunk, which is a branch of the aorta.

A similar but much smaller portal system exists between the hypothalamus and the anterior pituitary. The pituitary portal system governs the output of hormones from the anterior pituitary.

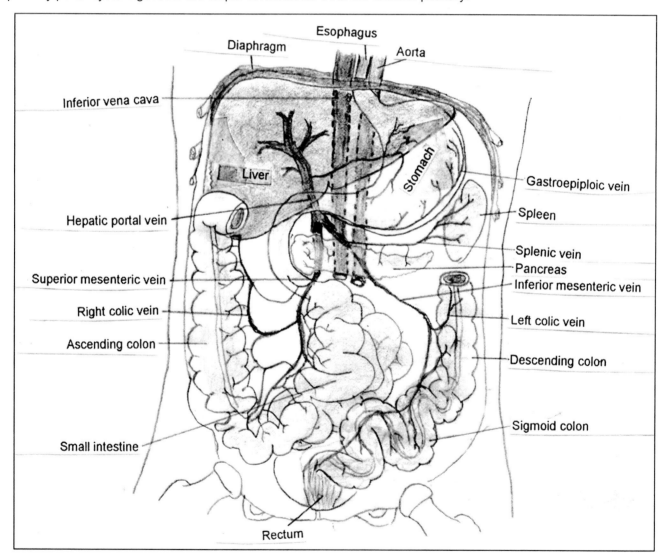

Above: The hepatic portal system. The hepatic portal vein drains the intestines, stomach, pancreas and spleen and takes blood to the liver. The liver also receives oxygen rich blood via the hepatic artery.

Fluid Mechanics

Dissolved gases (especially oxygen and carbon dioxide) cross the capillary wall by diffusion, moving from an area of greater concentration to an area of lesser concentration. Glucose, amino acids, vitamins and other relatively small molecules are assisted to cross the capillary wall by ***filtration***. Filtration occurs because the capillary pressure is higher than the tissue fluid pressure.

Edema is the accumulation of excess tissue fluid in the extracellular space. Edema can occur because the pressure differential between the capillaries and the tissue fluid is increased. An increased permeability of the capillaries will also cause edema. Congestive heart failure can cause poor venous return with subsequent increased intravenous and intracapillary pressure. Kidney failure can cause increased capillary pressure due to water retention. Hypertension can cause increased capillary permeability. Inflammation increases capillary permeability, which causes localized edema.

On the venous side of the capillary network, the reabsorption of tissue fluid back into the capillary may be reduced enough to cause edema. This situation may result secondary to a low level of plasma proteins (especially albumin) such as may occur in liver failure, starvation, and kidney disease with proteinuria (protein loss in the urine). Blocked lymphatic channels are another cause of edema. A block in lymphatic flow prevents the return of tissue fluid to the bloodstream. Lymphatic blockage is a common result of cancerous lymph nodes. Lymphatic blockage may also follow cancer surgery in which lymph nodes are removed. Edema fluid accumulation can reach fantastic proportions in elephantiasis, a tropical infectious disease that is caused by the larvae of *Filaria*, a type of roundworm that blocks lymphatic channels.

At the venous end of a capillary network, the blood pressure is decreased to the point that filtration is no longer a factor. Here the ***colloid osmotic pressure*** is responsible for pulling tissue fluid and waste materials into the capillary lumen. Plasma proteins (especially ***albumin***) establish most of the colloid osmotic pressure of blood.

Slightly more tissue fluid is formed at the arterial end of the capillary bed than is removed at the venous end. The excess tissue fluid enters the lymphatic system and is returned to the blood through lymphatic channels, the largest of which is the ***thoracic duct.*** The thoracic duct empties into the venous system at the base of the left subclavian vein. The ***right lymphatic duct*** is smaller; it empties into the right subclavian vein.

Blood is forced into the systemic arterial tree by ***contractions of the heart***. That force plus the ***volume of blood*** present, and ***peripheral resistance*** caused by the ***elasticity*** and ***smooth muscle contraction*** of the arteries create pressure within the arteries that is known as the ***systemic blood pressure***. The normal systemic blood pressure in Americans is regarded to be 120/80 mm Hg. 120 mm Hg is the systolic pressure, systole being the time when the left ventricle is contracting and blood is being pumped out of the heart through an open aortic valve. 80 mm Hg is the diastolic pressure, diastole being the time when the left ventricle is relaxing with the aortic valve closed. The diastolic pressure is maintained by the smooth muscle and elastic tissue in the tunica media of the arteries and arterioles. The greater the distance between the heart and an artery, the lower the blood pressure. The difference between the systolic and diastolic pressures gradually disappears as you proceed into the arterioles. At the arterial end of the capillary network, the blood pressure is about 30-35 mm Hg, which is high enough to allow filtration and low enough to prevent capillary rupture. The blood pressure falls to 12-15 mm Hg at the venous end of the capillary network. The blood pressure gradually decreases in the larger veins, and it approaches zero entering the right atrium.

Systemic hypertension is an elevated blood pressure, which is judged to be significant and worthy of treatment at levels above 140/90 mm Hg. Prolonged or severe hypertension contributes to arterial damage, which is especially damaging to the coronary arteries, the cerebral arteries, and the arterioles of the kidneys.

The major factors that ***influence systemic blood pressure*** are: (1) the force of the pump, which is created by ventricular contraction, (2) the ***peripheral resistance***, which is constriction of the arteries or any abnormal blockage of flow, and (3) the ***volume of blood*** in circulation. The blood pressure will be higher if the heart pumps with greater force, or if the arteries constrict more, or if there is a greater volume of blood in circulation.

The ***pulmonary blood pressure*** is the pressure of the blood in the pulmonary arteries. The normal pulmonary artery pressure is created by: (1) the pumping force of the right ventricle, (2) the blood volume, (3) smooth muscle in the tunica media of the pulmonary arteries and (4) elastic tissue in the tunica media of the pulmonary arteries.

Because the right ventricular wall is only 1/6 as thick as that of the left ventricle, the pulmonary blood pressure is considerably ***lower*** than the systemic blood pressure. The normal pulmonary artery pressure is only about 20/10 mm Hg, and it is even lower in the capillaries of the lungs. This relatively low blood pressure is necessary to prevent the filtration of fluid from the capillaries to the alveoli (air sacs) of the lungs. An elevated blood pressure in the pulmonary circuit is called ***pulmonary hypertension***, which can lead to right ventricular failure. Pulmonary hypertension can result from an increase in peripheral resistance in the lungs. Pulmonary fibrosis (scarring in the lungs) and pulmonary emboli (blood clots in the pulmonary arteries) cause pulmonary hypertension by increasing the resistance to flow.

Several factors are involved in the ***maintenance of normal systemic blood pressure:***
(1) The amount of venous return to the heart determines the amount of blood the left ventricle can pump into the aorta; the ventricles are able to pump only the amount of blood that they receive. A severe hemorrhage decreases venous return, decreases the stroke volume of the ventricles and decreases cardiac output. This is known as ***Starling's Law***.
Venous return is sensitive to gravity. It is highest when an individual is recumbent and lowest when he is standing erect and still. In the standing position venous return is dependant upon ***valves*** in the leg veins, ***muscle contractions*** in the legs (the skeletal muscle pump), and the ***respiratory pump*** (intrathoracic pressure changes caused by inhalation and exhalation).
(2) A significant hemorrhage with loss of a pint of blood or more will cause a temporary decrease in blood pressure, and it may cause dizziness or ***syncope*** (pronounced sink-o-pee, meaning to faint). A compensatory increase in the heart rate and increased vasoconstriction will increase the blood pressure to normal levels. These mechanisms will not be able to compensate if the hemorrhage is too great, and the result would be ***circulatory shock***, which is a blood pressure so low that it is life threatening because the tissues are not being adequately perfused. A greatly reduced cardiac output due to a low blood volume is one cause of shock.
(3) As the heart rate and force of contraction increase, so will the blood pressure. However, if the heart rate becomes too high, the ventricular output will decrease because the ventricles do not have time to fill between contractions, and consequently, the blood pressure would also decrease. An abnormally fast heart rate is called ***tachycardia.***
(4) The smooth muscle in peripheral vessels is normally slightly constricted, which maintains normal diastolic blood pressure. If vasoconstriction increases, the blood pressure will also increase. If vasodilatation occurs, the blood pressure will drop. Stressful conditions increase blood pressure through sympathetic stimulation, which causes vasoconstriction in the vessels of the skin and most organs. Vessels in the intestinal tract dilate after a heavy meal, and this can lower the systemic blood pressure.
(5) A considerable amount of elastic tissue is present in the walls of larger arteries, which has the ability to contract and stretch. This elasticity has the effect of lowering the systolic pressure and elevating the diastolic pressure.
(6) Blood has viscosity due to the presence of cells and proteins. Too many cells will raise the blood viscosity and the blood pressure. Anemia or decreased albumin content in the blood will decrease blood viscosity and lower blood pressure.
(7) Syncope is loss of consciousness associated with fainting. Syncope has several natural causes including urination with an overly full bladder (micturition syncope) and extreme coughing spells (tussive syncope). The most common cause of syncope is a ***vaso-vagal reaction***. Vaso-vagal reactions involve a sudden decrease in blood pressure and cardiac output associated with an emotional crisis. The sudden decrease in blood pressure is due to the shunting of blood to skeletal muscles (a sympathetic reaction) and sudden slowing of the heart rate (a vagal reaction).   A person who has fainted loses consciousness because he has insufficient blood flow to his brain. Treatment should include keeping the head low, which increases blood flow to the brain.
(8) Several hormones affect blood pressure. ***Catecholamines*** (epinephrine, norepinephrine and dopamine) secreted by the adrenal medulla cause vasoconstriction, a faster heart rate, and a greater force of contraction. These effects raise blood pressure. ***ADH*** (anti-diuretic hormone or vasopressin) from the posterior pituitary gland increases water reabsorption from the kidney tubules and increases blood volume, which increases blood pressure. ***Aldosterone*** is secreted by the adrenal cortex; it acts to increase sodium (Na+) reabsorption from the kidney tubules, which increases blood volume and increases blood pressure. ***ANH*** (atrial natriuretic hormone) is secreted by cardiac muscle cells in the right atrium of the heart. It opposes aldosterone in that it increases sodium and water loss by the kidneys, which decreases blood volume and decreases blood pressure. ANH is secreted in response to increased blood volume, which causes cells in the right atrium to stretch.

Intrinsic mechanisms for maintaining blood pressure affect the stroke volume of the heart, the blood volume and vasoconstriction. Starling's Law tells us that the more the ventricles are stretched (up to a physiological limit), the greater will be the cardiac output. When blood flow through the kidneys is reduced, less filtration into the urine occurs, which preserves blood volume. The kidneys secrete the enzyme, **_renin_,** in response to a fall in blood pressure. Renin stimulates a series of reactions that results in the formation of **_angiotensin II,_** an oligopeptide with multiple effects including vasoconstriction, increased aldosterone secretion by the adrenal cortex, increased ADH secretion by the posterior pituitary, and increased sodium reabsorption by the kidneys. All of these effects will increase the blood pressure. (See page 204.)

The nervous system exerts its effect on blood pressure through the **_autonomic nervous system_**, including the adrenal medulla. The **_adrenal medulla_** secretes **_catecholamines_**, which cause vasoconstriction and increase blood pressure. The **_medulla oblongata_** has a vasomotor center that can increase blood pressure by initiating **_sympathetic impulses_** that cause vasoconstriction. Correspondingly the medulla may reduce blood pressure by reducing the number of sympathetic impulses that it is sends out, thereby lowering the normal vascular tone and producing vasodilation. (The parasympathetic system does not innervate smooth muscle in the arteries.)

The Fetal Circulation

There are major differences in the pattern of circulation between the **_fetus_** and the infant. The placenta is the site for the diffusion of oxygen, carbon dioxide, nutrients and wastes between the fetus and the mother. The placenta is divided into two areas; one is connected to the fetal circulation, and the other is connected to the maternal circulation. Blood does not mix between the divisions. The umbilical cord of the fetus supplies oxygen-poor blood to the placenta via **_two umbilical arteries_**, which are branches of the right and left internal iliac arteries. The **_umbilical vein_** carries oxygen-rich blood from the placenta back to the fetus. The umbilical vein branches upon arriving to the fetus. The smaller of the two branches joins the fetal **_hepatic portal vein_**, which takes blood to the liver. The larger branch is the **_ductus venosus_**, which opens directly into the inferior vena cava. After birth, the umbilical vein, the umbilical arteries and the ductus venosus constrict and become fibrous cords.

Other differences between the fetal and the postpartum circulation involve the fetal lungs, which are deflated and nonfunctional prior to birth, thus requiring little blood supply. Two anatomical landmarks, the **_foramen ovale_** and the **_ductus arteriosus_**, shunt blood from the pulmonary circuit to the systemic circuit of the fetus. The **_foramen ovale_** is an opening in the interatrial septum through which blood flows from the right atrium to the left atrium. The **_ductus arteriosus_** is an artery-to-artery anastomosis that shunts blood from the pulmonary artery to the aorta. After birth, the lungs inflate and pull more blood into the pulmonary artery. The increased pressure in the pulmonary artery moves a flap on the left side of the interatrial septum, which closes the foramen ovale. The ductus arteriosus constricts and closes in response to higher oxygen content in the blood after the lungs fill with air.

Vascular Maladies

A **_thrombus_** is a blood clot.

An **_embolus_** is a clot or other substance that is carried through the circulation, but is not normally found in the blood stream. Emboli can lead to tissue necrosis by blocking an artery.

Atherosclerosis is the collection of cholesterol and other lipids in the walls of arteries. Lipids form plaques within arteries called atheromas. **_Stenosis_** is narrowing of a blood vessel or other tube. Stenosis of a blood vessel is typically caused by atherosclerosis. Atherosclerosis is the primary cause of myocardial infarcts (occlusions in the coronary arteries), strokes (occlusions in the cerebral arteries) and peripheral vascular disease (ischemia to the extremities). It is also a major factor in kidney disease.

Arteriosclerosis means hardening of the arteries. It includes atherosclerosis as its major component, and it also includes calcium deposits and a loss of elasticity in the walls of the arteries.

Thrombophlebitis, or phlebitis, is a clot with inflammation within a vein. It is tender and painful, but it does not tend to embolize (break off and travel through the vasculature).

__Phlebothrombosis__ is a clot that grows, worm-like, within a vein. It does not cause inflammation, and it is neither painful nor tender. However, this type of clot is in grave danger of causing one or repeated emboli to the pulmonary arteries, which can be fatal.

Study Guide
1. What was William Harvey's chief contribution to science?
2. Define artery, arteriole, capillary, sinusoid, venule and vein.
3. Understand the systemic circuit of circulation and compare it to the pulmonary circuit.
4. List the layers of an arterial wall. How do the walls of veins differ from the walls of arteries?
5. Trace the aorta from the heart to its bifurcation in the pelvis. List its major branches.
6. Define the following: anastomosis, aneurysm, varix, edema, and chyle.
7. What is circulatory shock?
8. Understand the processes involved in filtration and reabsorption by the capillaries.
9. Understand the hepatic-portal circulation and how it functions.
10. Understand the differences between circulation in the fetus and the adult.
11. Know the location and function of the ductus venosus, ductus arteriosus and foramen ovale.
12. What factors are involved in establishing blood pressure?
13. What parts of the body are most sensitive to prolonged hypertension?
14. What hormones affect the blood pressure?
15. Explain how the renin-angiotensin mechanism works.
16. Define arteriosclerosis, atherosclerosis, thrombophlebitis, and phlebothrombosis.
17. What is a thrombus? What is an embolus?

Chapter Twenty

The Heart

The heart is a muscular organ that pumps blood throughout the body. It is located in the ***mediastinum***, which is that part of the thorax between the two lungs. The ***base*** of the heart is located superiorly, which is where the great vessels enter and leave the heart. The ***apex*** of the heart is located inferiorly with a tilt to the left. The heart is surrounded by the ***pericardium***, a three-layered covering consisting of (1) an outer tough, fibrous, inelastic membrane, (2) a thin inner serosal membrane called the ***parietal pericardium***, and (3) a thin serosal membrane on the surface of the heart muscle called the ***visceral pericardium or epicardium***. The epicardium and the parietal pericardium secrete serous fluid into the pericardial sac, which prevents friction as the heart beats.

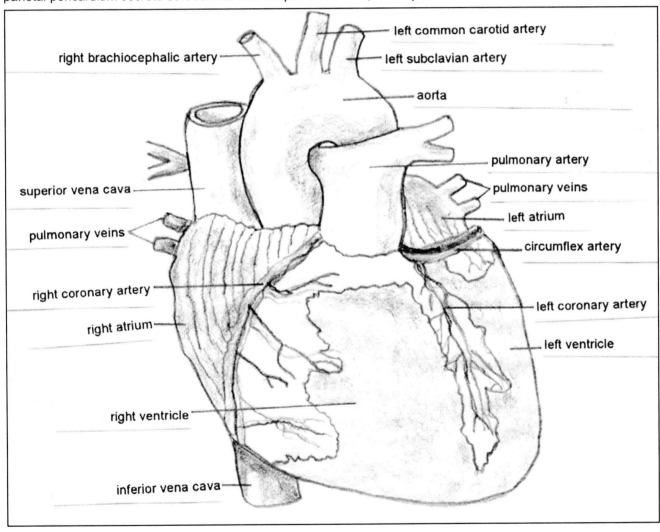

Above: The pericardium has been cut away in this drawing of the heart
and great vessels. The view is the anterior surface of the heart.

The walls of the heart are made up of cardiac muscle known as the ***myocardium***. The myocardium is filled with ***myocytes*** (cardiac muscle cells). The heart has four chambers, which are lined with a thin layer of simple squamous epithelium (the ***endothelium).*** Cardiac endothelium is continuous with the endothelium that lines the inner surface of blood vessels. The four chambers of the heart are the ***right and left atria*** and the ***right and left*** *ventricles.* The myocardial wall of the ventricles is much thicker than that of the atria, and the left ventricle, which pumps blood through all the body except the lungs, has the thickest muscular wall. The atria are separated by the **interatrial septum**, and the ventricles are separated by the **interventricular septum.** Each atrium has an ear-shaped appendage called an **auricle.**

The right atrium accepts blood from the body by way of two large veins, the **superior vena cava** and the **inferior vena cava**. Contractions of the right atrium push blood through the **tricuspid** valve into the right ventricle. When the right ventricle contracts, blood is forced through the **pulmonary valve** into the pulmonary artery trunk. The pulmonary artery divides into four main branches, which lead to the lungs. Blood flows through the pulmonary capillary bed into four pulmonary veins, which open into the left atrium. Contractions of the left atrium push blood through the **mitral** (bicuspid) valve into the left ventricle. When the left ventricle contracts, blood is forced through the **aortic valve** into the aorta. Blood travels from the aorta through the arterial tree of the systemic circuit to destinations throughout the body. Thus the right ventricle is the pump for the **pulmonary circuit**, and the left ventricle is the pump for the **systemic circuit.**

The four heart valves are constructed so as to direct the flow of blood in one direction. Valvular heart disease can result in **stenosis** (a rigid narrowing of the opening of a valve) or **insufficiency** (an inability of a valve to close completely -- also known as regurgitation).

Right: A drawing of the heart, (anterior view).
(1) Superior vena cava
(2) Aorta
(3) Pulmonary artery
(4) Pulmonary veins
(5) Pulmonary valve
(6) Left atrium
(7) Right atrium
(8) Left coronary vessels
(9) Papillary muscle
(10) Interventricular septum
(11) Aortic valve (hidden)
(12) Cusp of mitral valve
(13) Cusp of tricuspid valve
(14) Right ventricle
(15) Left ventricle
(16) Inferior vena cava
Blood returns to the heart through the venae cava.
It passes through the right atrium, tricuspid valve, right ventricle, pulmonary valve, pulmonary artery, lungs, pulmonary veins, left atrium, mitral valve, left ventricle, aortic valve and leaves through the aorta.

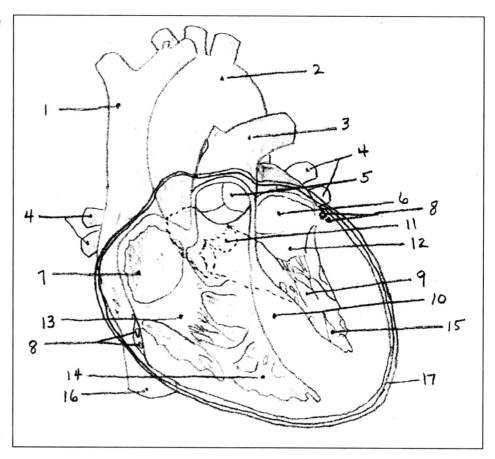

The **mitral** valve has two cusps (flaps); hence it is also called the bicuspid valve. The **tricuspid** valve has three cusps. The mitral and tricuspid valves are anchored to the left and right ventricles respectively by fibrous strands called **chordae tendineae**, which connect to columns of myocardium inside the ventricles called **papillary muscles**. The chordae tendineae are commonly known as the heartstrings. The mitral and tricuspid valves together are called the **AV valves** because they are located between the atria and the ventricles.
The pulmonary and aortic valves each have three cusps shaped like half-moons. Hence they are called **semilunar valves**.

Openings to the coronary arteries are located at the base of two of the three cusps of the aortic valve. There are two coronary arteries, and they supply the myocardium with arterial blood through their branches. The major branches of the left coronary artery are the ___anterior interventricular branch and the circumflex artery___. The major branches of the right coronary artery are the ___posterior interventricular branch and the marginal artery___. Venous blood from the myocardium drains into the ___coronary sinus___, which opens into the right atrium.

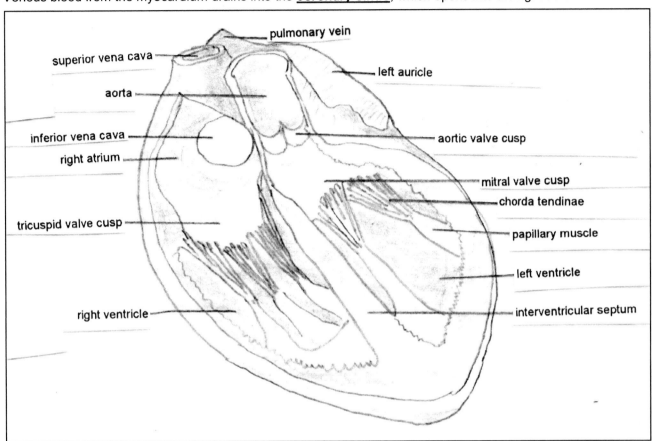

Above: This drawing of the interior of the heart shows the structure and locations of the heart valves, chambers and great vessels. The auricles are ear-shaped appendages of the atria.

The sequence of events of a single heartbeat is called a ___cardiac cycle___. The cardiac cycle begins with spontaneous depolarization involving cells in the ___sinoatrial (SA) node___. The SA node is a localized ___autorhythmic___ area of specialized cells in the right atrium that functions as the cardiac ___pacemaker___. The electrical nerve impulse from the SA node travels to myocardial cells in the right and left atria, and the atria contract simultaneously. The impulse then travels to the ___atrioventricular (AV) node___. The AV node is a locus of specialized autorhythmic cells located in the lower interatrial septum. The nerve impulse is retarded as it passes through the AV node, which gives the ventricles time to fill with blood following contraction of the atria. From the AV node the impulse travels quickly through a bundle of nerve fibers within the interventricular septum called the ___bundle of His___. The bundle of His splits into a ___right bundle branch and a left bundle branch___. Impulses reach the ventricles simultaneously and the ventricles contract at the same time. Upon reaching the ventricles, the nerve impulse first travels to the apex through the right and left bundle branches. Then it travels upward through the myocardium of the ventricles by nerve fibers called ___Purkinje fibers. Ventricular contraction begins at the apex___ and spreads upward, forcing blood out of the ventricular chambers.

Motor nerves to the heart are part of the autonomic nervous system. Most of the nerves to the heart are sympathetic, but the ___vagus___ nerve supplies parasympathetic fibers as well. Stimulation of the ___parasympathetic___ nerves to the heart affects the SA node and slows the heart rate. ___Sympathetic___ fibers to the heart arise from the upper thoracic spinal nerves and pass through the lower cervical and upper thoracic paravertebral ganglia. They are mostly **_beta adrenergic_** in classification. Sympathetic stimulation makes the heart rate increase, and it makes the heart beat with increased force. Beta adrenergic blocking drugs are capable of slowing the heart rate, decreasing the force of cardiac contractions, and thereby decreasing the blood pressure. **_Baroreceptors_** in the **_carotid sinus_** and the **_aortic arch_** monitor blood pressure. Signals from the baroreceptors are sent to the cardiac center in the medulla via the vagus cranial nerves. The cardiac center sends impulses through the sympathetic nerves and the vagus nerve to the heart to control the heart rate and force of contraction.

An effect on the heart rate is called a **_chronotropic_** effect. An effect on the force of contraction of the heart muscle is called an **_inotropic_** effect.

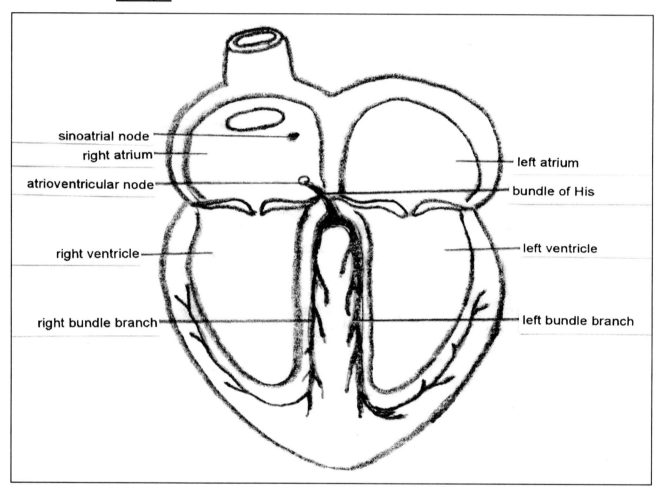

Above: The conduction of a nerve impulse through the heart. The impulse begins at the sinoatrial (SA) node. It travels through myocytes in the right atrium to the atrioventricular (AV) node and the bundle of His. The impulse then splits into a right and left bundle branch. Each bundle branch proceeds to the apex of the heart, after which the impulse travels upward through the outer walls of the ventricles. The speed of the impulse is enhanced by intercalated discs, which are electrical gap junctions between myocytes.

Diastole is the period during which the ventricles are filling with blood. In diastole the atria contract, the tricuspid and mitral valves open, the ventricles are relaxed and fill with blood, and the aortic and pulmonary valves are closed. **_Systole_** is the period of time when the ventricles contract, the aortic and pulmonary valves open, blood is forced into the aorta and pulmonary artery, and the tricuspid and mitral valves close.

The heart sounds can be described as a "lub-dup" sound. The "lub" is the first heart sound, or **_S-1_**.

_S-1_ represents the closure of the tricuspid and mitral valves. The second heart sound, or _S-2_, is the "dup" sound. _S-2_ represents the closure of the aortic and pulmonary valves. Listening to heart or other sounds is called _auscultation_. Sometimes turbulent blood flow will cause additional heart sounds. A _third or fourth_ heart sound can frequently be heard in cardiac failure. Third and fourth heart sounds occur in diastole. They have a low pitch and are often barely audible. A _murmur_ is a heart sound produced by the abnormal flow of blood through a valve or through a septal defect. Murmurs may be either very soft or quite loud, and they may have a low pitch or a high pitch. Murmurs of aortic stenosis and mitral insufficiency are audible in systole. Murmurs of aortic insufficiency and mitral stenosis are audible in diastole.

The inherent pacemaker in the SA node establishes the normal heart rate at 60-80 beats a minute. This _autorhythmicity_ exists due to a gradual leakage of sodium (Na+) ions into the myocytes of the SA node, which creates a gradual depolarization. The resting potential of these cells is -60 mV. When sodium ion leakage brings the potential to -40 mV, a spontaneous action potential ensues, which results in muscle contraction. The impulse travels through atrial myocytes from the SA node to the AV node.

The AV node and some areas of the myocardium of the ventricles also have spontaneous firing. The SA node fires at an average rate of _72 beats_ a minute; the AV node fires at about _40-50 beats_ a minute, and areas in the myocardium will fire at about _20-40 beats_ a minute. If the SA node is dysfunctional, the AV node will take over the duties of the pacemaker, but the heart rate will be slower as a result. If neither the SA nor the AV node is functional, the heart rate will slow to the rate of the myocardial autorhythmicity at 20-40 beats a minute, which may reduce the cardiac output to such an extent that life cannot be sustained. Occasionally _premature heartbeats_ will originate from an area of atrial or ventricle depolarization that is outside the nodes. These beats are called premature or ectopic beats. They are common, and they are usually not a serious problem unless they become too frequent. Artificial _pacemakers_ are electronic devices that have energy supplied by a battery, and they initiate an impulse periodically. Wires connect them to the atria and the bundle of His, and they are capable of making the heart beat regularly.

An electrocardiogram or _EKG_ is a paper recording of electrical signals from the heart. The primary waves of an EKG are the _P wave, the QRS complex and the T wave_. The P wave corresponds to atrial depolarization, the QRS complex corresponds to ventricular depolarization, and the T wave corresponds to ventricular repolarization.   An EKG can reveal many cardiac abnormalities including arrhythmias, cardiac ischemia and necrosis. When performing an EKG, leads are placed on both wrists and on the left ankle. A movable lead is placed across the chest. The test is quick and painless.

An EKG recording will reveal the cardiac rate, rhythm, strength of contraction and the path the impulse travels. Waves above the baseline represent electric impulses traveling toward the designated lead.   Waves below the baseline represent electric impulses traveling away from the designated lead. Areas of ischemia or damaged muscle cause aberrations from the normal direction of impulse flow through the heart.

Tachycardia is an abnormally fast heart rate; _bradycardia_ is an abnormally slow heart rate. _Fibrillation_ is constant twitching at a rate so high that true heartbeats do not occur. _Flutter_ is a heart rate of 200-400, a rate that is beyond the physiologic limits for the heart to act as a pump because the ventricles do not have time to fill. Fibrillation and flutter may involve the atria, the ventricles, or both.

The special, unique histology of myocytes is instrumental for the rapid spread of nervous impulses through the myocardium. These specialties include _gap junctions_ called _intercalated discs_, _interdigitating folds_ at cellular junctions, and _strong mechanical junctions_. The mechanical junctions include _desmosomes_ and the _fascia adherens,_ a protein that links the plasma membranes of adjacent cardiac cells. The mechanical junctions provide a framework that allows the myocardium to act effectively as a pump. The gap junctions and interdigitating folds increase communication between myocytes, and they increase the speed of electrical impulses through the myocardium.

A connective tissue framework called the _fibrous skeleton_ is present within the myocardium. It provides a framework of support for valves and great vessels, and it limits nervous impulses to established routes.

The heart begins beating when the fetus is but four weeks old, and the heart must contract about seventy-two times a minute for a lifetime. Myocytes utilize aerobic respiration almost exclusively to make ATP. Therefore, oxygen is a constant primary necessity for the heart. Cardiac myocytes have abundant large mitochondria that fill 25% of the cell. In contrast smaller mitochondria fill only two percent of a skeletal muscle cell. The myocardium is not particular regarding the fuel it burns; glucose, fatty acids, amino acids, ketones and lactic acid can all be metabolized for energy.

Right: Abbreviations for the waves seen on an EKG.
Below: Examples of EKGs.

R = R wave

S = S wave

ST = ST segment

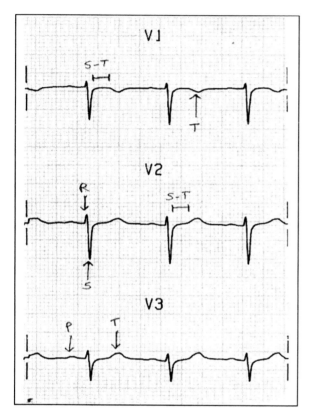

Above: A normal tracing.

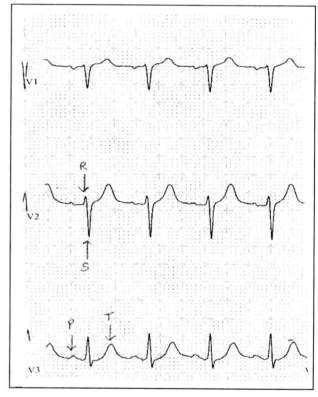

Above: Tachycardia, rate ca. 120. To determine the rate divide the number of units between like waves into 300.

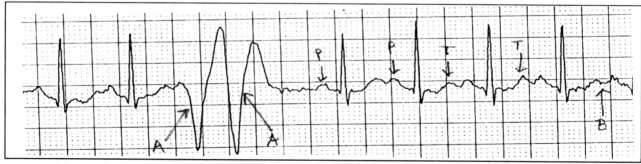

Above: Two premature beats are present at the places designated as "A." P waves are seen before normal contractions, but not before premature ventricular contractions. Skeletal muscle activity produced the irregular baseline at "B."

The first heart sound, S-1, represents closure of the mitral and tricuspid valves. This sound corresponds to ventricular contraction, and it occurs late in the QRS complex. The second heart sound, S-2, represents closure of the aortic and pulmonary valves. This sound occurs near the end of the T wave, when the ventricles have begun to relax and dilate.

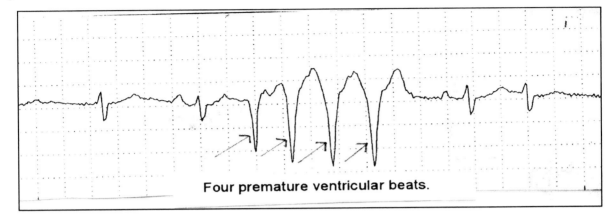

Four premature ventricular beats.

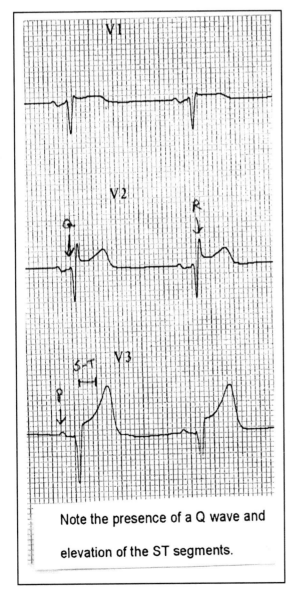

Note the presence of a Q wave and

elevation of the ST segments.

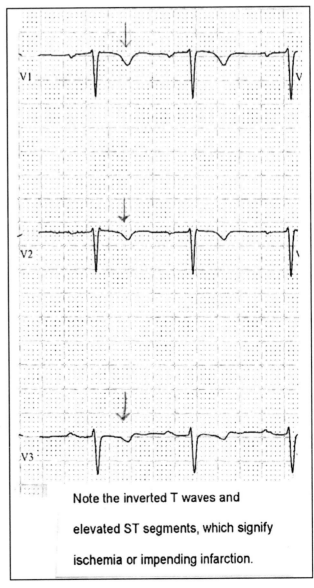

Note the inverted T waves and

elevated ST segments, which signify

ischemia or impending infarction.

Heart block is a cardiac arrhythmia that may be **supraventricular** (above the ventricles and in the atria). If a supraventricular block arises in the SA node, it is called a sinus block, and it produces a slow, irregular heartbeat with the AV node acting as the pacemaker (nodal rhythm). When the block is in the AV node, several types of arrhythmias are possible depending upon the degree of the block. For example in 2:1 block only one of every two impulses from the SA node makes it through the AV node to the ventricles. The EKG in 2:1 block will show two P waves for every QRS complex. Sometimes heart block is located below the AV node. In these cases the block is usually located either in the left bundle branch or the right bundle branch. The EKG in bundle branch block typically shows a wide spreading out of the QRS complex.

Drugs used to medically treat heart conditions include those with **chronotropic** effects (effects on the heart rate), those with **inotropic** effects (effects on the force of contraction), and effects on heart rhythm. Some of these drugs are:
Beta adrenergic blocking agents. These drugs decrease the heart rate and decrease the force of contraction.
Digitalis (digitoxin, digoxin, ouabain). Digitalis has many effects on the heart including increasing the force of contraction and increasing the speed of conduction through the AV node.
Quinidine and procaine amide. These two drugs have multiple similar effects including slowing conduction through the AV node. They have been used to prevent and treat atrial fibrillation. They are seldom used today because of toxicity.
Lidocaine. This drug is a local anesthetic that has been found to be useful in treating arrhythmias when used in an IV drip.

Stenosis (narrowing) of a coronary artery is usually due to **atherosclerosis,** which is the buildup of fatty deposits called atheromas in the arterial wall. Pain can result if a portion of the myocardium supplied by a narrowed coronary artery becomes **ischemic** (hypoxic due to an inadequate blood supply). Such pain is called **angina pectoris;** it may be localized over the left chest, or it may be referred to the left shoulder and inside of the left arm. If a section of myocardium becomes necrotic due to a lack of blood supply, it is called a **myocardial infarct** or MI. Infarcts may lead to electrical disturbances (**arrhythmias**) and **heart failure**, which is the failure of the heart as a pump. Heart failure results in a low cardiac output. A weakened heart muscle cannot force blood through the arteries with enough force, which causes the ventricles to dilate and the heart to enlarge. A third or fourth heart sound can be created by the reverberation of sound waves through dilated ventricles. When a third or fourth heart sound is present, it is described as a **"gallop"** rhythm. When the left ventricle fails as a pump, fluid backs up in the lungs and enters the alveoli. This is called **pulmonary edema**, and it results in shortness of breath. When the right ventricle fails to pump adequately, fluid collects in the ankles and other dependant parts of the body. Perfusion of the vital organs may become compromised with either right or left sided failure. **Cor pulmonale** is hypertrophy of the right ventricle with subsequent right-sided heart failure. Cor pulmonale is due to a lung disorder such as emphysema or pulmonary fibrosis.

Cardiac catheterization is a means by which some cardiac procedures are done, and it generally precedes any surgical procedure on the heart. Cardiac catheterization has proved to be an extremely useful tool, not only to the radiologist and the coronary vascular surgeon, but to other cardiac surgeons and cardiologists as well. Cardiac catheterization involves threading a catheter into the femoral artery or the femoral vein to the heart. If the catheter is placed in the femoral vein, it can be threaded up the inferior vena cava to the right side of the heart where the tricuspid and pulmonary valves can be evaluated. The coronary arteries, the aortic valve and the mitral can be evaluated by inserting the catheter into the femoral artery and passing it to the heart. Stenosis and insufficiency of a valve can be graded by measuring pressure differentials across the valve. The systolic pressure in the right ventricle corresponds to the systolic pressure in the pulmonary artery, so that pressure can be deduced. Another cardiac procedure that can be accomplished with cardiac catheterization is the ablation of abnormal electrical circuits that produce intermittent tachycardia.

If a radio opaque liquid is injected from a catheter into the coronary arteries, X-rays can show areas of narrowing. Surgical treatments for a narrowed coronary artery include a **coronary artery bypass**. In this procedure, a leg vein (usually the saphenous vein) is used to bypass a narrowed section of coronary artery. **Balloon angioplasty** is a procedure in which a balloon catheter is threaded into a coronary artery to the obstruction. The balloon is inflated, which stretches the narrowed section of artery. **Laser angioplasty** involves inserting a catheter into a coronary artery and vaporizing atheromas with a laser beam. A **stint** is a tube that can be placed in a narrowed section of artery to keep it open.

Cardiac disorders are not limited to the coronary arteries and arrhythmias. ***Pericarditis*** is inflammation of the pericardium; the Coxsackie B virus is a known cause of pericarditis. Inflammation of the pericardium can cause fluid to collect in the pericardial sac. The tough, fibrous outer layer of the pericardial sac is inelastic, and the presence of fluid in the pericardial sac will reduce cardiac output by not allowing the ventricles to completely fill. This is a condition known as ***cardiac tamponade***. Pericarditis can sometimes be diagnosed at the bedside if a friction rub is heard while listening to heart sounds. Cardiac tamponade can result from other disorders including trauma.

A ***cardiomyopathy*** may be of viral or toxic etiology (cause). This disorder effects the myocardial cells, which weakens the pumping action of the heart to the point of heart failure.

There are a myriad of congenital heart defects, some of which are benign (not serious) and some of which are serious. ***A septal defect*** is a congenital abnormality in which an opening in the interatrial or the interventricular septum exists. Septal defects allow blood to flow directly from one side of the heart to the other.

Mitral valve prolapse affects one in forty people in the U.S. It is genetically inherited, and it has a higher incidence in women. It involves prolapse of the mitral valve into the left atrium when the valve closes at the beginning of systole. Mitral insufficiency may also be present. Mitral valve prolapse is usually not a serious condition, but chest pain, fatigue, dyspnea (shortness of breath), and heart failure can follow. Careful auscultation of a heart with mitral valve prolapse frequently reveals a clicking sound in early diastole that represents opening of the prolapsed mitral valve.

Rheumatic fever is an inflammation of the joints that follows a ***streptococcal infection***, usually a strep throat. It is most common in children. In rheumatic fever the streptococcal infection triggers the body's immune system to produce an antibody that affects the joints and the heart valves. The joints recover without complications, but scarring of the heart valves may produce a life-long illness. Adults may suffer an increased fibrosis in their heart valves years after having an attack of rheumatic fever. ***Endocarditis*** is a bacterial infection of a heart valve; it occurs in valves that have been diseased, often due to rheumatic fever. Endocarditis is often subacute, meaning that it begins insidiously and progresses relatively slowly, but the infection can destroy the valve. The organism most often responsible for ***SBE (subacute bacterial endocarditis)*** is Streptococcus viridans, a type of bacteria that is otherwise harmless. This is NOT the same streptococcus that causes strep throat and rheumatic fever. Timely antibiotic therapy for strep throat has reduced the incidence of rheumatic fever dramatically. Valves that are seriously damaged can be surgically replaced with a valve from a pig or with an artificial valve.

Congenital (present at birth) ***heart defects*** are not infrequent, and they may cause symptoms in an infant and in an adult. The severity of the disorder varies with the type and severity of the defect. Congenital heart defects include atrial septal defects, ventricular septal defects, a patent ductus arteriosus, stenosis of the pulmonary artery, valvular defects, transposition of the great vessels, and the tetralogy of Fallot. Situs inversus is the congenital positioning of the heart and great vessels to the opposite side of the body (the heart is tilted to the right, and the aorta arches to the right.)

The ***tetralogy of Fallot*** includes a ventricular septal defect, pulmonic valvular stenosis, right ventricular hypertrophy and positioning of the aorta over the outflow of the right ventricle. This combination of defects is the most common cause of cyanosis in childhood.

Coarctation is a congenital stenotic section of the aorta. Coarctation may occur at any level of the aorta, but it is most frequently seen near the ductus arteriosus. An aortic valve defect often accompanies coarctation.

Hyperkalemia is an elevated serum potassium level. The normal level of potassium in the serum is 3.5-5.0 mEq/L. A level of 5.5-6.0 is considered mild; 6.1-7.0 is considered moderate, and over 7.0 is considered severe. ***Acute hyperkalemia*** comes on ***suddenly*** following severe contusions or hemolysis. These conditions are associated with cellular rupture and the release of intracellular K+ into the extracellular fluids. The extracellular potassium is pumped into cells of the nervous system and the muscular system where it lowers the neuromuscular threshold. Heartbeats become rapid, weak and irregular, and the heart may go into ventricular fibrillation. ***Ventricular fibrillation*** is a constant ineffectual twitching of the heart that is rapidly fatal because the heart is not functioning as a pump. ***Defibrillation*** is an electric shock given to the heart in ventricular fibrillation. Defibrillation causes all electric activity in the heart to stop for a brief time.   If successful, the SA node or AV node will then take over the heart rhythm.

An injection of potassium chloride is a method by which some states carry out the death penalty. The infusion of glucose and insulin is an effective emergency treatment for hyperkalemia because potassium enters the cell along with glucose.

Chronic, slow onset hyperkalemia occurs in renal failure and with the use of some diuretics. In this condition sodium channels gradually become inactivated and do not respond to impulses. Diminished excitability can lead to ***cardiac arrest.***

Hypokalemia exists if the serum potassium level is below 3.5 mEq/L. ***Acute hypokalemia*** results in hyperpolarization of the myocytes, which leads to bradycardia and failure of stimuli to create contractions. If severe, the heart will go into ***cardiac arrest*** and stop in diastole. ***Chronic hypokalemia*** activates Na+ channels and leads to hyperexcitibility, which can result in ventricular fibrillation. ***Hyperkalemia and hypokalemia are life threatening if severe.***

Skeletal muscles and cardiac myocytes react differently to abnormal levels of calcium in the blood. Skeletal muscles become less responsive in ***hypercalcemia,*** and they become more excitable in ***hypocalcemia.*** These differences are due to the ability of ***extracellular*** calcium ions (Ca++) to affect the polarity across the cell membrane. Low levels of Ca++ outside the cell will depolarize the membrane, and high levels will hyperpolarize the membrane. The threshold is lowered in hypocalcemia and skeletal muscle activity is excitable. Skeletal muscles are sluggish in hypercalcemia because the threshold is elevated.

The effects of hypercalcemia and hypocalcemia are ***reversed*** in cardiac muscle cells, presumably because calcium ions diffuse into cardiac muscle cells more easily than they do skeletal muscle cells. That means that it is the ***intracellular*** calcium levels that affect the response of ***cardiac myocytes***. In ***hypercalcemia*** an abundance of calcium ions enters cardiac muscle cells. That lowers the threshold and makes the heart more excitable to the point of ventricular fibrillation. Calcium diffuses out of the cardiac muscle cells in ***hypocalcemia***, which raises the threshold, and makes heart contractions weak. Hypocalcemia may cause the heart to stop beating (cardiac arrest).

Atrial fibrillation leads to an irregular heartbeat, but it usually does not cause severe symptoms because the ventricles keep beating. However, the cardiac output is lower when atrial fibrillation is present. Atrial fibrillation is best corrected by medication, electroshock or implantation of a pacemaker. A complication of atrial fibrillation is the formation of a blood clot in the right or left auricle. Auricular clots can embolize; clots in the right auricle embolize to the lungs; clots in the left auricle embolize throughout the systemic arterial circulation. Other causes of emboli that are of cardiac origin include subacute bacterial endocarditis and an atrial myxoma. An atrial myxoma is a benign tumor that grows within the atrium. Emboli from atrial myxomas are bits of tissue that have broken off from the main tumor mass. Most atrial myxomas occur in the left atrium.

Study Guide
1. Name the chambers of the heart, and tell whether each contains oxygenated or deoxygenated blood.
2. Describe the pericardium.
3. Describe each of the heart valves, and tell their location.
4. Where are the superior and inferior venae cava?
5. Follow the flow of blood from the venae cava to the aorta.
6. What are the papillary muscles? What are the chordae tendineae?
7. Describe the location of the coronary arteries.
8. Define angina pectoris, myocardial ischemia and a myocardial infarction.
9. Define left-sided and right-sided congestive heart failure and cor pulmonale.
10. Understand the workings of the sinoatrial (SA) node and the atrial-ventricular (AV) node.
11. Outline the course of an electric impulse through the heart.
12. Which nerve supplies parasympathetic innervation to the heart?
13. Define systole and diastole.
14. Define tachycardia, bradycardia, flutter and fibrillation.

15. What is the function of an intercalated disc?
16 Draw an electrocardiogram reading with three normal heartbeats. Identify the waves.
17. What is meant by a chronotropic effect and an inotropic effect on the heart?
18. Understand the relationship between rheumatic fever, mitral valvular disease and subacute bacterial endocarditis.
19. Understand atrial fibrillation, atrial flutter, ventricular fibrillation, premature contractions, heart block and cardiac arrest.

Chapter Twenty-one

The Reproductive Systems

Male

The male sexual organs are the **_testes_** (testicles), **_penis_**, **_prostate gland_**, **_seminal vesicles_** and associated structures. Sperm are produced in the testes; they mature in a long coiled tube called the **_epididymis_**. The right and left epididymides extend from the testes and are continuous with the **_vas deferens (ductus deferens)_**, which are tubes that merge with the **_urethra_** in the **_prostate gland_**. The prostate is immediately distal to the urinary bladder. The urethra is a single tube that extends from the bladder to the tip of the penis. The urethra is the conduit to the exterior for urine and semen.

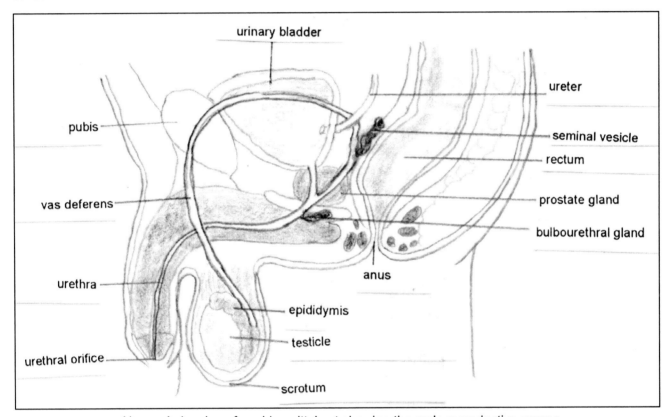

Above: A drawing of a mid-sagittal cut showing the male reproductive organs.

The testes are a pair of glands located in the **_scrotum_**, a cutaneous sac in the perineum. The **_primary spermatocytes_** undergo **_meiosis_** in the testes, and sperm cells are the product. This process is called **_spermatogenesis_**. Meiosis begins with a primary spermatocyte, which has a **_diploid_** number of chromosomes (46), and ends with four spermatids that contain a **_haploid_** number of chromosomes (23). Spermatids mature into spermatozoa. Because the sex chromosomes of human males consist of one X and one Y chromosome, each sperm has either one X or one Y chromosome. If the sperm that fertilizes the egg has an X chromosome, the fetus will be female. If the sperm that fertilizes the egg has a Y chromosome, the fetus will be male.

For the first 8-10 weeks of life a male fetus is indistinguishable from a female fetus. **_Testosterone_** and **_Mullerian inhibiting factor_** (MIF) are secreted by the primordial testes after that time. Those hormones stimulate growth of the phallus (penis), atrophy of primordial female organs (uterus and fallopian tubes), and differentiation of the sex organs into testes. Without the stimulus of testosterone, a fetus will develop female genitalia.

Androgens are steroid hormones that exert a masculinizing effect. The adrenal glands of infants with the **adrenogenital syndrome** secrete excessive amounts of androgens. Female infants with this syndrome develop external genitalia that resemble those of males.

Right: A histological section of a testis. Testes consist primarily of seminiferous tubules. Sperm cells are at the center of a seminiferous tubule in this drawing. Sperm cells in the tubules are immature. Spermatocytes, spermatogonia, sustenacular cells and interstitial cells are present in the area surrounding the lumen of the tubule. Interstitial cells secrete testosterone. Sustentacular (Sertoli) cells secrete inhibin, a hormone that inhibits FSH secretion by the pituitary gland.

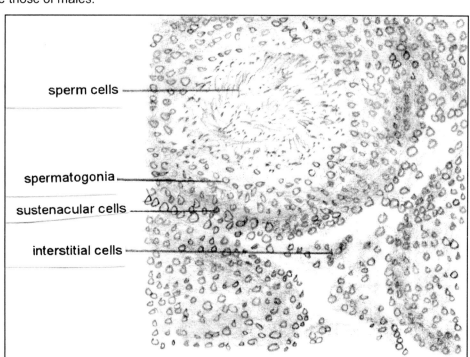

Right: A schematic drawing showing a sagittal section of a testicle. The primary spermatocytes undergo meiosis in the seminiferous tubules. Sperm pass into the efferent ductules (vasa efferentia) then to the epididymis where they mature. The vas deferens carries sperm toward the urethra.

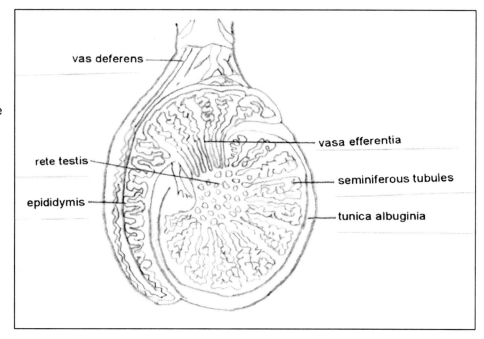

The sex organs (testes and ovaries) originate in **gonadal ridges** near the kidneys. By 7-8 weeks of **gestation** (pregnancy) they have differentiated into either testes or ovaries. By 6-10 weeks of gestation the testes have begun to descend into the **inguinal canals**, and they enter the **scrotum** around 28 weeks of gestation. It is necessary that the temperature of the testes be about **95 degrees F** for spermatogenesis to occur. This lower temperature is obtained by the testicles being in the scrotum outside the pelvic cavity.

Males with the normal XY karyotype, but with the rare ***androgen insensitivity syndrome,*** produce normal amounts of testosterone, but their target cells ***lack receptors for testosterone***. These individuals develop female external genitalia including a vagina, but not a uterus.   Breast development and other secondary sex characteristics are female.

The testes are surrounded by a fibrous capsule called the ***tunica albuginea***. The testes are divided into lobes, each of which contains ***seminiferous tubules*** that contain stratified cuboidal spermatogonia cells. Spermatogenesis takes place within these tubules. The seminiferous tubules merge to form the ***rete testis***, a complex tubular network containing cilia. Cilia propel spermatozoa through the rete testis to about a dozen or so ***vasa efferentia*** (efferent ductules), then to the ***epididymis*** and the ***vas deferens***. Other cells of the testes include ***interstitial cells***, which produce ***testosterone***, and ***Sertoli (sustenacular)*** cells, which produce the hormone ***inhibin***. Inhibin suppresses the secretion of ***FSH*** (follicle stimulating hormone) by the anterior pituitary. FSH promotes sperm production; thus inhibin indirectly suppresses sperm production.

Sperm mature in the ***epididymis,*** which is a long coiled tube that lies posterior to the testicle. When mature, sperm are propelled by smooth muscle in the epididymis to the ***vas deferens*** (ductus deferens). The vas deferens ascends from the scrotum and enters the ***inguinal canal***. The vas deferens and the testicular vessels and nerves enter the pelvic cavity through an opening in the abdominal wall. This opening in the abdominal wall is the most common site for herniation in males (inguinal hernia). The vas deferens, testicular blood vessels and nerves in the inguinal canal are contained in a connective tissue sheath called the ***spermatic cord***. A ***vasectomy*** is a sterilizing procedure that entails cutting the vas deferens inside the spermatic cord. The right and left vas deferens extend over the pubic arch and enter the pelvic cavity. Then they proceed in an inferior and posterior direction to a position behind the bladder. The vas deferentia receive the ducts of the ***seminal vesicles,*** after which they are known as the ***ejaculatory ducts***. The ejaculatory ducts are short ducts that open into the urethra within the ***prostate gland***. The prostate secretes a thin, milky fluid that makes up about 30% of the seminal fluid. This gland is located immediately anterior to the rectum, and it can be palpated through the rectum.
The Above: A mature spermatozoon.
bulbourethral glands are located distal to the prostate. They secrete an alkaline fluid into the urethra prior to ejaculation, which neutralizes the acidity of the urine and the female vagina.

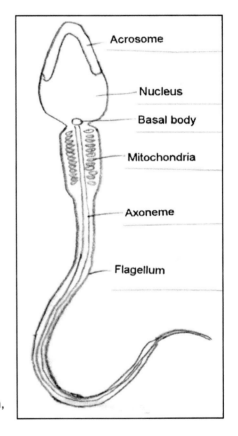

Acrosome

Nucleus

Basal body

Mitochondria

Axoneme

Flagellum

The urethra discharges urine and semen. ***Semen*** is a mixture of sperm cells and secretions of the prostate gland, seminal vesicles and bulbourethral glands. It has a pH of about 7.4. Ejaculation produces about 2-4 ml of semen with about 100 million sperm per ml. Sperm counts less than 25 million per ml are usually infertile. There is evidence that male fertility is decreasing. The average male sperm count in the United States has decreased from 113 million per ml in 1940 to 66 million per ml in 1990, and the average volume of semen has decreased 19% in that time. Concomitant to that has been an increase in congenital anomalies of male infants including ***cryptorchidism*** (undescended testicles) and ***hypospadius*** (a urethral opening in the shaft of the penis rather than the tip). The cause for these changes is obscure, but exposures to unknown chemicals that have an estrogen effect are suspected.

The penis contains three cylindrical bodies called corpora; they are the right and left ***corpora cavernosa*** and the ***corpus spongiosum***. The corpora are a ***spongy*** tissue surrounded by tough, fibrous connective tissue called the ***tunica albuginea.*** An erection is produced by filling the corpora cavernosa with blood. Erection occurs due to stimulation by parasympathetic impulses, which dilate the penile arteries and increase blood flow to the corpora. The engorged corpora compress venous outflow from the penis, which helps maintain an erection. The corpus spongiosum contains the urethra. It passes along the underside of the penis to the tip where it is expanded into the ***glans.*** The skin of the shaft of the penis is quite loose, but the skin of the glans is tightly adherent to the underlying corpus spongiosum. The glans contains numerous nerve endings, and it is protected by the ***prepuce or foreskin***, a fold of skin that is continuous with the skin of the shaft. Sebaceous glands in the foreskin produce a waxy secretion called ***smegma.*** Circumcision removes the foreskin. Ejaculation occurs due to sympathetic stimulation producing contractions of smooth muscle in the vas deferens, prostate gland and seminal vesicles.

When sexual stimulation occurs, ***nitric oxide*** (NO) is released. Nitric oxide activates an enzyme that catalyzes the formation of ***cGMP*** (cyclic guanosine monophosphate). Cyclic GMP causes dilation of the penile arteries. Sildenafil (***Viagra***) and similar drugs act to help create and prolong an erection by inhibiting the enzyme that degrades cGMP.

Men undergo a gradual reduction of testosterone secretion with age. ***Benign prostatic hypertrophy*** also develops with age and may cause urethral obstruction. ***Cancer of the prostate*** is second only to skin cancer as the leading cause of cancer among men. The incidence of ***prostatic cancer*** is far more common in men who are elderly; however, most cases of prostatic cancer progress quite slowly, and it usually is not the cause of death in these patients. ***Testicular cancer*** occurs more commonly in younger men, and it is the most common solid tumor in men between the ages of fifteen and thirty-five.

Female

The female reproductive system consists of a pair of ***ovaries***, a pair of ***fallopian (uterine) tubes***, the ***uterus***, the ***vagina*** and associated structures.

Right: Meiosis I and II. The result of meiosis is the production of the ovum, the first polar body and the second polar body. The polar bodies degenerate.

There are hundreds of potential egg cells in the primary follicles of the ovaries at birth, but only 300-400 of these follicles will produce a mature ovum. Each primary follicle contains an ***oocyte,*** which is surrounded by ***follicle cells***. ***FSH*** (follicle stimulating hormone secreted by the anterior pituitary) is required for a primary follicle to mature into a mature follicle, which is known as a ***graafian follicle***. ***LH*** (luteinizing hormone secreted by the anterior pituitary) causes ovulation, which is expulsion of a secondary oocyte from an ovary. After ovulation, the follicle cells become the ***corpus luteum***, which secretes ***estrogen*** and ***progesterone***. Estrogen is a general term used for several female hormones, the most common being ***estradiol.***

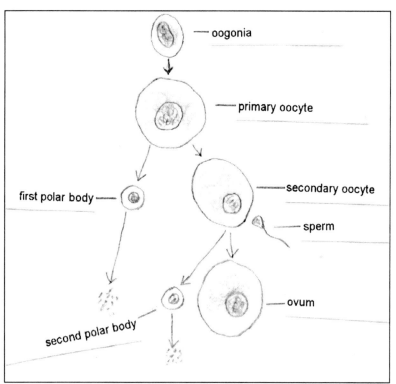

oogonia

primary oocyte

first polar body

secondary oocyte

sperm

second polar body

ovum

Primary ovarian cells destined to produce ova are called **_oogonia_**. Oogonia differentiate into **_primary oocytes_**. Both oogonia and primary oocytes are diploid. In meiosis I a primary oocyte divides into a secondary oocyte and a first polar body. **_Meiosis II is suspended in metaphase_** and is not complete until after ovulation has occurred and a sperm cell has penetrated the plasma membrane of the secondary oocyte.   Then the secondary oocyte completes meiosis II by dividing into the ovum and the second polar body.   Oogonia and primary oocytes are diploid. The secondary oocyte, first polar body, second polar body and the ovum are haploid. The fertilized ovum is a zygote, and it is diploid.

Ovulation is expulsion of the secondary oocyte from the ovary into the pelvic cavity. The ovary is partially surrounded by feathery projections called **_fimbriae_** at the dilated end of a fallopian tube. The fimbriae contain smooth muscle that waves material into the fallopian tube. Epithelial cells on the inner surface of the fallopian tubes contain **_cilia_** that beat toward the uterus. Movements of the cilia and the fimbriae usher the oocyte into the fallopian tube.

After the expulsed oocyte reaches the fallopian tube, it travels toward the uterus. Fertilization usually takes place in the fallopian tube. The **_zygote_** (fertilized egg) usually implants in the wall of the uterus. If it implants elsewhere, such as the fallopian tube or on the abdominal peritoneum, it is called an **_ectopic pregnancy_**. It is rare for an ectopic pregnancy to result in a live birth, and the mother's health is frequently endangered by the existence of an ectopic pregnancy.

Right: Two primordial egg cells are visible in this drawing. The primordial egg on the left is a primary oocyte within a primary follicle. The primordial egg (ovum) on the right is a secondary oocyte that is larger and more mature. Granulosa cells (follicular cells) surround ova. Inside the layer of follicular cells is a clear area called the zona pellucida. The large follicular cavity (antrum) is filled with fluid. In time multiple ovarian follicles bulge on the surface of an

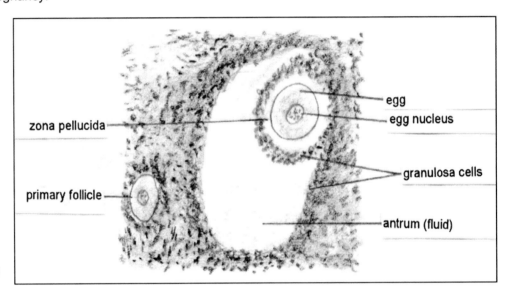

ovary and make the ovary appear cystic. When an oocyte is fully developed, it is extruded from the ovary and enters the fallopian tube.

The **_uterus_** is an organ of smooth muscle with simple columnar epithelium. The **_fundus_** of the uterus is the upper part; the **_body_** is the central portion, and the **_cervix_** is the narrow lower end that opens into the vagina. The fallopian tubes enter the uterus between the fundus and the body. The **_endometrium_** is the inner lining of the uterus. The endometrium becomes increasingly vascularized under the influence of estrogen and progesterone secreted by the corpus luteum. The increased vasculature of the endometrium allows for implantation of the zygote and development of the **_placenta._** **_Endometriosis_** is an abnormal growth of endometrial tissue on the abdominal peritoneum. Despite its ectopic location, this tissue responds to ovarian hormones much like the endometrium of the uterus. Proliferation and bleeding from ectopic endometrial tissue can lead to abdominal pain and discomfort.

The **_vagina_** is a muscular tube that extends from the perineum to the cervix. A thin membrane called the **_hymen_** usually covers the vagina in the perineum. The hymen is ruptured by the first sexual intercourse or by the use of tampons. The vagina is the depository for sperm during sexual intercourse. It is a conduit for the drainage of menstrual flow and for the birthing of the fetus. The mucosa of the prepubertal vagina is simple columnar. It undergoes **_metaplasia_** to nonkeratinized stratified squamous during puberty due to the influence of estrogen.

The external genitalia of the female are called the **_vulva_**. The vulva consists of the **_labia majora_**, which are two lateral folds of cutaneous tissue, and the **_labia minora_**, which are two inner folds of skin. The **_clitoris_** is a small mass of erectile tissue anterior to the urethral orifice; it is the counterpart of the male penis. **_Bartholin glands_** are located inside the labia minora; their secretions keep the mucosa moist and lubricated during intercourse.

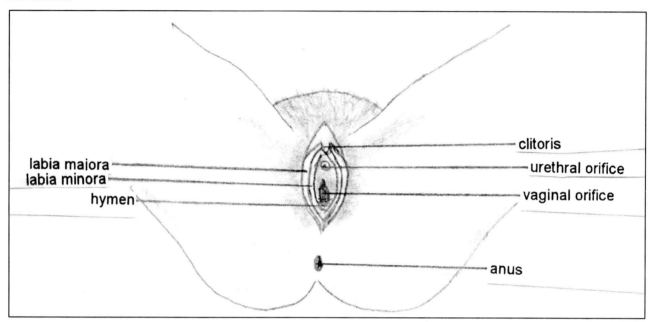

Above: The female external genitalia.

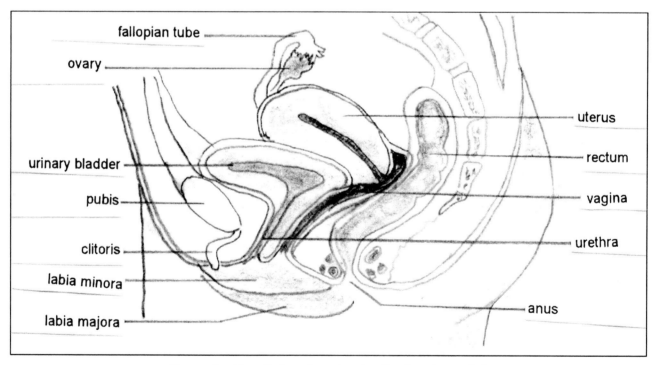

Above: A midsagittal section showing the female genitalia.

Mammary glands develop as a response to the secretion of estrogen and progesterone. The anterior pituitary secretes the hormone, *prolactin,* following delivery of the fetus. Prolactin promotes milk production.

The *menstrual cycle* typically lasts 28 days, the same length of time as a lunar cycle. The fourth and last phase of the menstrual cycle is the *menstrual phase.* This phase coincides with the menstrual flow, and it usually lasts 3-6 days. The *follicular phase* is the first phase of the menstrual cycle, and it follows the menstrual phase. *FSH* is secreted by the anterior pituitary gland during the follicular phase. FSH causes the ovarian follicles to develop and the follicle cells to secrete estrogen. *LH* secretion by the anterior pituitary increases during the second, or *ovulation*, phase, and LH stimulates ovulation. The third phase, the *luteal phase*, follows ovulation. In the luteal phase LH influences the *corpus luteum* to secrete progesterone and estrogen. Progesterone and estrogen stimulate the growth of blood vessels in the *endometrium*. If a zygote does not become implanted in the endometrium, the secretion of LH, estrogen and progesterone decrease, the vascular endometrium sloughs off, and the cycle begins anew.

Menarche is the age of onset of menstrual periods and the beginning of fertility in the female. It occurs at the time of *puberty*. Puberty begins with secretions of FSH and LH by the anterior pituitary. FSH stimulates the growth of ovarian follicles, which secrete estrogens. *Androgens* (male hormones) are secreted by the ovaries and the cortex of the adrenal glands. Estrogen stimulates the development of the breasts, and androgens stimulate terminal hair growth in the pubic and axillary regions. Those are secondary sex characteristics of the female.

Studies have shown that the average age of menarche has been steadily decreasing. This finding is suspected to be due to exposure of young girls to dietary or environmental estrogens. *Precocious puberty* is puberty that occurs at an unusually early age. Black females have a genetic tendency to undergo puberty at a younger age than White females.

Menopause marks the end of ovulation and menstrual periods. A sharp reduction in the secretion of estrogen occurs during menopause, and symptoms such as hot flashes are common.

The incidence of *breast cancer* is second only to skin cancer in women; breast cancer occurs in 10% of all American females. Some families carry a gene that predisposes to breast cancer, but most cases are not hereditary. Estrogen stimulates some breast cancers to grow. The incidence of breast cancer is significantly higher in the United States than it is in less developed countries. The cause for this appears to be in the American diet. Breast cancer also occurs in males; the incidence is low, but the mortality is higher in males than females.

Pregnancy

In the *first trimester* of pregnancy (first three months), *human chorionic gonadotropin* (HCG) is secreted by the *blastocyst* (early embryo) and by the fledgling *placenta*. Pregnancy tests measure the amount HCG in the urine. HCG and LH stimulate the growth of the corpus luteum, and the *corpus luteum* secretes estrogen and progesterone.

Estrogen and progesterone levels increase during the second half of pregnancy, and the *placenta* becomes the chief source for these hormones. *Estrogen* stimulates growth of the uterus and the breasts, and it also stimulates growth of the fetus. *Progesterone* suppresses uterine contractions, and it stimulates growth of the endometrium and the breasts.

Pregnancy causes major changes to the mother's body. Skeletal changes include an increase in width and flexibility of the pubic symphysis and an increase in mobility of the sacroiliac joints. Pregnant females are subject to nausea and intolerance to some foods, a condition commonly known as "morning sickness." If vomiting becomes severe it is termed *hyperemesis gravidarum*. The uterus increases in size from 50 grams to 900 grams during pregnancy. The enlarged uterus can interfere with digestive functions, and it can cause constipation and heartburn. Extra calories and nutrients are needed to support the fetus. Oxygen demand rises, and ventilation increases. The skin is stretched, and striae (stretch marks) may appear over the abdomen. The pituitary gland increases in size by 50%, which reflects an increased production of ACTH and TSH. There is an increased production of melanin in the skin secondary to an increased MSH (melanocyte stimulating hormone) secretion by the pituitary.

The period of pregnancy is known as **_gestation_**; the normal gestation is 40 weeks or 9 months as measured from the beginning of the mother's last menstrual period until the birth of the baby. By the seventh month the fetus turns to a head down or vertex position in the womb (uterus) and most deliveries are head first. Breech deliveries (feet first) have a higher complication rate. The seven-month fetus (28-29 weeks) is considerably undersized, but it usually is viable outside the womb. The fetus who is only six months of age at the time of delivery rarely survives, and birth defects are common in these infants.

Expulsion of the fetus is accomplished by contractions of the uterus. Contractions of the abdominal muscles (a **_Valsalva_** maneuver) are also helpful in expelling the fetus. Uterine contractions begin as a result of rising estrogen secretions and the secretion of **_oxytocin_** by the posterior pituitary. Both of these hormones stimulate uterine contractions.

Weak, ineffectual uterine contractions occur all during pregnancy. These are called **_Braxton-Hicks contractions._** With the onset of true labor, stronger contractions begin about thirty minutes apart. These contractions increase in strength and frequency until they are occur every minute or so prior to delivery. The intermittent nature of uterine contractions allows the placenta to refill between contractions. Stretching of the cervix triggers a **_positive feedback_** that causes more **_oxytocin_** release, and oxytocin stimulates contractions of the body of the uterus.

Pain associated with childbirth is due to ischemia of the uterus and stretching of the vaginal canal. An **_episiotomy_** is an incision done with scissors through the vagina and the labia to widen the birth canal. Episiotomies are done to prevent the vagina from lacerating. An episiotomy is sutured following delivery.

A woman is termed **_primagravida_** when she is in her first pregnancy. Successive pregnancies deem that she is **_multigravida_**. A **_primipara_** woman is in her first delivery. A **_multipara_** woman has had more than one delivery. Labor is typically longer in a woman's first delivery (primipara), and the length of time for labor decreases with subsequent deliveries (multipara). The progress of labor is measured by **_dilation_** and **_effacement_** (thinning) of the cervix. **_Crowning_** is the term for an infant's head that is visible in a dilated cervix.

Following delivery of the fetus, the uterus continues to contract. The **_placenta_** subsequently separates from the uterine wall and is delivered. About 350 ml of blood is lost when the placenta is delivered. The mothers of many animal species ingest the delivered placenta, presumably to obtain the hormones found there.

The **_puerperal period_** is the six week period following delivery. During this time the uterus involutes to its former size. Lochia is a vaginal discharge that is normal and lasts for about 10 days post partum (after delivery).

The mammary glands become distended with secretions in late pregnancy. The first secretions are a liquid called **_colostrum_**. Colostrum is much lower in fat than is true breast milk, which is not secreted until several days after delivery. Colostrum and breast milk are high in **_immunoglobulins_**, which protect the infant from infections.

Problems with pregnancy, labor and delivery include the following:
(1) **_Hyperemesis gravidarum_** is severe nausea and vomiting during pregnancy.
(2) **_Gestational diabetes_** is diabetes mellitus appearing only during pregnancy; it is related to relative insulin insensitivity.
(3) **_Eclampsia, pre-eclampsia, and toxemia_** are terms for the occurrence of severe hypertension with fluid retention and proteinuria during pregnancy. Toxemia is most common in the third trimester. Eclampsia is the term used if the disorder is complicated by seizures. Eclampsia can be fatal.
(4) **_Abortion_** is the expulsion of a nonviable fetus; it is associated with vaginal bleeding. Spontaneous abortions occur because of fetal abnormalities, placental abnormalities and uterine insufficiency.

(5) *Abruptio placenta* is premature separation of the placenta from the wall of the uterus. In this condition an emergency Caesarian section may be required to save the life of the infant.
(6) *Placenta praevia (previa)* is the condition where the placenta is placed low in the uterus near the cervix. If the placenta blocks the cervical canal, the infant cannot be born unless a Caesarian section is done.
(7) *Puerperal fever* is a streptococcal infection of the mother's birth canal following delivery.

A number of diseases are transmitted through sexual intercourse. These diseases are known as sexually transmitted diseases (STD) or venereal diseases (VD). *Syphilis* (or lues) is caused by *Treponema pallidum*, a corkscrew shaped bacterium that is classified as a spirochete. *T. pallidum* is capable of penetrating the skin of the penis and the mucosa of the female vagina. Syphilis has three stages, and symptoms typically disappear between stages. The first stage is manifest by a *chancre*, which is a visible skin or mucous membrane ulceration that contains active spirochetes. The second stage lasts 3-5 weeks and involves a distinctive rash, fever, arthritic pains and alopecia (hair loss). The third stage involves damage to heart valves, blood vessels and the nervous system; it often results in paralysis and dementia.

Gonorrhea is an infectious disease caused by *Neisseria gonorrhea*, a gram negative diplococcus. Gonorrhea typically produces a *purulent* (yellow pus) *urethral discharge* in the male. In the female the gonococcus tends to infect the uterus and fallopian tubes and cause what is known as *PID* (pelvic inflammatory disease). Scarring can cause urethral obstruction in the male and sterility in the female.

Chlamydia, Mycoplasma and Ureaplasma are other causes of infectious urethritis in the male.

Genital Herpes is caused by the HSV-2 virus (*Herpes simplex* virus type 2). HSV-1 causes fever blisters in humans, and HSV-1 is a close relative of HSV-2. Herpes viruses travel through axons of sensory nerves to the dorsal root ganglia, where they become dormant. They can later multiply and migrate along the nerves to cause cutaneous lesions. HSV-2 has been found to be a risk factor in causing cervical cancer.
Genital warts are caused by human papillomaviruses (HPV). These warts may occur on the skin of the genitalia or near the genitalia, and on the mucosa of the vagina or cervix. They have also caused lesions on the ovaries. Chronic HPV infections are closely associated with cervical cancer, and the virus can be found in the cervix in *90% of cases of cervical cancer.* A vaccine that immunizes against HPV is now available.
Hepatitis B and *hepatitis C* viruses can be transmitted sexually. They cause severe and often fatal liver infections.

The most important epidemic of our time is *AIDS* (acquired immunodeficiency syndrome), which is caused by *HIV* (human immunodeficiency virus). This virus apparently escaped from a reservoir in African monkeys and chimpanzees to humans in the mid twentieth century. It is estimated that since that time AIDS has been responsible for the deaths of 25 million people, and 38.6 million people are currently suffering from the disease. Between 21.6 million and 27.4 million of those presently afflicted are in Sub-Saharan Africa. It takes an average of 9-10 years to develop full blown AIDS after an initial infection with HIV.
AIDS was first reported in several homosexual men in Los Angeles in 1981. Retrospectively it has been found in preserved plasma taken from a man in the Democratic Republic of Congo in 1959. The first case in the United States to be proven from preserved tissue was a 15 year old African-American boy who had been to Haiti, but died in St. Louis. Preserved serum from a Norwegian sailor who died in 1976 has also tested positive for HIV.
HIV preferentially infects *helper T cells* (T-H). T-H counts between 600 and 1200 per microliter are normal; T-H counts less than 200 cells per microliter signify that an HIV-infected individual has progressed to AIDS and is vulnerable to the complications of AIDS. The loss of T-H cells reflects a loss of cellular immunity and humoral immunity, and AIDS patients lose the ability to fight HIV and other pathogenic organisms.
HIV can be transmitted through blood, semen, vaginal secretions and breast milk. It can also be transmitted through the placenta and cause a congenital infection. The most common means of transmission in adults are sexual intercourse, the administration of contaminated blood products, and the use of contaminated needles.
No cure is presently available, but a growing number of expensive new drugs are now available to suppress HIV multiplication, reduce the complications of AIDS and prolong the life of the AIDS patient. It is hoped that an effective AIDS vaccine will be forthcoming, but none is available at present.

Study Guide
1. Name the organs of reproduction in the male, and understand their location.
2. Name the organs of reproduction in the female, and understand their location.
3. Define haploid and diploid. Know which cells are haploid and which are diploid.
4. What are androgens and what glands secrete them?
5. What are estrogens and what glands secrete them?
6. What is the function of FSH and ICSH in the male?
7. What is the function of FSH and LH in the female?
8. Define cryptorchidism.
9. Define hypospadius.
10. Understand the physiology of a penile erection.
11. Know that the most common cancer in men and in women is skin cancer. What is the second most common cancer in men? ....in women?
12. Acquaint yourself with the following sexually transmitted diseases: syphilis, gonorrhea, HIV, genital Herpes and hepatitis B.
13. Review the menstrual cycle.
14. What is the corpus luteum, and what hormones does it produce?
15. Understand the anatomical relationship between the ovary and the fallopian tube.
16. Define zygote, embryo and fetus.
17. Define ectopic pregnancy.
18. Define endometrium and endometriosis.
19. Describe the prepubertal and the postpubertal epithelium of the vagina.
20. What is prolactin?
21. What is colostrum?
22. Define menarche and menopause.
23. What hormones are secreted by the placenta?
24. What are Braxton-Hicks contractions?
25. What is oxytocin?
26. Define primipara, multipara, crowning, dilation and effacement as they relate to pregnancy and delivery.
27. Define the puerperal period.
28. What is puerperal fever?
29. Define toxemia, eclampsia and pre eclampsia.
30. Define abruptio placenta and placenta praevia.

Chapter Twenty-two

Life in Utero

In utero means within the uterus.

Mitosis is cell division by somatic cells. Somatic cells are all the cells of the body except the germ cells. Mitosis produces two daughter cells that are exact genetic replicas of one parent cell. *Meiosis* is cell division that becomes sperm and egg cells, which are known as *gametes*. The genetic material of gametes is unlike that of other cells; gametes contain only half as much genetic material as the cells from which they are derived. In other words, mitosis results in the production of somatic cells, which are diploid (they have 46 chromosomes), and *meiosis* results in the production of the sperm and egg cells, which are *haploid* (they have 23 chromosomes).

Meiosis differs from mitosis in four important ways:
(1) Meiosis occurs only in the production of sperm and egg cells.
(2) Whereas mitosis results in a cell with a diploid number of chromosomes, meiosis results in a cell with a haploid number of chromosomes.
(3) Mitosis results in new cells that have the exact genetic make up as the parent cell. In meiosis the DNA within each chromosomal pair is mixed in a process known as crossing over. Crossing over creates a new chromosome that is not a copy of an original chromosome. Instead the new chromosome contains a new combination of DNA with material from both the maternal parent and the paternal parent.
(4) In mitosis a parent cell produces two cloned diploid daughter cells. In meiosis four haploid daughter cells are produced from one parent cell. Each of the daughter cells has different genetic material.

A review of meiosis (See chapter four)

In meiosis as in mitosis, DNA is first replicated. This step creates twice the amount of DNA in the nucleus. Each chromosome then consists of two *chromatids* joined by a *centromere.* Each chromatid has an amount of DNA equal to that of the chromosome before DNA replication. The cell is still diploid, and it has 46 chromosomes, but each chromosome has twice as much DNA as it had before.

The process of meiosis is divided into two stages, *meiosis I and meiosis II. Prophase, metaphase and anaphase* of meiosis I are similar to the phases in mitosis, except that in meiosis I the maternal and the paternal chromosomal pair line up side by side, creating a *tetrad*. Each tetrad contains four chromatids. *Crossing over* is the mixing of genetic material within a tetrad, and it occurs in prophase of meiosis I.

In *telophase* of meiosis I the tetrad splits, but the centromeres do not disappear. As a result each chromosome contains two chromatids. Therefore, the daughter cells of meiosis I contain only 23 chromosomes and they are haploid. Each of the 23 chromosomes of these cells contains two chromatids, so the nuclei of these cells contain an amount of DNA equal to that of the parent cell before DNA replication.

In *Meiosis II* the chromatids break apart and each daughter cell receives one chromatid from each chromosome. These daughter cells remain haploid, but now they have only half the DNA material of a diploid cell before DNA replication. This is the final product of meiosis. Each sperm cell and each egg cell has 23 single stranded chromosomes when meiosis II is complete.

The production of *sperm* cells begins with *spermatogonia* cells in the testes. Spermatogonia cells are *diploid* (they have 46 chromosomes), and they divide by *mitosis* to reproduce themselves. Some spermatogonia cells (called "Type B") develop into *primary spermatocytes*, which then divide by meiosis. Four sperm cells are formed from the meiotic division of one primary spermatocyte. Potentially four egg cells could be formed from the meiotic division of one *primary oocyte*, but that does not happen. The first meiotic division results in the formation of a *secondary oocyte* and the *first polar body*. The first polar body degenerates, and the secondary oocyte *remains suspended in metaphase* of meiosis II until fertilization occurs. Then the secondary oocyte divides into the *egg* cell and the *second polar body*, which degenerates.

Each egg cell contains 22 *autosomes* and one X (*sex) chromosome*. The sperm cells contain 22 autosomes and either one X chromosome or one Y chromosome. Thus it is the sperm cell that determines whether the child will have an XX karyotype (chromosomal make up) and be female, or have an XY karyotype and be male.

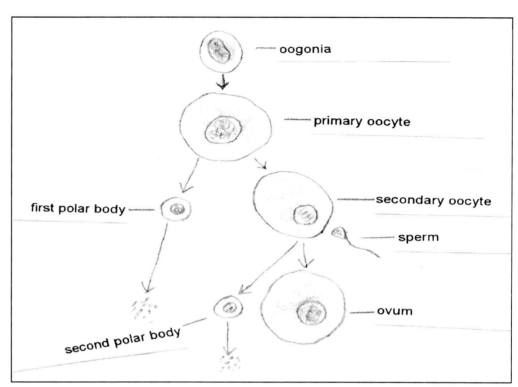

Right: Meiosis I and II. The result of meiosis I is the production of the secondary oocyte and the first polar body.
The second polar Meiosis II is not complete until fertilization of the secondary oocyte has occurred. Then the secondary oocyte divides into the ovum and the second polar body.
Both polar bodies degenerate.

Faulty meiosis may result in the sperm or the egg having an abnormal amount of genetic material. In such a case the **_zygote_** (fertilized egg) and every cell of the embryo, fetus and infant would have an abnormal amount of genetic material. For instance there are syndromes in which there is an extra chromosome. In these syndromes either the sperm or the egg would have had an extra chromosome, and therefore, the embryo would have 47 chromosomes--twenty-two pair and one triplet. These syndromes are thought to be caused by failure of a centromere to disappear during anaphase II of meiosis. The result is one germ cell with an extra chromosome and one germ cell lacking a chromosome.

The most common of these syndromes is **_Down's syndrome_**. In Down's syndrome there is an extra chromosome #21, and it is called **_trisomy 21_**. Symptoms of Down's syndrome include mental retardation, prominent epicanthal folds (hence the previous name, "Mongoloid"), short stature, short fingers and hands, retarded physical development, a large protruding tongue and low set ears. Heart, kidney and immune disorders are common. Seventy-five percent of individuals with Down's syndrome die before birth, but a few survive past sixty years, although many of these people have developed senile dementia by the age of forty.

Not all cases of Down's syndrome are of equal severity. Some lack many of the usual physical characteristics and are much brighter than others. Most of those who die prior to being born truly have an extra chromosome, but milder cases of Down's syndrome may have 46 chromosomes. In these people one of the #21 chromosomes contains an extra amount of genetic material and can be seen to be longer than normal. This genetic snafu occurs during prophase I as the result of faulty crossing over of genetic material, which results in an unequal distribution of chromatic material between the #21 chromosomes.

Trisomy 13 and **_Trisomy 18_** result in severe fetal malformations. Most infants with either of these karyotypes die before birth and are spontaneously aborted. Both disorders are invariably fatal no later than early infancy.

There are no known syndromes whereby a fetus lacks an autosome because these cases are invariably fatal prior to delivery. However, if the fetus lacks a sex chromosome, the symptoms are less severe, and the fetus may survive. In addition there are several syndromes with trisomy of the sex chromosomes in which survival is possible or even probable. One is **_Klinefelter's syndrome_**, in which the individual has an XXY karyotype. These people are male, but the have undeveloped testes, low testosterone levels, and they are usually sterile.

Individuals with Klinefelter's syndrome tend to be taller than average. They have long limbs, they are often overweight, and their secondary sex characteristics fail to develop at puberty. They have high pitched voices and sparse body hair. They sometimes have enlarged breasts (gynecomastia). Learning problems are common in people with Klinefelter's syndrome.

The XYY karyotype was initially identified in the French male prison population in 1961. This led to the conclusion that XYY males were antisocial and violent. Further studies have shown that the mental capacities and motor skills of XYY boys develop more slowly than normal; they tend to have learning problems and minor speech problems. Their tendency for violence appears to have been overstated; however, they have elevated testosterone levels, which may produce violent behavior. XYY males average three inches taller than other males, and most have pronounced acne as teenagers. Despite learning problems, their intelligence is usually within the normal range. Most are regarded as normal males, and they are often fertile despite the presence of abnormal, immature appearing sperm cells on microscopic examination.

Females with triploid sex chromosomes have an XXX karyotype. These women are usually fertile, and they lead relatively normal lives. They tend to be tall with long legs, and they tend to be in the low normal range of intelligence. They are often referred to as emotionally immature, and they frequently are regarded as troublemakers.

Additional sex chromosomes (XXXX, XYYY, etc.) lead to more severe forms of the above syndromes.

The only viable syndrome that is due to the lack of a chromosome is ***Turner's syndrome***. About three percent of all fetuses with Turner's syndrome are born alive and survive to adulthood. They have 45 chromosomes and the XO karyotype ("O" designating the lack of the second sex chromosome). Individuals with Turner's syndrome are short, infertile females. They are mentally retarded, and they have a webbed neck, widely spaced nipples and a wide carrying angle (coxa valga). Their ovaries are atrophic and nearly absent; secondary sexual characteristics fail to appear at puberty.

A few individuals have been discovered who possess two kinds of somatic cells, each with its own type of genetic material (DNA). These people are normal in all respects, and they are only discovered when their DNA is analyzed. They are essentially two individuals in one body, and they are called ***chimera.*** It is known that the secondary oocyte is suspended in metaphase of meiosis II until fertilization occurs. How a human chimera forms is not known, but one theory claims that it comes about due to simultaneous fertilization of the secondary oocyte by two different sperm. This could result in fertilization of both the potential egg nucleus and the potential second polar body, which would not degenerate after fertilization. The double zygote would undergo cytokinesis with each of the two daughter cells containing a different genetic makeup.

Sperm cells are deposited in the vagina during sexual intercourse. The number of sperm deposited averages 66 million, and over 100 million is common. If less that 20 million are ejaculated, the male is usually infertile. Spermatozoa are motile due to their flagella, and in order to fertilize an egg, they most migrate from the vagina through the uterus to a fallopian tube. They must choose the correct fallopian tube and ascend it to the proximal 1/3 where fertilization takes place.

An egg (actually a secondary oocyte that is suspended in metaphase) is released from an ovary of a fertile female approximately every 28 days. The egg must enter the fallopian tube (there is no direct connection here, only a wide opening to the tube) and travel down the tube. If the egg encounters sperm in the upper part of the tube, fertilization may take place. The window for fertilization to occur must take into account a maximum of 24 hours during which the egg is fertile after its release from the ovary, and a 48 hour period during which the sperm are fertile after ejaculation. This period is reduced by about ten hours because the sperm must undergo a process called capacitation before they can penetrate the egg. ***Capacitation*** involves the removal of cholesterol from the head (***acrosome***) of the sperm. This exposes enzymes necessary for penetration of the egg.

Around the egg is a blanket of ***granulosa cells*** called the ***corona radiata*** and a gelatinous layer called the ***zona pellucida***. The presence of hundreds of sperm and their enzymes is required to open a path through the granulosa cells and the zona pellucida, so that one sperm will reach the plasma membrane of the egg. After one spermatocyte has penetrated the egg cell membrane, additional sperm cannot enter due to the opening of sodium channels in the egg cell membrane, which depolarizes the membrane and prevents other sperm from binding with the membrane and entering the egg. Spermatic penetration also increases calcium penetrability of the egg cell membrane, which creates an area of swelling under the zona pellucida that pushes other sperm away from the egg.

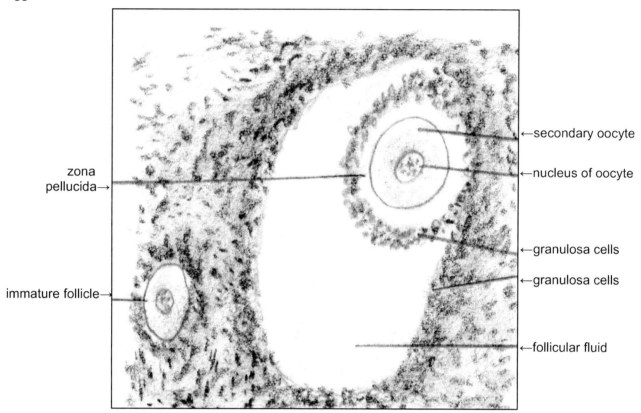

zona pellucida→

immature follicle→

←secondary oocyte

←nucleus of oocyte

←granulosa cells

←granulosa cells

←follicular fluid

Above: Granulosa cells and the zona pellucida surround the secondary oocyte.

Only the head and midpiece of the sperm enter the egg; the flagellum is left behind. The mitochondria of the sperm are destroyed within the egg. Only maternal mitochondrial DNA is passed on to offspring.

Before **_fertilization_** (penetration of a sperm cell through the plasma membrane of the egg), the meiotic process of the egg is suspended in metaphase II. It is not until after fertilization that the secondary oocyte completes meiosis II. After fertilization, the egg and the sperm each form a **_pronucleus_**. Each pronucleus contains twenty-three chromosomes. The pronuclei swell and unite into a single nucleus with a diploid number of chromosomes. The fertilized egg has then become a **_zygote._**

The zygote begins to undergo mitosis about thirty hours after fertilization. When it is three days old, it consists of sixteen cells or more, and it is called a **_morula_** (mulberry).

Identical or monozygotic twins result from a division into two cellular masses at the morula stage or before. Dizygotic or fraternal twins result from the concomitant release of two secondary oocytes, each of which is fertilized by a different sperm.

The morula loses the zona pellucida and granulosa cell coverings; it becomes a hollowed-out sphere call a **_blastocyst_**. A blastocyst contains an outer layer of cells called the **_trophoblast_** and an inner mass of cells called the **_embryoblast_**. The trophoblast becomes the fetal part of the **_placenta_**, and the embryoblast becomes the **_embryo._**

At about six days the blastocyst attaches to the inner lining of the uterus (the **_endometrium_**) and begins to implant itself. The term "pregnancy" or "gestation" refers to the presence of an implanted blastocyst, embryo or fetus. If the blastocyst attaches to the wall of a fallopian tube and implants there, it is called an **_ectopic pregnancy_**. Ectopic pregnancies may also occur on the peritoneum of the abdominal or pelvic cavity. Ectopic pregnancies are a serious threat to the mother's life. Tubal pregnancies usually result in rupture of the fallopian tube within twelve weeks. Abdominal pregnancies are rarer; they usually require an abortion, but a few have resulted in a live birth following a Caesarean delivery. The most common cause of an ectopic pregnancy is a stricture in a fallopian tube.

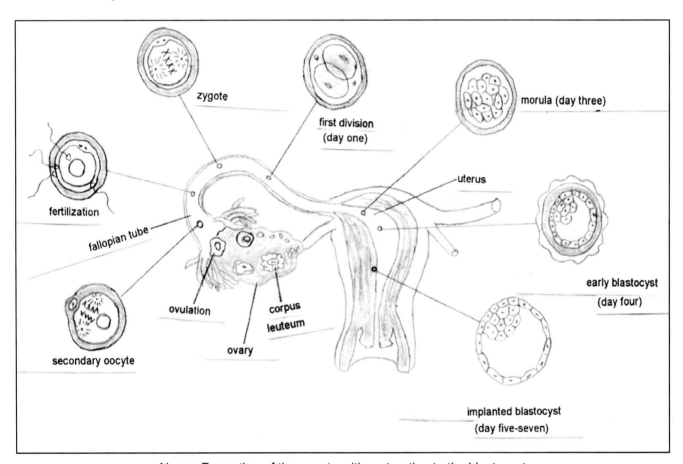

Above: Formation of the zygote with maturation to the blastocyst.

The embryo stage begins at one week gestation and continues until the end of the second month. The embryo stage is characterized by the gradual change from an amorphous cellular mass into an identifiable organism. The embryo begins as a disc with two cell layers, **_ectoderm_** and **_endoderm._** **_Mesoderm_** forms by an invagination of ectodermal cells into the space between the ectoderm and the endoderm. Ectoderm, mesoderm and endoderm are the **_primary germ cell layers_**. Ectoderm develops into the epidermis and the nervous system. Endoderm develops into the epithelium of the GI tract and its associated glands (liver, pancreas, and smaller glands) and the epithelium of the lungs and respiratory tract. Epithelial tissues contain a basement membrane and are derived from either ectoderm or endoderm. Mesoderm develops into muscle tissue and the various connective tissues of the body including bone, cartilage, and blood.

The early embryo is a tiny disc in the blastocyst. Four membranes develop with the embryo: (1) A _**yolk sac**_ and (2) an _**amniotic membrane**_ develop from cells of the embryonic disc. Cells of the yolk sac eventually form part of the digestive tract, the first blood cells, and future germ (sperm and egg) cells. The amnion protects the embryo by completely surrounding it with fluid. Amniotic fluid initially forms by filtration from the mother's plasma; later the fetus urinates into the amniotic cavity.

(3) The _**allantoic membrane**_ forms from the yolk sac. The allantois becomes the foundation for the umbilical cord and a portion of the urinary bladder.

(4) The fourth fetal membrane is the _**chorion**_, which develops _**chorionic villi**_ from the _**trophoblast**_ and functions as the fetal portion of the _**placenta**_. The placenta has begun to develop by the eleventh day, and it continues to develop until the twelfth week. The trophoblast divides into the _**syncytiotrophoblast**_ and the _**cytotrophoblast.**_ Chorionic villi are extensions of the syncytiotrophoblast that penetrate deeply into the endometrium of the uterus and stimulate the maternal circulation to pool into sinuses. These sinuses surround chorionic villi. The diffusion of gases, nutrients and waste products takes place across the placental membrane between the chorionic villi of the fetus and the placental sinuses of the maternal circulation. The fetal and the maternal circulation are kept separated by the membranes of the placenta. Materials crossing the placental membrane to the fetus include oxygen, fatty acids, amino acids, steroids, vitamins, minerals, glucose and electrolytes. Waste products that cross the placental membrane to the mother include carbon dioxide, urea, ammonia, uric acid and creatinine.

The placenta functions as the lungs, kidneys and digestive system of the fetus and it is responsible for the production of _**HCG**_ (human chorionic gonadotropin), a hormone that is detectable by pregnancy tests.

By _**eight weeks**_ of age all the organ systems are present. At this time the embryo is three cm. long, and it is classified as a _**fetus.**_ In the early fetus bones have begun to ossify, muscles exhibit tiny, feeble contractions, and the heart beats and circulates blood. The head is half as long as the total embryo, and the heart and liver are proportionately large.

The fetal stage of development begins at the eighth week and lasts until birth. The circulation of the fetus depends upon the fetal heart, and the placenta serves the respiratory, digestive and urinary functions of the fetus. Two _**umbilical arteries**_ arise from the fetal internal iliac arteries and lead to the placenta. A single umbilical vein leads from the placenta to the fetus. The umbilical vein branches into the future _**hepatic portal vein**_, which goes to the liver, and the _**ductus venosus**_, which empties into the inferior vena cava. The ductus venosus is larger than the fetal portal vein; however, the ductus venosus closes at birth. The umbilical vein closes becomes the round ligament of the liver, which extends from the liver to the umbilicus. The ductus venosus becomes the ligamentum venosum, which is on the inferior surface of the liver. The median umbilical ligaments of the abdominal wall and the superior vesical arteries, which supply the bladder, are derived from the umbilical arteries.

The umbilical vein and the ductus venosus bring blood that is rich in oxygen and nutrients from the placenta to the inferior vena cava of the fetus. This blood goes to the right side of the heart. But the fetal lungs are not functional, and most of this oxygen-rich blood bypasses the lungs by two routes: (1) Blood is shunted from the right atrium to the left atrium through an opening between the atria called the _**foramen ovale**_. (2) Blood is shunted from the pulmonary artery to the aorta through a connecting channel called the _**ductus arteriosus**_. Both the foramen ovale and the ductus arteriosus close after birth when the lungs have filled with air.

Congenital (present at birth) circulatory problems include the failure of the foramen ovale or the ductus arteriosus to close. These openings are called _**patent**_ when they do not close at birth. When the ductus arteriosus or the foramen ovale is patent, the left ventricle is required to work harder to pump blood into the systemic circuit because a left-to-right shunt (systemic circuit to pulmonary circuit) develops after birth. Pulmonary hypertension, pulmonary edema and cardiomegaly (an enlarged heart) are side effects to look for in this situation.

If a patent ductus arteriosus is complicated by valve defects and pulmonary hypertension caused by constricted pulmonary vessels, the shunt may become a right-to-left shunt (pulmonary to systemic circuit). The result would be the circulation of oxygen-poor blood through the systemic circuit, and the patient's skin would be cyanotic.

A defect in the interventricular septum (interventricular septal defect) would create a left-to-right shunt because the left ventricle is more powerful than the right ventricle; consequently the blood in the left ventricle is under higher pressure. Eventually pulmonary hypertension, pulmonary edema and cardiomegaly could result.

The fetus usually assumes a **_vertex_** (head down) position by the seventh month, and most vaginal deliveries are head first. When the fetal feet present first, the position is called **_breech_**. Breech deliveries are more difficult and have more complications than vertex deliveries. When vaginal delivery of the fetus is expected to be difficult and inadvisable, delivery may be carried out by a surgical incision into the abdominal wall and into the uterus. This is called a **_Caesarean section_**.

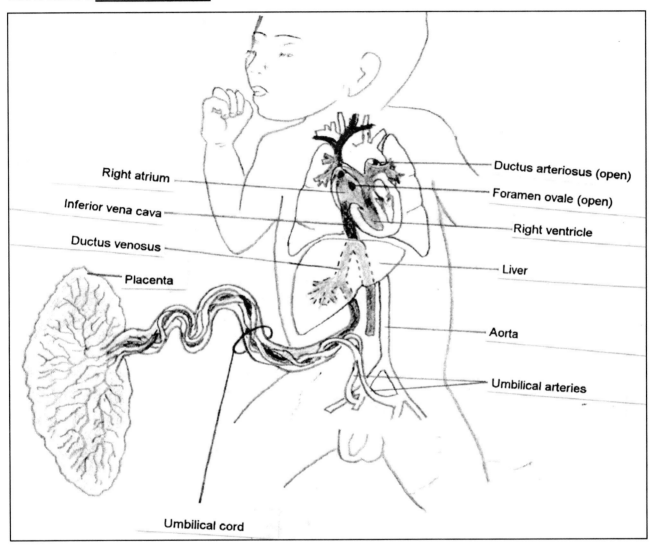

Above: The pattern of blood circulation in the fetus.

Prematurity

Gestation time is measured from the beginning of the last menstrual period (LMP) to the birth of the baby. The LMP begins about two weeks before fertilization and implantation so that gestational measurements overstate the length of pregnancy by about two weeks. The LMP is used because most women remember the time of their menstrual periods, and there are no useful ways to determine the time of fertilization or implantation.

Forty weeks is the normal length of time for a measured gestation. Prematurity is regarded as a gestation less than **_37 weeks_**. Prematurity often leads to complications due to the immature status of the infant's organs. The **_kidneys_** may not be able to concentrate the urine or resorb electrolytes adequately. The **_liver_** has a decreased capacity to conjugate bilirubin or synthesize bile salts and clotting factors. And the liver may not produce enough albumin to prevent edema. The infant may be unable to take feedings well enough to prevent hypoglycemia or hypocalcemia.

Breathing problems are frequently encountered in premature infants ("premies"), and they are the leading cause of death in the premature. This is called ***respiratory distress syndrome or hyaline membrane disease.*** Immaturity of the lungs leads to a ***lack of surfactant***, without which the ***alveoli collapse***. Oxygen and positive pressure ventilation may be necessary.

Premies are prone to develop ***retinopathy of prematurity (retrolental fibroplasia)***, which entails the growth of blood vessels and fibrous tissue on the surface of the retinas and into the vitreous cavities of the eyes. Infants with respiratory distress syndrome who have been given oxygen are most susceptible to develop retinopathy of prematurity.

Cardiac abnormalities, especially a patent ductus arteriosus, are common in premature infants.

The shorter the gestation of a premature infant, the more likely it is that the infant will have problems. Infants with a gestation ***less than 32 weeks*** (seven months) are especially likely to have major complications, and many will not survive. 12% of all births in the U.S. are premature, and 25% of all neonatal deaths are due to prematurity. Premature babies who survive have a higher incidence of developmental delay, mental retardation, cerebral palsy, behavioral problems, mental depression and reduced vision and hearing.

The youngest recorded premie to survive had a gestational period one day short of 22 weeks. The smallest premie to survive was a 25 week fetus who weighed only 8.6 ounces (244 grams) and was eight inches long. These cases who survived are extreme exceptions, and they required a lengthy hospital stay before they could be released.

Generally speaking, the newborn that is less than 32 weeks or has a birth weight less than 2 1/2 pounds (1400 gm) is in a high risk category for complications of prematurity and neonatal death. It is uncommon for a baby to survive who has a birth weight less than one pound ten ounces (700 grams).

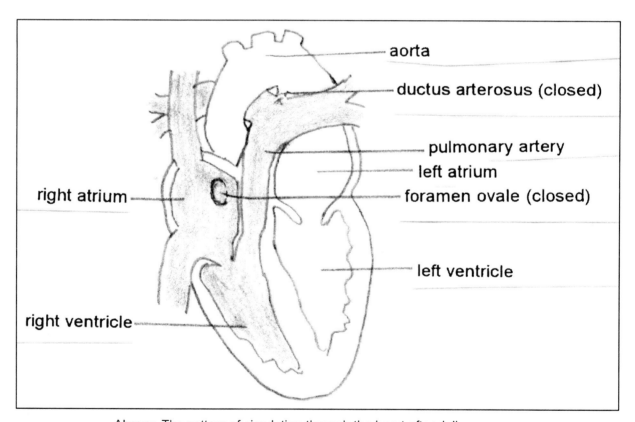

Above: The pattern of circulation through the heart after delivery.

Postmaturity

A postmature baby has a gestation that exceeds **_42 weeks_**. Postmature births account for about 7% of all births in the U.S. After 42 weeks, the **_placenta functions less efficiently_**, and the fetus may stop gaining weight or even lose weight. The fetus may become hypoxic and hypoglycemic as a result of poor placental function.

The volume of amniotic fluid may decrease in the postmature fetus, and meconium (the stool of a fetus or newborn) may enter the amniotic fluid. When a postmature newborn first breathes, he may aspirate amniotic fluid containing meconium, which would create respiratory problems.

The postmature baby may exhibit dry, peeling skin, overgrown nails, abundant hair and creases on his palms and soles. Meconium in the amniotic fluid may stain his skin brown, green or yellow.

It is possible that the fetus sends chemical messages that stimulate uterine contractions signifying that it is ready to be delivered, but the fetus is a passive participant in the labor process. The fetus is expulsed by contractions of the uterus and the maternal abdominal muscles.

Following delivery of the fetus, the placenta and fetal membranes (collectively called the "after-birth") are delivered, and the umbilical cord is clamped. Uterine contractions limit maternal blood loss, but about 350 cc of blood is typically lost by the mother during placental delivery.

The first secretion of the mammary glands following delivery is colostrum, an antibody-rich, protein-rich, low fat liquid. Breast milk, which has a high fat content, begins to be secreted three or four days post-partum.

The six week period after delivery is called the **_puerperal period_**. The uterus rapidly involutes during this period by diminishing in size and cellularity. **_Puerperal fever_** is a streptococcal infection of the mother's uterus and birth canal that occurs in the puerperal period. Puerperal fever was the cause of death for thousands of women until 1847, when a Viennese physician named Ignatz Semmelweiss accused his colleagues of spreading the infection by failing to wash their hands between deliveries. Semmelweiss was proved to be correct, and his insight led to a marked decline in maternal morbidity and mortality.

During the time an unborn child lives in his mother's womb, he is shielded from outside stimuli. He is in a protective cocoon, and unless he is he is exposed to toxic substances in his mother's blood or physical trauma to her abdomen, his life would be placid and serene. That completely changes with the shock of being born. Uterine contractions forcefully push him out of his home, and he is squeezed through a narrow channel that mashes his head into a misshapen deformity that persists for days. He is suddenly deprived of his life line, the umbilical cord. His respiratory system, urinary system and digestive system must now perform on their own. He is hypoxemic and cyanotic when he is delivered. He is spanked and frightened in order that his first breaths will be deep and forceful in order to fill his lungs with air. His young liver has not matured enough to furnish an adequate amount of glucose for his metabolic needs, and he must utilize stored fat for energy. He may suffer from hemolysis and become jaundiced because his liver cannot excrete an adequate amount of bilirubin into the bile. He is in danger of becoming dehydrated because his young kidneys are not yet able to concentrate urine adequately.

Changes in his heart and blood vessels must occur soon after birth. The umbilical arteries shrink and fibrose to become the median umbilical ligaments and the superior vesical arteries of the bladder. The umbilical vein and the ductus venosus fibrose and become ligaments attached to the liver. After the lungs inflate and more blood flows through the pulmonary circuit, two flaps close the foramen ovale in the interatrial septum. The ductus arteriosus gradually begins to close due to the increased oxygen level in the blood and the release of bradykinin by the newly inflated lungs. The ductus arteriosus becomes the ligamentum arteriosum, a fibrous cord between the ascending aorta and the pulmonary trunk.

Failure of the foramen ovale or the ductus arteriosus to close produces a left to right shunt and an increased work load on the heart.

Study Guide

1. Understand the processes of mitosis and meiosis.
2. Know the chromosomal content of somatic cells and gametes.
3. What are the products of meiosis?
4. Understand what is meant by haploid, diploid, tetrad, and crossing over.
5. Understand how the X and the Y chromosomes determine the sex of an individual.
6. Be familiar with the development of the zygote, morula, blastocyst, embryo and fetus.
7. Know the significance of the trophoblast, chorionic villi and placenta.
8. Understand the formation and function of the embryonic membranes (chorion, amnion, allantois and yolk sac).
9. Trace the route of blood circulation in the fetus.
10. Know the anatomy and functions of the placenta.
11. List the differences between the fetal circulation and the circulation in a normal two day old infant.
12. Know that the placenta is by far the major source of estrogen and progesterone in the pregnant female who has past 8 weeks gestation.
13. Know what substances normally cross the placenta and the direction they travel.

Chapter Twenty-three

The Lymphatic Immune System

Lymph nodes, the spleen, bone marrow and the thymus gland are organs that belong to the lymphatic-immune system. **_Lymph_** is tissue fluid contained in lymph vessels. Tissue fluid collects because filtration from the arterial end of the capillary network exceeds the osmotic reabsorption of fluid into the venous end of the capillary network. The excess tissue fluid enters small, permeable, fragile, dead-end lymph capillaries. **_Lacteals_** are lymph capillaries in the mucosa of the small intestine. Lacteals absorb digested fatty materials.

Lymph capillaries merge to form larger vessels, and lymph travels in a proximal direction. The movement of lymph is relatively slow; it is accomplished by **_muscle contraction_** and by pressure changes in the chest created by **_inspiration and expiration_**. The endothelial cells of a lymphatic capillary are not tightly bound, and they overlap, which acts as a one-way **_valve._** The basement membrane of the lymph endothelium is incomplete or absent, which facilitates the transit of material into a lymph vessel.

Lymph vessels are absent in areas that lack a blood supply (epithelial tissues, cornea, lens, and cartilage), and they are also absent in bone marrow and the CNS. Lymphatic vessels that are larger than capillaries contain true valves. Most lymphatic vessels parallel arteries and veins.

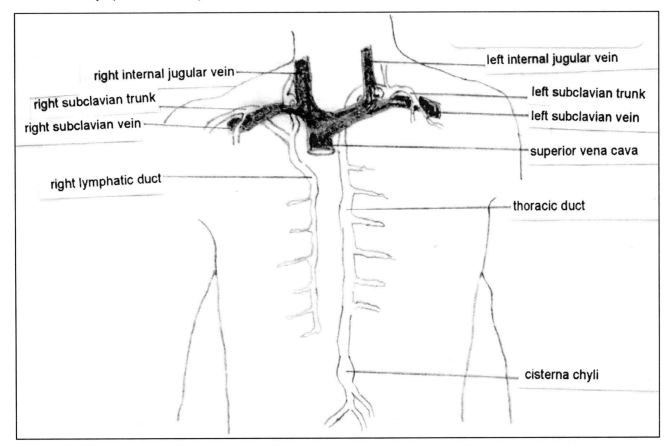

Above: Lymph drainage. Note the positions of thoracic duct and the right lymphatic duct.

Lymph vessels from the lower extremities, lower abdomen and pelvis unite at the L-2 level to form the **_thoracic duct_**, the largest lymph channel in the body. The thoracic duct is located anterior and to the left of the vertebral column. **_Lacteals_** from the small intestine drain into the **_cisterna chyli_**, a dilatation of the thoracic duct in the abdomen. Lymph travels in an upward direction in the thoracic duct to the left supraclavicular space. The thoracic duct also collects lymph from the left side of the head, neck and thorax, and it empties into the left subclavian vein.

The **_right lymphatic duct_** collects lymph from the right arm, right side of the head and neck and the right side of the thorax; it empties into the right subclavian vein. Flaps at the mouths of the thoracic duct and right lymphatic duct prevent backflow from the subclavian veins.

Right: The lymph drainage pattern of the body.

f

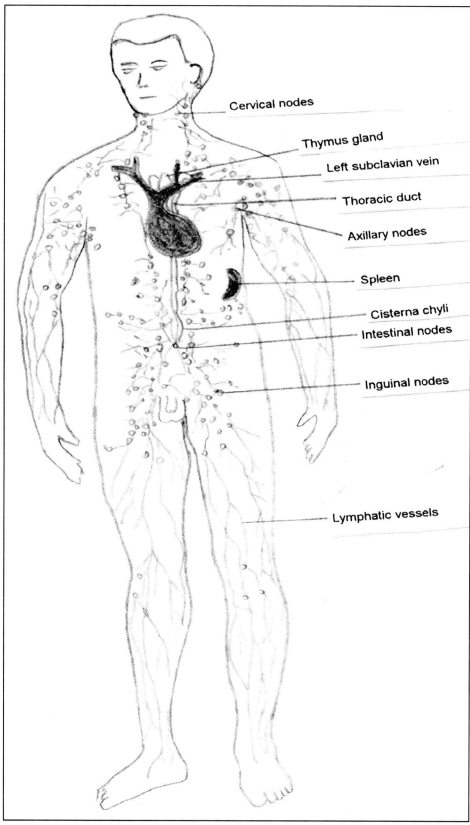

Cervical nodes

Thymus gland

Left subclavian vein

Thoracic duct

Axillary nodes

Spleen

Cisterna chyli

Intestinal nodes

Inguinal nodes

Lymphatic vessels

Lymph nodes are small organs that are frequently called "glands." They consist of masses of **lymphatic tissue**, a hemopoietic tissue that **produces some of the body's lymphocytes and monocytes**. Lymph nodes are concentrated in certain areas along lymph channels where they act as filters for the lymph. Each node has several afferent and several efferent channels by which lymph enters and leaves the node. Lymph nodes contain lymphocytes, monocytes, macrophages and plasma cells. These cells attack pathogens (microorganisms that cause disease) and foreign matter that travels to the node through the lymph vessels.

A lymph node is a bean-shaped organ with a **hilum** or indentation on one side. The **stroma** is made of **reticular connective tissue**. Reticular cells are branched cells that contribute to the stroma. The **parenchyma** is divided into an **outer cortex and an inner medulla**. The **cortex** consists mainly of ovoid lymphatic **nodules**. When the lymph nodes are actively fighting a pathogen, these nodules contain **germinal centers** where **B cells** are multiplying and producing **plasma cells**. The medulla contains cords of lymphoid and reticular cells.

When a lymph node is actively fighting an infection, it enlarges and may become tender. This condition is called **lymphadenitis**. (Aden- refers to a gland). Cancerous nodes are usually enlarged, firm and nontender. Lymphadenopathy is a term for enlarged nodes of any etiology (diagnostic cause).

Lymph nodes are found in many places in the body. They are especially plentiful in the anterior and posterior cervical areas, axillae, mesentery, and inguinal areas. Pathogens enter the body through breaks in the skin of the extremities or through air that is inhaled. Note that lymph nodes are concentrated at the junctions of the head and extremities with the trunk, and their location can prevent pathogens from progressing to the trunk.

Right: A drawing of a section of A lymph node. Lymph enters the node through the afferent lymphatics. Lymph filters through the node and exits at the hilum through efferent lymphatics. The germinal centers are sites of mitosis for lymphocytes.

Lymph nodules are less organized than lymph nodes. They small masses of lymphatic tissue beneath the epithelium of all mucous membranes. They are found in the respiratory tract, digestive tract, urinary tract and reproductive tracts. **Peyer's patches** are prominent lymph nodules in the small intestine. The **palatine tonsils** are lymph nodules in the oral pharynx; the **adenoids** (pharyngeal tonsils) are lymph nodules in the nasopharynx. The **lingual tonsils** are under the base of the tongue.

The **spleen** is located under the rib cage in the left upper quadrant (LUQ) of the abdomen. It functions to produce erythrocytes in the fetus, but not in adults. The spleen has three functions after birth: **(1)** It produces some of body's lymphocytes and monocytes. **(2)** It is a site for plasma cells to reside and produce antibodies, and **(3)** macrophages in the spleen phagocytize pathogens, foreign material and spent erythrocytes. Other organs can take over the functions of the spleen, so the spleen is not necessary for life; however, people become more susceptible to some infections following a splenectomy (removal of their spleen).

The **thymus gland** is located in the superior mediastinum. It is quite prominent in the young, but it gradually shrinks in size; adults retain very little thymus tissue. Thymic hormones stimulate the production of **T lymphocytes** from lymphoblasts. **T lymphocytes govern the production of antibodies by B lymphocytes and plasma**

cells. T lymphocytes differentiate into **_helper T_** cells, **_suppressor T_** cells and **_cytotoxic T_** cells. T cells of the immune system are not fully immuno-competent until the age of two years, and children younger than two are more susceptible to some infections. (*Hemophilus influenzae* are bacteria that are associated with severe illnesses in the young.) Some immunizations, including the measles vaccine, should be delayed until immune competency is established.

Immunity is the body's ability to destroy pathogens and foreign material and thereby prevent infections. Cancer cells are regarded as foreign and most are destroyed by the immune system. Transplanted donor organs are also foreign, and they are attacked by the immune system. Prior to organ transplantation, tissue and blood markers are checked to get the closest possible match between the donor and recipient, so as to limit antibody formation against the transplant. Drugs given to the recipient may be effective in suppressing his immune system and subverting a transplant rejection.

Right: Blood cells and immune cells.

Top row left to right:
Neutrophile, eosinophile, basophile

Second row left to right:
Red cells and platelets
Monocyte
Lymphocyte

Bottom row:
Plasma cell

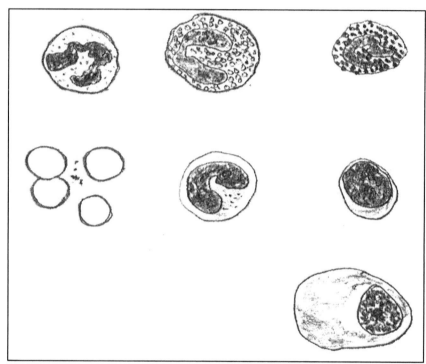

Inflammation accompanies infections and the immune response. There are four cardinal signs of inflammation, **_rubor, calor, dolor and tumor_**, or in English, **_redness, heat, pain and swelling_**. Inflammation is denoted by the suffix -itis, as in lymphadenitis. The Inflammatory response to an infection may result in a **_purulent exudate_**, which is the yellow fluid commonly known as pus. It consists of millions of polys (neutrophiles), bacteria, proteins and debris. Bacterial infections caused by staphlylococci, pneumococci and other bacteria lead to the formation of a purulent exudate. An **_abscess_** is exudate surrounded by a wall of fibrous tissue. Other infections, such as tuberculosis, cause an immune response known in histology as a **_granuloma._** **_Exudates_** tend to be thick and cloudy. A **_transudate_** is a **_clear_** effusion of fluid that is colorless to straw-colored. Whereas exudates are indicative of an infection, transudates suggest irritation or the pooling of an excessive amount of fluid.

Pyrogens are circulating proteins that **_raise the body temperature_**. Active macrophages and leukocytes secrete a pyrogen called interleukin-1, which is capable of setting the hypothalamic thermostat at a higher level. High body temperatures inhibit some viruses and bacteria. High temperatures also increase metabolism so that more heat is produced, reactions occur faster, and cells move more quickly. For each one degree Centigrade rise in temperature, the metabolic rate increases by ten percent.

Lymphocytes are at the center of **_antibody_** production. They develop from **_lymphoblasts_**, which are stem cells that are derived from **_hemocytoblasts_** in the bone marrow. Some lymphoblasts are converted to **_T cells_** under the influence of thymic hormones in the thymus gland. T cells then migrate to the spleen and lymphoid tissues. There are three types of mature T cells: **_helper T cells_**, **_cytotoxic T cells_** and **_suppressor T cells_**.

B cells (lymphocytes) mature from stem cells in the bone marrow, and they migrate to the spleen and lymphoid tissues. **B cells are activated by T cells**. Most activated B cells become **plasma cells**, which are prolific producers of antibodies. Some activated B cells become **memory B cells**, which are responsible for long term immunity. (See page 213.)

Natural Killer Cells (NK cells) are large lymphocytes that destroy cancer cells, virus-infected cells, and transplanted cells. They also destroy bacteria and viruses. NK cells are neither T cells nor B cells, but a separate class of lymphocytes. NK cells will attack any cell with foreign antigens on its surface. NK cells act by secreting vesicles containing **perforins**, which are proteins that poke holes in the cell membrane of the target.

Macrophages (also called **histiocytes**) are tissue phagocytes that develop from **monocytes**. **Neutrophiles** and **eosinophiles** are phagocytes, and they are called **microphages**. Neutrophiles are quick to arrive at the site of inflammation, and they are quick to phagocytize bacteria and debris. Eosinophiles phagocytize material that has been coated with antibodies. Macrophages and microphages can move through capillary walls by squeezing between endothelial cells. This movement is called **diapedesis**. **Kupffer** cells are fixed macrophages (histiocytes) around sinusoids in the liver. **Microglia** cells are fixed macrophages (histiocytes) in the central nervous system.

Antigens are substances that are subject to attack by antibodies of the immune system. **Pathogens** are bacteria, viruses, fungi, and other microorganisms that are capable of causing disease. Pathogens have markers on their surface that act as antigens for the immune system. The immune system is capable of recognizing self-antigens, and it normally does not produce antibodies to self-antigens. But the immune system will produce antibodies to infectious microorganisms, donor transplants and cancer cells, which it recognizes as foreign.

Antibodies are proteins that act as **immunoglobulins**. Antibodies are produced by **plasma cells** and **memory B cells** in response to foreign antigens. **Immune globulins** and **gamma globulins** are terms used for antibodies. Each antibody attaches itself to **one specific** foreign antigen and tags it for destruction by macrophages.

Classes of antibodies include the following:

(1) *IgG* (immunoglobulin G) antibodies are located in the blood and tissue fluid; they provide long term immunity to a disease.

(2) *IgA* (immunoglobulin A) antibodies are in tears, saliva, breast milk and mucous membranes; they protect against pathogenic invasion.

(3) *IgM* (immunoglobulin M) antibodies are the first to ward off an infection (IgG follows).

(4) *IgD* (immunoglobulin D) antibodies function as receptors for antigens on B lymphocytes.

(5) *IgE* (immunoglobulin E) antibodies are manifest in allergic reactions; they cause mast cells and basophiles to release histamine.

Cytokines are a diverse group of polypeptides and small proteins that are secreted by leukocytes, macrophages, mast cells and several other cell types. **The cytokines function to bolster the immune response.** The cytokines include pyrogens, interferons, interleukins, tumor necrosis factor, chemicals that regulate phagocytic activities (chemotactile factors), and colony stimulating factors. Some of their functions follow:

(1) *Interleukins* are secreted by leukocytes and macrophages. They draw macrophages to an area of inflammation; they make T cells more sensitive to antigens; they stimulate B cells and plasma cells; they help produce fever, scar formation, and mast cell formation. They also stimulate the anterior pituitary gland to secrete ACTH. **Pyrogens** are interleukins that affect the hypothalamus to raise the body temperature.

(2) *Interferons* are secreted by activated lymphocytes, macrophages and tissue cells that have been invaded by a virus. Interferons trigger the production of antiviral proteins, which interfere with viral replication within the cell. Interferons attract and stimulate NK cells and macrophages. The NK cells and macrophages can then destroy virus-infected cells before the virus can multiply within the cell.

(3) *Tumor necrosis factors* are secreted by activated macrophages and cytotoxic T cells. They slow tumor growth, kill some tumor cells, stimulate granulocyte production (neutrophiles, eosinophiles and basophiles), induce fever, and increase the sensitivity of T cells to interleukins.

(4) *Chemotactile factors* attract macrophages and microphages and prevent their premature departure from a wound.

(5) *Colony stimulating factors* are produced by active T cells, macrophages, endothelial cells and fibroblasts. They stimulate erythropoiesis and lymphopoieses.

The three subgroups of T cells are *__helper T cells__*, *__suppressor T cells__* and *__cytotoxic T cells__*. *__Helper T cells__* attract and stimulate phagocytes, and they activate B cells when foreign material is detected. *__Cytotoxic T cells__* recognize a pathogen after it has been labeled by a macrophage or other cell. They kill diseased or foreign cells by delivering cytotoxic chemicals to the target cell. *__Suppressor T cells__* stop the immune response by releasing interleukins that inhibit T and B cell activity.

Helper T cells, cytotoxic T cells, suppressor T cells, natural killer cells and complement (see below) are all involved in *__cell mediated immunity__*. Cell mediated immunity does not involve antibodies; instead *__lymphocytes directly attack infected cells__*. Cell mediated immunity begins with phagocytosis of foreign material by a macrophage. The phagocyte presents an antigen of the foreign material on its surface, and this antigen is recognized by T cells. *__Helper T cells and cytotoxic T cells__* are activated by the antigen. They divide and multiply, and some become long-lived *__memory T cells__*. Memory T cells are responsible for the *__T cell recall response__*, which quickly produces an immune response if the same antigen is encountered in the future. *__Cytotoxic T cells__* destroy microorganisms and foreign cells by chemically disrupting their cell membranes. Cytotoxic T cells and helper T cells also produce interleukins, which draw macrophages toward sites of activity. After an infection has passed, *__suppressor T cells__* secrete inhibiting interleukins that halt the immune response.

__Humoral immunity__ (blood-borne antibody mediated immunity) involves antibodies produced by activated B cells and plasma cells. Both humoral immunity and cell mediated immunity entail macrophages engulfing an antigen and presentation of the foreign antigen on the surface of the macrophage. The antigen is recognized by T cells; helper T cells become activated, and they present the antigen on their surface. Then the two types of immunity differ. In *__humoral immunity B cells__* are activated by the *__activated helper T cells__*. The activated B cells divide and multiply forming *__plasma cells and memory B cells__*. Plasma cells and memory B cells produce *__antibodies__* against the specific antigen. An *__antigen-antibody complex__* forms, which results in *__opsonization__* and *__complement fixation.__* *__Opsonins__* are *__antibodies__* that bind to bacteria or other pathogens and label them for phagocytosis by macrophages and neutrophiles. *__Complement__* is not an antibody; it is a group of about twenty plasma proteins. When "fixed," these proteins bind to the antigen-antibody complex and to each other, forming an enzymatic ring around the foreign antigen that punches holes in the membrane of the target and destroys it. If the foreign antigen is a pathogen, complement fixation promotes chemotactile factors (including one called properdin) that attracts phagocytes and stimulates phagocytic activity. Complement also promotes inflammation by inciting mast cells to release histamine.

After the foreign antigen is destroyed, *__suppressor T cells__* stop the immune response. Without suppressor T cells, excessive antibody production could trigger an autoimmune response that could result in antibodies attacking the individual's own cells.

The immune system produces about two million antibodies, each specific for one antigen. *__Antibodies__* work in four different ways to destroy pathogens: **(1)** They *__bind__* to active sites on pathogens, **(2)** they *__agglutinate__* pathogens, **(3)** they *__precipitate__* agglutinated clumps of antibodies and pathogens, and **(4)** they *__fix complement__*. Antibodies do not destroy pathogens by these processes; they render active sites (antigens) on the pathogens harmless either by covering them or by the agglutination process, and they mark the pathogen for destruction by phagocytes or complement.

When a foreign antigen is first presented to the immune system, antibody production is often too slow to prevent the illness. After recovery from a disease, residual antibodies and memory cells specific for that pathogen remain, and they give a quick response to any future exposure to that antigen. The quick response by memory cells is called the secondary or *__anamnestic__* (not forgetting) response; in this response plasma cells can be formed from memory B lymphocytes within hours.

Here is a chronological summary of the immune response. *__(1) Neutrophiles, macrophages and NK cells__* migrate to the area and begin destroying the invading pathogens. *__(2) Cytokines__* draw more phagocytes and lymphocytes to the area. (3) *__T cells__* are activated by the presence of antigens on the surfaces of phagocytes, and the activated T cells multiply. They include *__helper T cells__*, *__cytotoxic cells__* and *__memory T cells__*.. (4) *__Helper T cells activate B cells__*, which transform into plasma cells and memory B cells. (5) *__Plasma cells__* increase the level of circulating antibodies.

Below is an outline of cell mediated immunity and humoral immunity.

Cell mediated immunity
1. Phagocytes engulf an invading microorganism and display an antigen on their surface. This display activates helper T cells.
1. NK cells and cytotoxic cells attack and destroy the invading pathogen.
2. Some helper T cells are transformed into memory T cells. Memory T cells provide the T cell recall response, which is part of long term immunity.
3. Suppressor T cells stop the immune response when the infection has been controlled.

Humoral immunity
1. Phagocytes engulf an invading microorganism and display an antigen on their surface. This display activates helper T cells.
2. Activated helper T cells activate B cells.
3. Activated B cells transform into plasma cells and memory B cells.
4. Plasma cells and memory B cells produce antibodies against the antigen.
5. Opsonins react with the antigen and label them for destruction by phagocytes.
6. The antigen-antibody complex fixes complement. Fixed complement destroys the pathogen.
7. Suppressor T cells stop the immune response when the infection has been controlled.

Autoimmune diseases are caused by *autoantibodies*, which are antibodies against one's own tissue cells. The resulting antigen-antibody reaction causes inflammation and damage to the body's own cells. Examples of autoimmune diseases include the collagen vascular diseases. These related diseases include *rheumatoid arthritis, scleroderma, periarteritis nodosa and systemic lupus erythematosis (lupus).* A collagen disease may entail an antibody attack against connective tissues in the joints, skin, kidneys and the heart valves. Scleroderma is a generalized disease with prominent cutaneous involvement; periarteritis nodosa is characterized by inflammation of small and medium sized arteries. Other examples of autoimmune diseases include *Graves disease* and *diabetes mellitus*. Grave's disease is a type of thyroiditis caused by antibodies attacking thyroglobulin, a thyroid hormone precursor. Antibodies attack and destroy the insulin-producing beta cells in the islets of Langerhans of the pancreas in type I diabetes mellitus.

A specific antigen has been identified in some autoimmune disorders. Rheumatic fever and acute glomerulonephritis are caused by autoantibodies that follow a streptococcal infection. The autoantibody of rheumatic fever attacks the joints and the heart valves; the autoantibody of acute glomerulonephritis attacks the glomeruli of the kidneys. Reiter's syndrome is an arthritic condition that is caused by an autoantibody that follows an infection with a *Shigella* bacillus (bacillary dysentery). Reiter's syndrome often includes inflammation of the urethra (especially in males) and the conjunctivae.

Vaccines serve as the body's first exposure to an antigen; antibody production and memory cells are created in the immune response. A vaccine may contain antigens from infectious particles that have been killed or attenuated (weakened), or vaccines may be made from part of a pathogen such as the capsule. Vaccines can also be a toxoid, which is an inactive derivative of a toxin that is produced by a specific type of bacteria. Toxoids to tetanus and diphtheria are examples of this type of vaccine.

Allergies and autoimmune disorders make up *hypersensitivity,* which is an abnormal reaction by the immune system that may be harmful. An allergy is part of the immune response, and an allergen is like an antigen. But allergens (allergic antigens) are not usually harmful. It is the response of the immune system that causes discomfort and morbidity in allergic conditions.

There are *four types of allergic reactions*.
(1) Type I or immediate hypersensitivity is *IgE* mediated, and it includes most common allergies. The hypersensitivity response occurs quickly after exposure to the allergen. It may take the form of asthma, which is characterized by constriction of the bronchioles, or it may take the form of anaphylaxis, which is an immediate and severe type I reaction that produces circulatory shock and may be fatal.

(2) Type II hypersensitivity involves *IgG* or *IgM* antibodies. Type II hypersensitivity can occur with blood transfusions and some drug allergies.

(3) Type III hypersensitivity involves the precipitation of _**IgG**_ or _**IgM**_ antibody complexes, which causes intense inflammation.

(4) Type IV hypersensitivity is a cell-mediated reaction that includes allergies to poison ivy and graft rejections. Contact allergies occur when the skin or a mucous membrane comes in contact with the allergen. Histamine release in the skin produces erythema (redness), pruritis (itching) and vesiculation (blisters). Some food allergies can produce a contact allergic reaction in the pharynx and epiglottis, which may lead to marked swelling and interference with breathing.

**Genetic immunity or innate immunity** does not involve antibodies or the immune system. Rather the pathogen is not attracted to the host, or the host does not support the growth of the pathogen. Humans and dogs suffer from different viral pathogens for example. Measles, distemper and rinderpest are similar viruses, but only humans are infected with the measles virus; only dogs get distemper, and only cattle get rinderpest.

**Passive immunity** is obtained from a source other than one's own immune system. For example a mother passes immune globulins to her fetus through the placenta. These globulins afford immunity for the infant to the same diseases to which the mother is immune. This type of immunity typically lasts until about nine months of age, but immune globulins are present in breast milk, and passive immunity for the infant can be prolonged by breast feeding. Artificially acquired passive immunity is obtained by the administration of injections of gamma globulin. This is not a vaccine, and it does not stimulate the immune system, but it can give some degree of temporary protection against rabies, hepatitis A, hepatitis B, botulism and rubella (German measles).

**Active immunity** is the production of one's own antibodies. Naturally acquired immunity follows recovery from a disease. Artificially acquired immunity is the result of a vaccine. The length of time that memory T cells can be expected to afford immunity following a vaccination depends on the vaccine.

**Stress** is a frequently used and misused term that is best applied to a situation that causes increased ACTH production by the pituitary, which then causes the adrenal glands to secrete an increased amount of cortisol and other glucocorticoid hormones. These hormones suppress the inflammatory response, decrease the activity and number of phagocytes, and inhibit the production and effects of interleukins.

The immune system functions less well in the _**elderly;**_ cancer cells are not destroyed as efficiently, infections are not fought as effectively, and auto antibodies that attack one's own cells are formed more readily. Thus the elderly may be more susceptible to cancer, infectious diseases and autoimmune disorders such as rheumatoid arthritis.

**Severe combined immunodeficiency disease** (SCID) is a group of related disorders caused by different recessive alleles. These diseases result in a scarcity of T cells and B cells. Children with SCID are highly vulnerable to infections because they cannot mount an effective defense. These are the "bubble babies" who must be kept isolated in a sterile environment to survive. None has lived past the age of twelve.

**AIDS** (acquired immunodeficiency syndrome) is a twentieth century disease in humans that is caused by _**HIV**_ (the human immunodeficiency virus). The HIV virus is a retrovirus, a group of RNA viruses that use RNA and a transcriptase enzyme to synthesize DNA. The newly formed DNA is inserted into the host cell's DNA where it may lay dormant, or it may activate and produce new viral RNA particles. The HIV virus _**preferentially attacks helper T cells**_; the severe depletion of helper T cells explains the inability of a person with AIDS to fight infections.

Study Guide
1. What is lymph?
2. Describe the following, and tell where each is found: lacteals, thoracic duct, and right lymphatic duct.
3. Describe the gross and microscopic anatomy of a lymph node.
4. Tell where you could find the following lymphatic tissues: Peyer's patches, palatine tonsils, adenoids, lingual tonsils, spleen, and thymus gland.
5. Define immunity

6. List the classes and subclasses of lymphocytes, and understand the role of each in immunity.
7. Define allergy.
8. What cell type may be markedly increased in allergic disorders?
9. Define inflammation.
10. Define pyrogen.
11. Define cytokine, and name six types.
12. What is an antigen?
13. What is an antibody?
14. What is a plasma cell? What cell is the precursor to a plasma cell?
15. Name five types of immunoglobulins, and describe the function of each.
16. Understand complement fixation and opsonization.
17. What is an autoimmune disease? Give examples.
18. What is passive immunity?
19. How dos HIV affect the immune system?

Chapter Twenty-four

The Digestive System

All the energy that anyone receives must come from the food he eats. Food must contain **_carbohydrates, fats, proteins, minerals and vitamins_**, all of which are necessary for life. In order to be utilized, the food that is eaten must be broken down **_mechanically_**. The physical action of teeth and the musculature of the stomach and intestines accomplish that feat, so that molecules of fat, carbohydrates and proteins can be acted on **_chemically_** by enzymes. The mechanical and chemical actions on food are known as **_digestion_**.

The Mouth

Mechanical digestion begins in the mouth by the action of **_teeth_** and the **_tongue_** to break down food and mix it with saliva. There are twenty deciduous teeth (baby teeth) and 32 permanent teeth. The deciduous teeth include eight incisors, four canines and eight molars. The permanent teeth include eight incisors, four canines, eight premolars and twelve molars. Each tooth sits in an **_alveolus_**, or socket, which is a depression in the maxilla or the mandible. Each tooth has one to four **_roots_**, which are extensions of the tooth buried deeply in the bone. Teeth are made up of a covering of **_enamel,_** which is nonliving and will not replace itself. Enamel is comprised of calcium and magnesium salts crystallized tightly into microscopic cylinders. Enamel covers **_dentin_**, which is a living, cellular tissue with fibers and canaliculi in a calcified matrix. Dentin surrounds the **_pulp cavity_**, the sensitive center of the tooth that contains nerves and blood vessels. Vessels and nerves enter the pulp cavity through an opening at the tip of a root. The **_crown_** is that part of the enamel and dentin that is above the gum line. All the enamel is in the crown. Dentin below the crown is surrounded by **_cementum_**, a thin layer of bone-like tissue. Cementum is surrounded by the **_periodontal ligament_** (periodontal membrane), which is periosteum that covers the inside of the alveolus. There are fibers between dentin and cementum, between cementum and the periodontal ligament, and between the periodontal ligament and bone. These fibers hold the tooth securely in place in a synarthrotic joint called a **_gomphosis._**

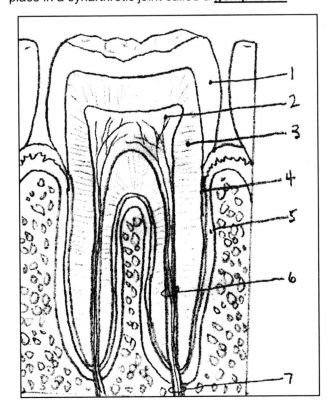

Left: A lower molar tooth embedded in bone of the mandible.
(1) Enamel
(2) Pulp
(3) Dentin
(4) Cementum
(5) Periodontal ligament
(6) Root canal
(7) Branches of alveolar vessels and nerves

273

Dental caries involves the formation of a cavity in the enamel of a tooth. Cavity formation begins with food residue, especially sticky sugars, collecting on the teeth. ***Plaque*** is a build up of carbohydrates and bacteria on the surface of a tooth. Bacteria metabolize the sugars and produce acidic by-products that dissolve the enamel. If not repaired, the destruction can invade the dentin and pulp, resulting in severe pain and loss of the tooth. ***Gingivitis*** is inflammation of the gums due to bacterial invasion. The most common cause of tooth loss in adults is ***periodontitis***, an infection that destroys the periodontal ligament.

There are three pairs of major salivary glands, the ***parotid, submandibular and sublingual***. The secretions of the parotid glands are serous; those of the sublingual glands are mucous, and those of the submandibular glands are mixed. The submandibular and sublingual glands are innervated by the facial nerves; the parotid glands are innervated by the glossopharyngeal nerves. Saliva contains two enzymes, ***salivary amylase and salivary lipase***. Salivary amylase acts to break down starch to sugars in the mouth, but salivary lipase does not function until it is activated by acid in the stomach. Salivation is triggered by the smell of food and the presence of food in the mouth. The nucleus for salivation is in the medulla.

Chewing food and mixing it with saliva produces a slurry that can be swallowed. The muscles of the pharynx, tongue, epiglottis, larynx and hyoid bone are involved in swallowing, which is completed by a reflex action coordinated in the medulla and the pons. The actions of these muscles push the bolus of food into the esophagus, a muscular tube with stratified squamous epithelium. The esophagus stretches from the pharynx to the stomach. During swallowing, the larynx is elevated and is covered by the epiglottis; the pharynx is elevated, which allows the soft palate to occlude the posterior opening of the nasopharynx, and the tongue initially is retracted. These movements assure that food is directed into the esophagus and not into the larynx or the nose.

The Esophagus

The esophagus, stomach and intestines form a continuous tube called the ***alimentary canal*** (or the gut), which lies between the pharynx and the anus. The wall of the alimentary canal consists of four layers, which are:

(1) The ***mucosa*** (mucous membrane) surrounds the lumen. The inner lining of the mucosa is epithelial tissue that is derived from endoderm. The epithelium is stratified squamous in the esophagus; it changes to simple columnar in the stomach and intestines. Connective tissue surrounds the epithelium. The mucosa contains goblet cells and larger mucus producing glands. Lymph nodules, macrophages and smooth muscle (the ***muscularis mucosae***) are present in the deeper parts of the mucosa.

(2) The ***submucosa***, or ***lamina propria***, surrounds the mucosa. This layer is areolar connective tissue, and it contains blood vessels and lymphatic vessels. Nerves of the autonomic nervous system form a plexus in the submucosa called ***Meissner's plexus***. Parasympathetic impulses from the vagus nerves increase secretions and muscular action of the gastro-intestinal tract. Sympathetic impulses from thoracic and lumbar spinal nerves inhibit secretions and muscular action.

(3) The ***external muscle layer*** surrounds the submucosa. Most of this layer contains an inner circular and an outer longitudinal layer of smooth muscle. Exceptions to this rule exist in the esophagus and in the stomach. In the upper one-third of the esophagus the external layer is composed of striated muscle rather than smooth muscle, and this portion of the esophagus is under voluntary control. The stomach contains an additional layer of smooth muscle with an oblique orientation inside the other two layers. When a food bolus has reached the stomach and been partially digested, it becomes known as ***chyme.*** Sequential contractions of the external muscle layer and the muscularis mucosae propel chyme through the gastrointestinal tract. The activity of these muscles is called ***peristalsis***. Peristalsis is a sequential wave of constriction down the alimentary canal that pushes chyme toward the anus. ***Auerbach's plexus*** (also called the myenteric plexus) is a nerve plexus in the external muscle layer that supplies parasympathetic and sympathetic innervation to smooth muscle of the external muscle layer.

(4) The outermost layer is a connective tissue membrane known as the ***visceral peritoneum*** or the ***serosa.*** The serosa is a thin serous membrane that is continuous with the parietal peritoneum that lines the walls of the abdominal cavity. The ***mesentery*** is a portion of the visceral peritoneum that is folded over the intestines anteriorly, forming an apron-like covering called the ***greater omentum***. The ***lesser omentum*** is a smaller fold of mesentery between the stomach and the liver.

The **_esophagus_** passes through the posterior thorax behind the trachea, and it passes through the esophageal hiatus of the diaphragm. The **_cardiac sphincter_** of the esophagus is immediately below the diaphragm. It marks the junction of the esophagus and the stomach, and it prevents stomach contents from regurgitating into the esophagus. Vomiting occurs as a result of irritation or excessive stretching of the wall of the stomach. The emetic center in the medulla signals the cardiac sphincter to relax, and it signals the diaphragm and the abdominal muscles to contract spasmodically. These muscles squeeze the abdomen and force the contents of the stomach up into the esophagus.

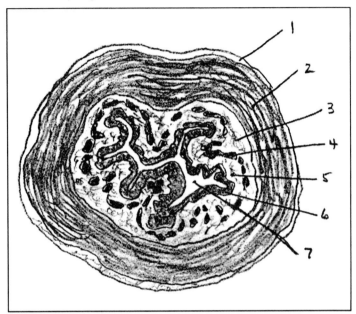

Left: A transverse cut through the esophagus. The lumen is collapsed in this drawing.
(1) Connective tissue adventitia
(2) Muscularis externa
(3) Submucosa (lamina propria)
(4) Muscularis mucosa
(5) Connective tissue of the mucosa
(6) Stratified squamous epithelium
     of the mucosa
(7) Lumen

The Stomach

The **_stomach_** is a pouch in the LUQ (left upper quadrant) of the abdomen; it is shaped like a large comma. The left side of the stomach is called the **_greater curvature_**; the right side, facing the liver, is called the **_lesser curvature_**.

The areas of the stomach are the cardiac, fundus, body, antrum and pylorus. The **_cardiac_** portion of the stomach is a small area adjacent to the cardiac sphincter. The **_fundus_** is the upper portion of the stomach; the body is the central portion; the **_antrum_** is the upper portion of the **_pylorus,_** which is the lower area of the stomach that leads to the duodenum (the upper portion of the small intestine). The **_pyloric sphincter_** is situated between the stomach and the duodenum.

The mucosa of an empty stomach is drawn into folds called **_rugae_**. When the stomach fills, these folds smooth out, which allows the stomach to stretch. The gastric mucosa is filled with tiny tube like depressions called **_gastric pits_**. These pits contain an assortment of **_gastric epithelial cells_** that secrete substances necessary for digestion. The cells of the gastric pits include:
  (1) _Mucous cells_. These cells are **_goblet cells_**; they produce mucus, which aids in propelling chyme through the gastro-intestinal tract and provides a protective coating over the mucosa. Mucus producing cells are especially numerous in the cardiac and pyloric areas of the stomach.
  (2) _Stem cells_. Cells of the gastric mucosal epithelium are short-lived; their life expectancy is only three to six days. Stem cells are capable of undergoing frequent and rapid **_mitosis,_** and they are able to differentiate into the various cells of the gastric pits to replace cells that are lost.
  (3) _Parietal cells_. These cells are found especially in the upper half of the stomach (fundus and upper body regions). They secrete **_hydrochloric acid_** (HCl) and **_intrinsic factor_**. HCl is a strong acid that lowers the pH of the stomach contents to as low as 0.8. This extremely acidic environment serves to break down food, activate some enzymes and destroy bacteria. The mucosa is protected from the acidity by its coating of mucus. Tight

junctions between epithelial cells prevent gastric juice from penetrating the mucosa. ***Intrinsic factor*** combines with ***vitamin B12*** and thereby allows that vitamin to be absorbed in the ileum (the distal portion of the small intestine).   A lack of vitamin B12 leads to ***pernicious anemia*** and neurological defects (***combined system disease***). Gastric secretions are decreased in the aged. Pernicious anemia is caused by a lack of intrinsic factor secretion, which leads to the failure of vitamin B12 absorption.

   (4) ***Chief cells***.   These are the most numerous cells in the gastric pits of the fundus and body of the stomach. They secrete ***enzymes*** including chymosin, which curdles milk proteins, lipase and pepsinogen (an enzyme precursor that is converted to the enzyme, pepsin, by hydrochloric acid). Enzymatic action in the stomach partially digests proteins, fats and carbohydrates.

   (5) ***Enteroendocrine cells***. These cells secrete ***gastric hormones*** and ***paracrine*** messengers, both of which regulate the digestive system. ***Gastrin*** is one of these hormones; gastrin stimulates the secretion of HCl, intrinsic factor and stomach enzymes.

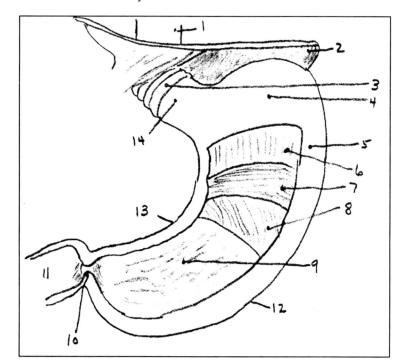

Left: A drawing of the stomach. The outer layers have been cut to reveal inner structures.
(1) Esophagus
(2) Diaphragm
(3) Cardiac sphincter
(4) Fundus area
(5) Body area
(6) Outer longitudinal muscle
(7) Middle circular muscle
(8) Inner oblique muscle
(9) Antrum
(10) Pyloric sphincter
(11) Duodenum
(12) Greater curvature
(13) Lesser curvature
(14) Cardiac area

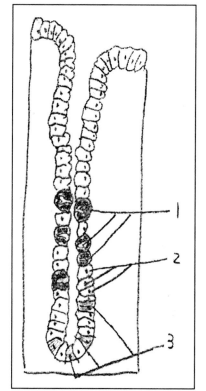

Right: A drawing of a gastric pit. The lumen of the stomach is at the top of the drawing.
(1) Parietal cells. These cells secrete hydrochloric acid and intrinsic factor.
(2) Chief cells. These cells secrete the enzymes chymosin, lipase and pepsinogen.
(3) Enteroendocrine cells. These cells secrete gastric hormones and paracrine molecules that regulate digestion.
The undesignated cells are goblet cells and stem cells.

Sensations received by the smell or the sight of food are sent to the hypothalamus, which sends signals to the vagus nerve nuclei in the medulla. Vagal stimulation initiates the secretion of gastric mucus, acid, enzymes and hormones. Secretions accelerate when food enters the stomach. Acetylcholine and histamine are neurotransmitters that stimulate gastric secretions. Inhibition of these neurotransmitters will inhibit gastric secretions. Cimetidine (Tagamet) and famotidine (Pepcid) are pharmacological antihistamines that inhibit hydrochloric acid secretion.

 After food has been present in the stomach for approximately thirty minutes, churning of the gastric musculature begins to propel the chyme to the pyloric sphincter. The pyloric sphincter allows only about three cubic centimeters of chyme to pass into the duodenum at a time. Overfilling the duodenum inhibits gastric motility, which gives the duodenum time to empty.

The Small Intestine

 The ***small intestine*** is divided into three parts, the ***duodenum, the jejunum and the ileum***. The ***duodenum*** is about ten inches in length. Most of it is retroperitoneal (behind the posterior parietal peritoneum). The ***common bile duct*** and ***the main pancreatic duct*** empty into the duodenum at a common orifice called the ***ampulla of Vater***. A band of smooth muscle called the ***sphincter of Oddi*** guards this opening. An accessory pancreatic duct is often present; it opens separately into the duodenum. Enteroendocrine cells in the duodenum secrete several hormones that control the digestive system including ***secretin, cholecystokinin and gastric inhibiting peptide***. These hormones suppress gastric secretions and gastric motility, and they stimulate gall bladder contractions and pancreatic secretions. The result is a pouring out of bile from the gall bladder to the common bile duct, and a pouring out of enzymes and bicarbonate from the pancreas to the pancreatic duct. The bile and pancreatic secretions enter the duodenum.

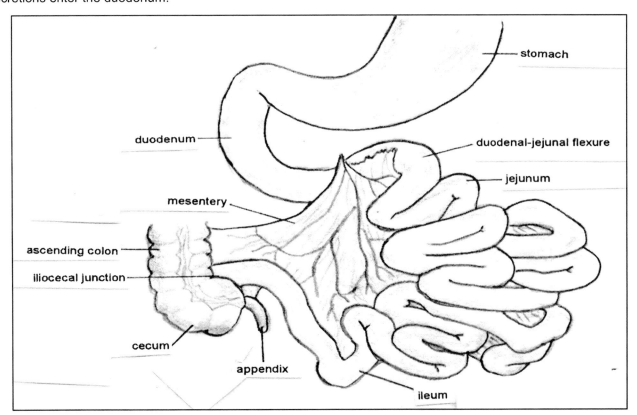

Above: A drawing of the small intestine. The small intestine is a long convoluted tube about twenty-one feet in length. The duodenum is the first part; it receives the common bile duct and the pancreatic duct. Bicarbonate secretions into the duodenum neutralize stomach acidity. The duodenum is mostly retroperitoneal, and it is about ten inches in length. The second part of the small intestine is the jejunum, which averages about eight feet in length. The third part is the ileum, which averages about twelve feet in length. Most absorption takes place in the jejunum and the ileum.

The Digestive System   Chapter Twenty-four

Bile contains *bile salts*, which are amphiphilic and serve to emulsify fat, which is necessary for fat digestion. Bilirubin and its breakdown products are excreted in the bile. The liver *conjugates* some toxins and excretes them into the bile. Conjugation is the linkage of an amino group or glucuronic acid (an acid based on glucose) to another compound. *Pancreatic enzymes* include precursors ("zymogens") of the *proteolytic* enzymes, trypsin, chymotrypsin and carboxypeptidase. Other pancreatic enzymes break down carbohydrates (pancreatic *amylase*); or fats (pancreatic *lipase)*, and two pancreatic enzymes break down nucleic acids (ribonuclease and deoxyribonuclease). *Brunner glands* in the duodenal mucosa secrete mucus rich in *bicarbonate*, which counteracts the acidity of the stomach and allows the pancreatic enzymes to function. Pancreatic enzymes are not effective in acid environments. Bicarbonate in the pancreatic juice helps to raise the pH of chyme in the duodenum to about 7.5.

The pancreas and most of the duodenum are *retroperitoneal* (behind the parietal peritoneum). The *jejunum* begins at a sharp bend of the duodenum that enters the peritoneal cavity, and the jejunum and ileum are within the peritoneal cavity. The jejunum is about eight feet long; it ends inconspicuously at that point and becomes the ileum. The *ileum* is about twelve feet long and ends at the *ileocecal junction*, where a flap of tissue called the *ileocecal valve* denotes the connection of the ileum to the *cecum* of the large intestine.

Most absorption of food substances takes place in the jejunum and the ileum. The surface area of the mucosa of these areas is increased by folds called *plica semilunaris*; the surface area is further increased by projections of the mucosa called *villi*, which give a velvet-like appearance to the surface. *Microvilli* are tiny projections of the plasma membranes of the columnar epithelial cells of the small intestine; these tiny projections form the "brush border," which further increases surface area.

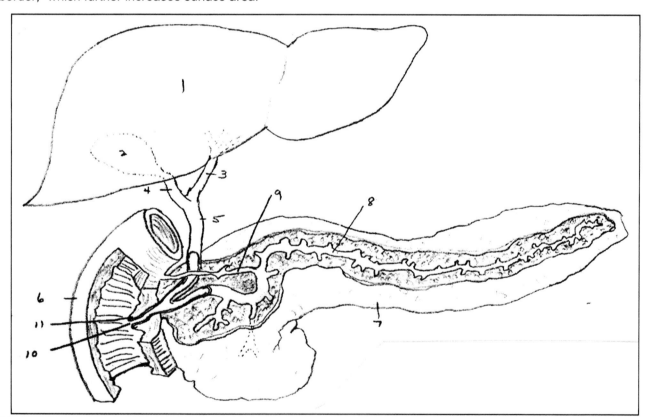

Above: This is a schematic drawing showing the relationships of the bile duct and the pancreatic duct. (1) liver; (2) gall bladder; (3) hepatic duct; (4) cystic duct; (5) common bile duct; (6) duodenum; (7) pancreas; (8) pancreatic duct; (9) accessory pancreatic duct; (10) ampulla of Vater; (11) sphincter of Oddi.

The epithelial lining of each villus contains *absorptive cells* and *goblet cells*. A capillary network and a *lacteal* (a dead-end lymph vessel) are located centrally in the villus. Sugars, amino acids, sodium, potassium, chloride, bicarbonate, other ions, water, water soluble vitamins (vitamin C and the B family of vitamins), fats and fat soluble vitamins are taken into the absorptive cells either by active transport, passive transport, diffusion or pinocytosis. Once absorbed into the cell, fatty acids are recombined with glycerol to form _**triglycerides**_. The triglycerides are then covered with protein to produce _**chylomicrons and lipoproteins,**_ which circulate in the blood. The absorption of fat soluble vitamins depends upon the presence of fat in the chyme. They will be poorly absorbed if the chyme lacks fat. Most nutrients leave the absorptive cells and enter the capillary network of the villus, but fats and fat soluble vitamins (vitamins A, D, E and K) enter the lacteals.

Do not confuse villi with microvilli. Microvilli are finger-like extensions of the plasma membranes of small intestine epithelial cells. They contain enzymes called "brush border enzymes," which carry out the final stages of enzymatic digestion.)

Numerous pores called _**crypts of Lieberkuhn**_ or intestinal crypts are present in the epithelial mucosa of the small intestine. These crypts contain mucous cells, stem cells, absorptive cells and a few Paneth cells, which produce enzymes that destroy bacteria and protect against bacterial infection. _**Peyer's patches**_ are nodules of lymphatic tissue in the mucosa and submucosa of the ileum that also guard against bacterial infection of the wall of the intestine.

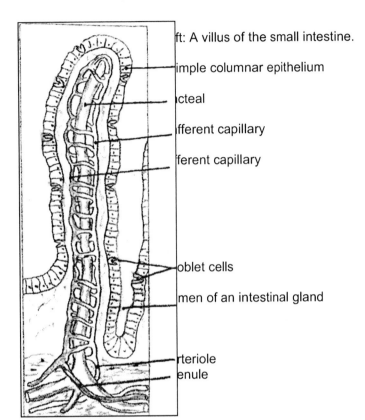

ft: A villus of the small intestine.

imple columnar epithelium

cteal

fferent capillary

ferent capillary

oblet cells

men of an intestinal gland

rteriole

enule

The Large Intestine

The _**large intestine**_ is also known as the _**colon**_. It is about 2.5 inches in diameter and totals about five feet in length. The large intestine begins at the ileocecal valve in the right lower quadrant of the abdomen. The _**cecum**_ is the first area of large intestine beyond the ileum of the small intestine. The cecum is relatively short, being only a few inches in length. The _**appendix**_ is a worm-like blind tubular appendage of the cecum in the RLQ (right lower quadrant) that contains lymphatic tissue.

Following the cecum are the _**ascending colon, transverse colon, descending colon, sigmoid colon, rectum and anus.**_ The _**ascending colon**_ begins in the RLQ and proceeds upward to the RUQ, where it makes a ninety degree bend to become the transverse colon. The _**transverse colon**_ proceeds to the LUQ where it makes another ninety degree turn to become the descending colon. The _**descending colon**_ enters the pelvic cavity and becomes the sigmoid colon. The _**sigmoid colon**_ makes an "S" shaped curve, leaves the peritoneal cavity and descends to the _**rectum**_, which is a six inch long muscular tube above the anus.

The external muscle layer of the colon consists of an inner circular layer and an outer longitudinal layer. The longitudinal layer of the colon is shaped into three relatively narrow strips of muscle on the outer surface of the colon called _**taenia coli**_. The taenia coli "gather" or pinch the colon into puckers and pockets. _**Haustra**_ are dilated areas of large intestine between the areas that are pinched by taenia coli.

Digestion does not take pace in the colon; however, **_water_** and some electrolytes, notably **_potassium,_** are absorbed. About 80% of the water that enters the colon is absorbed. The absorption of water is reduced in diarrhea; dehydration and hypokalemia can result. If diarrhea is accompanied by vomiting, the loss of electrolytes and acid from the stomach can lead to additional pH, water and electrolyte imbalances.

Trillions of bacteria live in the colon; so many that 30% to 80% of the dry weight of the stool is bacteria, depending upon the diet. Bacteria produce some vitamins that are necessary for human life, including vitamin K, riboflavin (B2), thiamine (B1), biotin (a B vitamin), and folic acid (a B vitamin). Air that is swallowed is a major source of intestinal gas, but bacteria in the colon also produce gases including hydrogen, hydrogen sulfide and methane, all of which are flammable. Indole and skatole are gaseous amines that are produced by colonic bacteria. Hydrogen sulfide, indole and skatole produce noxious odors.

The anus contains an **_internal anal sphincter_** of smooth muscle and an **_external anal sphincter_** of skeletal muscle. The defecation reflex is elicited when the rectum is stretched by fecal material, and the internal sphincter relaxes. The external sphincter is under voluntary control and can overcome this reflex.

Right: A drawing of the large intestine.
(1) Cecum
(2) Haustra
(3) Ileum of the small intestine
(4) Taenia coli (longitudinal muscle)
(5) Ascending colon
(6) Transverse colon
(7) Descending colon
(8) Sigmoid colon
(9) Rectum
(10) Anal sphincter
(11) Appendix

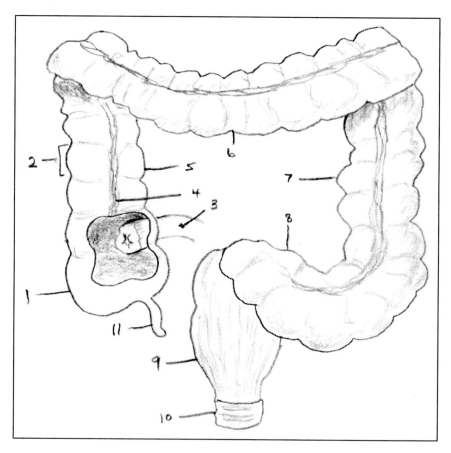

The Liver

Hepatic refers to the liver. The **_liver_** develops from endoderm as an outgrowth of the alimentary tube. It is the largest gland in the body, and it is second only to the skin as the largest organ in the body. The liver is reddish brown in color due to the presence of copious amounts of hemoglobin and bilirubin. It is located just below the diaphragm. It is divided into a right lobe in the RUQ and a left lobe in the LUQ. The right lobe is considerably larger than the left.

Liver cells are called hepatic cells; they are epithelial cells that surround blood filled channels called sinusoids. Hepatic-portal blood is venous blood from the intestines, stomach, pancreas and spleen that flows into the sinusoids of the liver before entering the inferior vena cava. Nutrients that are absorbed into capillaries in the gut enter the hepatic portal vein and go directly to the liver. The liver also receives well oxygenated arterial blood from the aorta by way of the hepatic artery.

The primary digestive function of the liver involves the production of **bile salts.** Bile salts (bile acids) are amphiphilic, and they cause fats to emulsify, which is necessary for fat digestion. Bile salts are synthesized by the liver from cholesterol, which is also synthesized in the liver. The secretion of bile salts is the only effective way that the body can excrete cholesterol; however, bile salts are largely reabsorbed and reutilized, thereby reducing the efficacy of this method of cholesterol excretion. The presence of pectins (soluble fiber) in chyme creates a colloidal gel that locks in bile acids and prevents their reabsorption.

The liver has a myriad of other functions including those listed below:

(1) The liver contains macrophages called **Kupffer cells**. Bacteria in the colon sometimes are able to enter the mucosa of the colon and the portal circulation. Kupffer cells function to phagocytize and destroy any bacteria that make it to the liver. Kupffer cells also phagocytize worn out erythrocytes and convert the **heme portion of hemoglobin into bilirubin.**

(2) **Bilirubin** that has been produced in the spleen and red marrow is removed from the blood by the liver. The liver conjugates bilirubin with glucuronic acid to make it water soluble; then the liver excretes it into the bile duct, which leads to the duodenum and subsequent excretion in the stool. Bilirubin and its breakdown compounds, stercobilin, urobilin and urobilinogen, are responsible for the normal brown color of the stool. The concentration of bilirubin increases in the blood in liver disease and in hemolytic states. This leads to an increase of bilirubin in the skin, which gives the patient a yellow color called **jaundice** (also known as **icterus**). The liver of a newborn with an Rh factor incompatibility and excessive hemolysis cannot excrete all the excess bilirubin into the bile, and jaundice results. If the bilirubin concentration exceeds a critical level, it precipitates in the tissues. The precipitation of bilirubin in the CNS is called **kernicterus**; it can result in permanent brain damage or death.

(3) The liver synthesizes **glycogen** from glucose, and it stores glycogen, which it can break down into glucose. The liver is, therefore, instrumental in maintaining a normal blood glucose level.

(4) The liver is able to synthesize twelve of the twenty **amino acids** that are used in protein synthesis. The other eight amino acids are called "essential," and they must be supplied by the diet. When an amino acid is in excess, it cannot be stored, but it can be converted into glucose or fat by the liver. That conversion removes an amino group (NH2) from amino acids, and ammonia (NH3) is formed. Ammonia is a highly alkaline toxin that must be quickly detoxified and excreted. The liver detoxifies ammonia through a series of metabolic reactions known as the **ornithine cycle**. In this cycle two ammonia molecules are combined with carbon dioxide to form **urea** (NH2CONH2). Urea is excreted in the urine. Ammonia is also produced by bacteria in the colon. Ammonia is water soluble; it is easily absorbed into the portal circulation, and the liver must quickly detoxify it.

(5) Hepatic cells synthesize the **proteins** of the blood (albumin and globulins), and they synthesize **clotting factors** including prothrombin, fibrinogen, factor eight and factor nine.

(6) The liver synthesizes **cholesterol** and other fats, and it combines them with proteins to form **lipoproteins,** which are carried in the blood. The liver and most other tissues are capable of the catabolism of fatty acids to produce energy in the form of ATP.

(7) The liver is a **storage facility** for fat soluble vitamins (vitamins A, D, E and K), and for vitamin B12, iron and copper.

(8) The smooth endoplasmic reticulum (SER) of hepatic cells is the main place where toxins and drugs (including ethyl alcohol) are chemically **detoxified.**

Cirrhosis. The hepatic cells of the liver, like the epidermal cells of the skin, have the ability to regenerate. After liver cells have been killed by a viral infection such as hepatitis or by a toxin such as ethyl alcohol, remaining cells can reproduce themselves by mitosis. However, scar tissue will form following severe or repeated insults to the liver, and scarring results in cirrhosis. A cirrhotic liver is a scarred, shrunken, nodular liver. Cirrhosis caused by alcoholism is called **Laennec's cirrhosis**. An obstruction of the common bile duct can cause **biliary cirrhosis**. Causes for obstruction of the common bile duct include its failure to develop in the fetus (biliary atresia) and blockage of the duct by gall stones (cholelithiasis). Scar tissue interferes with bile drainage; it causes an increase in pressure in the hepatic portal venous system, and it restricts the area where hepatic cells can regenerate. When the liver fails as an organ, the individual becomes jaundiced due to the build up of bilirubin. **Bilirubin** is normally excreted in the bile after the liver has conjugated it with glucuronic acid to form a glucuronide. Bilirubin is relatively insoluble before conjugation, and unconjugated bilirubin must bind to albumin to be transported in the blood. Unconjugated bilirubin blood levels are elevated when the liver is failing as an organ. A high concentration of conjugated bilirubin in the blood indicates an obstruction in the flow of bile. Ammonia builds up in the body when the liver can no longer convert it to urea satisfactorily. Ammonia is toxic to all tissues including the CNS; it can cause uncoordinated muscle contractions (called a liver "flap"), and it can cause coma and death.

Immediately above the anal sphincters are plexuses of hemorrhoidal veins. These veins are called **_hemorrhoids_** when they are dilated to the extent that they become varices. Hemorrhoids protrude into the anal canal and they can extrude through the anus. Hemorrhoids are caused by increased pressure in the hemorrhoidal veins, which can result from cirrhosis of the liver or chronic constipation with straining at the stool. Dilated veins (varices) also develop around the esophagus in cirrhosis. The hemorrhoidal veins and the esophageal veins are anastomoses between the portal venous system and the systemic veins; they shunt blood into the systemic circuit in patients with advanced cirrhosis. **_Esophageal varices_** and hemorrhoidal varices can be under high pressure in patients with cirrhosis. These vessels are thin-walled and subject to rupture, which can lead to massive bleeding.

The liver conjugates bilirubin and excretes it in the bile. If the liver is diseased, it may not be able to excrete enough bilirubin to give the stool its normal, brown color. The stools of people with hepatitis or blockage of the bile duct may be a light clay color due to the lack of bilirubin in the bile.

Active bleeding into the stomach or small intestine will produce a black, tarry stool called **_melena_**. The presence of as little as 50-60 ml of blood can produce a melanotic stool. The blackness is due to the oxidation of hemoglobin. The stool can be tested for occult blood by a simple test that uses gum guaiac, which tests for the presence of heme. Bleeding into the large intestine usually produces visible red bloody streaks in the stool.

Hepatitis is an inflammation of the liver that can have many etiologies. Virus infection is a major cause of hepatitis; it includes infections caused by hepatitis viruses A, B and C. When the destruction of hepatic cells is prolonged as it usually is in hepatitis C or chronic alcoholism, the hepatic cells attempt to regenerate. The regeneration of normal liver tissue is typically incomplete, and scar tissue forms. A scarred liver is a cirrhotic liver, and the presence of cirrhosis can disrupt normal blood and bile flow and prevent future regeneration. The outcome may be liver failure with jaundice, poor digestion, abnormal blood clotting, nutritional defects and anemia. **_Ascites_** is the accumulation of fluid in the peritoneal cavity; it is a common finding in patients with chronic cirrhosis of the liver.

The Gall Bladder

The **_gall bladder_** is a sac about 3-4 inches in length in the RUQ on the under side of the right lobe of the liver. The gall bladder stores bile. Bile enters and leaves the gall bladder through the **_cystic duct,_** which connects the gall bladder to the **_common bile duct_**. Contractions of the gall bladder are stimulated by the secretion of duodenal hormones following the entry of fat into the duodenum. Gall bladder contractions send stored bile into the duodenum through the common bile duct. **_Gall stones_** (cholelithiasis) are concretions of cholesterol, calcium carbonate and bilirubin in the gall bladder. Gall stones can cause pain when the gall bladder contracts following a fatty meal. Gall stones can obstruct the common bile duct, which can result in jaundice and liver damage. Gall stones are usually treated by surgical removal of the gall bladder (cholecystectomy).

The Pancreas

The **_pancreas_** is an elongated retroperitoneal gland about six inches in length. It is both an **_exocrine_** gland and an **_endocrine_** gland. The pancreas functions as an exocrine gland by secreting various **_enzymes_** into the **_pancreatic duct_**, which empties into the duodenum. The endocrine functions of the pancreas involve the secretion of the hormones, **_insulin_** and **_glucagon,_** into the bloodstream. **_Somatostatin_** is a paracrine secretion by the pancreas that inhibits insulin and glucagon secretion. Somatostatin also inhibits some digestive functions. Glucagon, insulin and somatostatin are secreted by different cells in the islets of Langerhans -- glucagon by the alpha cells, insulin by the beta cells, and somatostatin by the delta cells. **_Pancreatitis_** is an inflammation of the pancreas. Pancreatitis can be caused by several viruses including the mumps virus. It can also be caused by trauma to the pancreas. But most cases of adult pancreatitis are caused by either gall stones blocking the outlet of the pancreatic duct or by chronic alcoholism. Blockage of the pancreatic duct results in the backup of enzymes produced by the pancreas. These enzymes flood the pancreatic cells and begin to digest the pancreas itself. Pancreatic amylase and pancreatic lipase enter the blood stream where they can be detected by laboratory tests. Pancreatitis secondary to alcoholism is due to the build up of acetaldehyde to toxic levels. Acetaldehyde is a breakdown produce of ethyl alcohol. The patient with pancreatitis is acutely ill with frequent vomiting and severe pain radiating to the back.

Intestinal Disorders

Gastrointestinal infections have always been a scourge to mankind, and they continue to be. The causative agent is usually a bacterium, virus, amoeba, protozoan or a nematode (worm). The bacteria species *Salmonella* typically causes a febrile illness with vomiting and diarrhea. One strain of *Salmonella* causes typhoid fever. *Shigella* bacteria cause the severe diarrhea known as bacillary dysentery. *Vibrio comma* is a small bacterium that causes epidemics of cholera. Most viral gastrointestinal infections are self limited and without sequelae, however, the polio virus may cause permanent paralysis due to damage to motor neurons in the brain and spinal cord. Amoebae and several protozoa are capable of causing diarrhea (dysentery), which may be chronic and difficult to cure. Nematodes that cause disease include roundworms such as hookworm, and segmented worms such as the tapeworms.

Crohn's disease, or *regional ileitis*, is a chronic inflammatory disease of the intestines. The cause is unknown. Painful granulomas and abscesses with draining fistulas are common.

Ulcerative colitis is a chronic inflammatory disease of the colon. It results in diarrhea that is characterized by the presence of mucus, pus and blood in the feces. The cause is unknown. A total colectomy is often indicated due to the high incidence of colon cancer in patients with ulcerative colitis.

Appendicitis is an inflammation of the appendix that is usually caused by an obstruction of the lumen of the appendix by impacted fecal material (a fecolilth). The obstruction leads to a bacterial infection in the wall of the appendix, which can perforate and cause peritonitis. Appendicitis typically causes pain and tenderness in the RLQ.

One cause for pain in the LLQ is *diverticulitis*, which is inflammation of a diverticulum. *Diverticuli* are thin-walled dilated out-pockets of mucosa that herniate through the muscular wall of the sigmoid or descending colon. Diverticuli are caused by chronic constipation associated with a low fiber diet, which leads to increased pressure in the sigmoid colon.

Peptic ulcers are erosions of the wall of the duodenum or the stomach. The ulcerations can perforate the gut and lead to peritonitis, or they can erode into a blood vessel and cause massive bleeding. It was previously thought that peptic ulcers were caused by stomach acid and spicy foods, but it has now been found that a specific bacterium, *Helicobacter pylori*, can break down the mucous layer protecting the mucosa and invade the wall of the stomach or duodenum. Antibiotics against these bacteria are now a mainstay of the treatment for peptic ulcers. Drugs like aspirin and ibuprofen fit in the category of NSAIDS or nonsteroidal anti-inflammatory drugs. These drugs irritate the gastric mucosa, and they can produce ulceration and bleeding.

Celiac disease and nontropical sprue are intestinal disorders associated with diarrhea and malabsorption. Celiac disease is the pediatric form; sprue is the adult disease. The cause of these disorders is a hypersensitivity to *gliadin*, a protein component of *gluten*, which is present in wheat, barley and rye grains. Totally removing these grains from the diet cures the disorder. A hypersensitivity to a specific food or chemical may be the cause of other intestinal disorders that are of unknown etiology.

Whipple's disease is a rare intestinal disorder characterized by diarrhea, malabsorption, arthritis and abnormal skin pigmentation. Enlarged mesenteric lymph nodes and large macrophages in the submucosa (lamina propria) of the intestines characterize this disease. Whipple's disease was previously fatal, but now its cause has been found to be an infection by the bacteria *Tropheryma whippelii*. Antibiotic therapy is usually effective.

Carcinoma of the colon is one of the most common malignancies in America. It is associated with infrequent bowel movements, constipation, a diet that is high in chemicals that produce free radicals, and a diet that is low in antioxidants and fiber. ***Polyps*** are growths on the epithelial surface of the gastro-intestinal tract (most often the colon) that project into the lumen. Most polyps are benign; however, their removal is recommended because they are often malignant or premalignant.

Carcinoma of the stomach was the most common type of cancer in Americans in the early twentieth century, but its incidence has fallen dramatically. Cancer of the stomach has been linked to several things including diet, a genetic predisposition, gastric atrophy and peptic ulcer disease.

The liver is a common site for ***metastatic malignancies*** (malignant tumors arising elsewhere and spreading through the blood stream or lymphatic channels). Tumors of the colon are especially prone to metastasize to the liver via the hepatic portal circulation. Primary tumors of the liver are called ***hepatomas***. Hepatomas are much more common in people with cirrhosis, and they also have been associated with exposure to vinyl chloride, an industrial chemical. ***Hemangiomas*** commonly occur in the liver; they are typically benign, but they have been known to grow locally and cause obstructive jaundice or hemorrhage. Tumors originating in the pancreas and the esophagus have exceptionally poor prognoses.

Study Guide
1. What nutritional substances must be in the food you eat?
2. Draw and label a tooth.
3. Define gingivitis, caries and periodontal disease.
4. Name the major salivary glands.
5. Name two enzymes secreted by salivary glands.
6. Identify the histological type of epithelium in the mouth, pharynx, esophagus, stomach, intestines and anus.
7. What is Meissner's plexus? What is Auerbach's plexus?
8. Define mesentery, greater omentum, lesser omentum, parietal peritoneum, and visceral peritoneum.
9. Name the regions of the stomach, and know where they are located.
10. List the different cell types in the gastric pits, and tell the function of each.
11. What is intrinsic factor, and how does it relate to anemia?
12. Name the three divisions of the small intestine.
13. Locate the ampulla of Vater, sphincter of Oddi, cardiac sphincter, pyloric sphincter and ileocecal valve.
14. Describe the anatomic relationships of the common bile duct, cystic duct and pancreatic duct.
15. In which quadrant(s) will you find the following: stomach, appendix, gall bladder, pancreas, liver, sigmoid colon, cecum, and spleen?
16. List the pancreatic enzymes. Is the pancreas an exocrine gland or an endocrine gland? Explain.
17. Name three or more hormones secreted by the stomach and the duodenum, and give their actions.
18. Name two substances normally found in bile.
19. What digestive function do bile salts perform?
20. Define plica semilunaris, villi, microvilli, chyme, lacteal, chylomicron and lipoprotein.
21. Define Peyer's patches and crypts of Lieberkuhn.
22. Name the regions of the colon.
23. Describe taenia coli and haustra.
24. What are the two most important substances absorbed in the colon?
25. What are the differences between the internal sphincter and the external sphincter of the anus?
26. List seven functions of the liver.
27. Describe hemorrhoids, esophageal varices, hepatitis, cirrhosis, cholecystitis, cholelithiasis, pancreatitis, Crohn's disease, ulcerative colitis, appendicitis and diverticulitis.
28. How are hemorrhoids and esophageal varices a danger to patients with cirrhosis of the liver?
29. What is the significance of Helicobacter pylori?
30. What is the cause of nontropical sprue and celiac disease?
31. What is the cause of Whipple's disease?

Chapter Twenty-five

Metabolism

Metabolism includes all the reactions whereby the body breaks down or synthesizes molecules. Anabolism is the building up of molecules, which requires energy. Catabolism is the breakdown of molecules, which releases energy.

The *metabolic rate* represents the amount of energy dispelled by an organism in a given amount of time, and it is, therefore, the rate at which metabolic reactions are taking place. The *basal metabolic rate, or BMR*, is the metabolic rate while resting or sleeping. It can be measured in kilocalories of heat produced or in the amount of oxygen consumed per unit of time.

Appetite is hunger for foodstuffs; *anorexia* is lack of appetite. Appetite is controlled by a feeding center and a satiety center, both of which are in the hypothalamus. A low blood sugar stimulates the feeding center; a high blood sugar stimulates the satiety center and inhibits the feeding center. Hormones that suppress the appetite include *leptin* and *cholecystokinin*. Leptin is secreted by adipose tissue; high levels of body fat result in more leptin secretion. Cholecystokinin is secreted by the duodenum when amino acids and fat are present in chyme.

After the ingestion of a meal, sugars and amino acids are absorbed through the walls of the small intestine. These substances travel through the hepatic portal circulation to the liver. If sugars are in excess, they are converted to glucose and stored as the polysaccharide, *glycogen*, in the liver and in skeletal muscles.

Triglycerides are broken down into fatty acids and glycerol by lipase enzymes in the stomach and intestines. The fatty acids and glycerol are taken up by the absorptive cells, which resynthesize triglycerides. The absorptive cells place a protein-phospholipid coating around droplets of fat to create *chylomicrons*, a type of lipoprotein. Other types of lipoproteins are produced in the liver. They include *VLDL* (very low density lipoproteins), *LDL* (low density lipoproteins), and *HDL* (high density lipoproteins). *LDLs* contain a great deal of cholesterol, and high LDL levels in the blood are undesirable. *HDLs* are desirable because they pick up cholesterol from the blood, which the liver excretes into the bile.

Chylomicrons travel through lymph channels and the blood to the liver and to adipose tissue, where they are taken up by adipocytes. Free fatty acids and glycerol can enter capillaries of the hepatic portal circulation. *Fatty acids* are long carbon chains with a carboxyl group at one end. Three fatty acids (linoleic, linolenic and arachidonic) are called *essential fatty acids* because the body cannot synthesize them; they must be in the diet. They are used in phospholipid and eicosenoid (prostaglandin) synthesis. Each of the essential fatty acids is *unsaturated* (has double C=C bonds). Unsaturated fatty acids are more likely to be of plant origin, and saturated fatty acids are more likely to be of animal origin.

Amino acids circulate in the blood and are taken up by all cells of the body. They are used in peptide and protein synthesis. The body utilizes twenty different amino acids to manufacture proteins. Eight amino acids are *essential* and must be in the diet. The other twelve can be synthesized from other amino acids. Amino acids exist in the cytosol, but there is no mechanism for their storage. If they are not needed soon after their absorption in the intestines, they are converted to glucose or fat, or they are broken down to produce ATP.

Above: The structure of glycogen.

Above: A triglyceride.

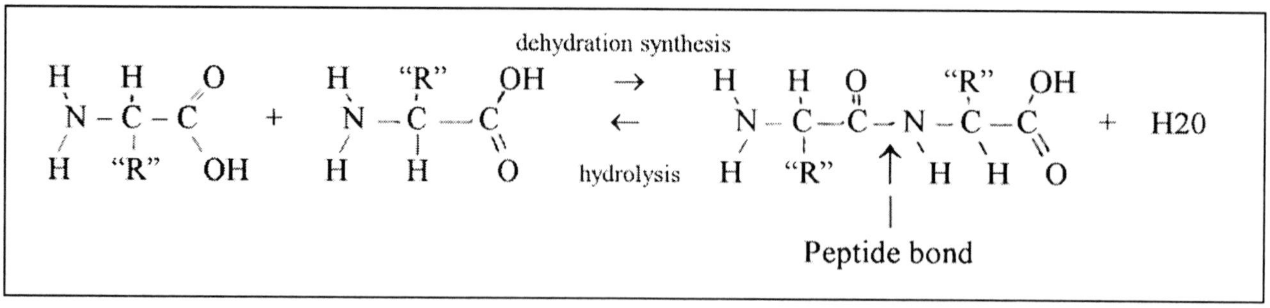

dehydration synthesis

Above: The synthesis of a dipeptide from two amino acids.

The body synthesizes ATP from the catabolism (breakdown) of carbohydrates, fats and proteins. Catabolic reactions produce heat, and the breakdown of ATP produces heat and energy to do the body's work.

Polysaccharides and disaccharides that are ingested are broken down into simple sugars (monosaccharides). Fructose and galactose are converted to glucose in the liver before they enter the systemic circulation. Other sugars used by the body, such as ribose and deoxyribose, are synthesized from glucose. Some simple sugars including mannitol and xylose cannot be metabolized, and they are excreted in the urine unchanged.

Glucose is stored in muscles and in the liver as glycogen; liver glycogen is a ready source of blood glucose.

An **_enzyme_** is a protein that catalyzes a reaction. Enzymes that have been named in the last few decades have names that end in **_-ase._**

Examples: Phosphokinase - adds a phosphate
Dehydrogenase - removes water and synthesizes
Hydrase - adds water and splits a molecule
Carboxylase - adds CO2
Carbonic anhydrase - splits carbonic acid
($H_2CO_3 \rightarrow H_2O + CO_2$)
ATP synthase - synthesizes ATP from ADP + phosphate

Oxidation - Reduction Reactions ("redox")

When a substance is oxidized, electrons are removed, and the molecule loses energy. When a substance is reduced, electrons are gained, and the molecule gains energy. The electron loss or gain in redox reactions is often in the form of hydrogen atoms; consequently, in these reactions one electron and one proton are simultaneously lost or gained.

A **_coenzyme_** usually functions as an electron "carrier." Coenzymes are electron donors (reducing agents) which are oxidized to become electron acceptors (oxidizing agents). Coenzymes work in conjunction with an enzyme and are necessary for the reaction to take place. Coenzymes usually **_are not specific_** for just one reaction. **_Enzymes are reaction specific._**

Examples of Coenzymes:

1. **_Coenzyme Q_** is an integral ingredient of the cytochrome chain.

Right: Coenzyme

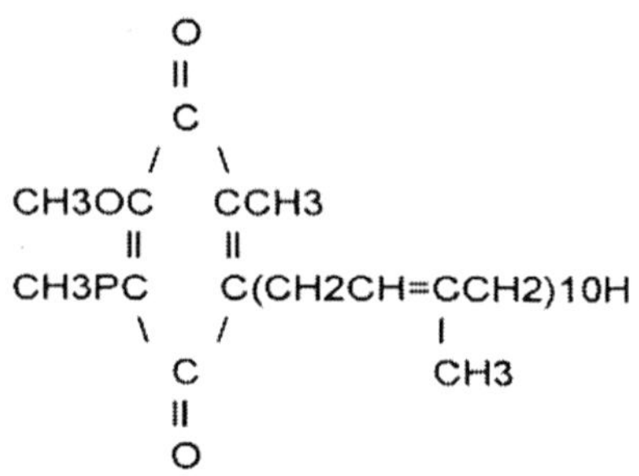

Coenzyme Q

Q.

2. **_NAD_** (nicotinamide adenine dinucleotide). NAD is derived from niacin (vitamin B3). NAD + 2 H $\longleftrightarrow$ NADH + H NAD is the low energy, oxidized form. NADH + H is the high energy reduced form. The reduced form has gained electrons (and protons) and has gained energy. The reduced form is written NADH + H because one of the hydrogen atoms is ionized.

3. *FAD* (flavin adenine dinucleotide). FAD is derived from riboflavin (vitamin B2).
$$FAD + 2\,H \longleftrightarrow FADH2$$
FADH2 is the reduced form which has gained electrons, protons and energy. NAD and FAD are *dinucleotides,* meaning that each contains two nucleotide moieties.

4. *Coenzyme A*, which is derived from vitamin B5 (pantothenic acid). Coenzyme A reacts with an acetate ion to form acetyl CoA. Acetyl CoA begins the Krebs cycle.

5. Iron (Fe), sulfur (S), copper (Cu), magnesium (Mg) and atoms of other elements can act as electron donors/acceptors and can be coenzymes for a reaction.

Energy Storing Nucleotides

A *nucleotide* is a molecule with three moieties, a *nitrogenous base, a sugar and one or more phosphate* groups. Nucleotides in man contain either ribose or deoxyribose as the sugar. The nitrogenous bases in nucleotides include the *purines, (adenine and guanine)*, and the *pyrimidines, (thymine, cytosine and uracil).* Purines are molecules with two carbon rings; pyrimidines have only one carbon ring. Nucleotides are the basis for DNA, RNA and ATP. DNA is the basis for our genetics; RNA is a template for protein synthesis, and ATP is the primary mechanism for energy storage. If a reaction requires energy to take place, that energy usually is supplied by ATP. ATP is *adenosine triphosphate*. Adenosine equals adenine + ribose.

Guanosine triphosphate, or *GTP,* is occasionally used by the body in place of ATP. Guanosine is guanine + ribose. GTP consists of guanine, ribose and three phosphate (PO4) moieties).

ATP contains three phosphate groups and two high energy phosphate bonds; adenosine diphosphate (ADP) has two phosphate groups and one high energy phosphate bond. Adenosine monophosphate (AMP or 3'5'cyclic AMP) has one phosphate group and no high energy phosphate bonds.
AMP is utilized as a second messenger for some cellular reactions.

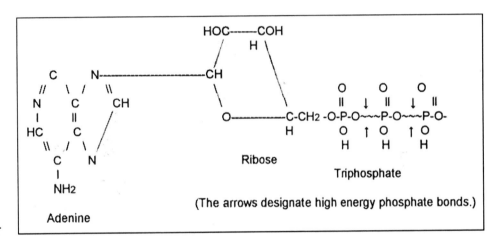

Above: The structure of ATP, a nucleotide.

Pathways in Carbohydrate Metabolism

Carbohydrates consist of sugars and starches. Carbohydrates are required in the diet in greater quantities than fats or proteins because they are rapidly and preferentially metabolized. The brain utilizes only glucose. The primary simple sugars (monosaccharides) in the diet are glucose, fructose and galactose. These sugars are often in the form of the disaccharides maltose, lactose and sucrose. Maltose consists of two glucose monomers; lactose consists of galactose plus glucose, and sucrose consists of glucose plus fructose.

Glycogen is animal starch; it is a polymer of glucose. Glycogen and digestible plant starches are broken down into glucose in the GI tract.

Glycogenolysis is the breakdown of glycogen into glucose.

Glycogenesis is the synthesis of glycogen from glucose. The liver and muscles can synthesize glycogen and later break it down to utilize the glucose.

Gluconeogenesis is the production of glucose from proteins and fats.

Aerobic refers to the presence of oxygen; *anaerobic* refers to the absence of oxygen.

Anaerobic glycolysis is the metabolism of glucose to produce two molecules of pyruvic acid. Oxygen is not required for glycolysis to take place.

__Anaerobic fermentation__ involves the conversion of pyruvic acid to lactic acid.

__Cellular Respiration__ is the further breakdown of pyruvic acid to CO2 and H2O. Cellular respiration requires oxygen, and it is, therefore, *__aerobic.__*

The metabolism of glucose involves both anaerobic and aerobic pathways. When oxygen is not present, only the anaerobic pathways can take place.

Glucose is also known as *__dextrose or levulose__*, depending upon how the molecule is oriented and will bend a light beam. In nature glucose is always dextrose. Galactose and fructose are *__isomers__* of glucose, meaning they have the same formula but different structures. dietary glucose is burned within a few hours after ingestion. Galactose, fructose, proteins, fats and lactic acid all have pathways by which they can be converted into glucose.

↓ *Carbon # 6*

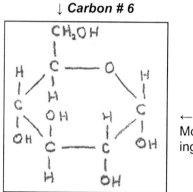

← *Carbon # 1*
Most
ingestion.

Above: The formula for glucose.

Anaerobic Glycolysis

The metabolism of glucose begins in the *__cytosol__*, and the process is anaerobic until the formation of *__pyruvic and lactic acids__* has taken place. Therefore, glucose is first broken down by an anaerobic process that does not require the presence of oxygen.

This process is called anaerobic glycolysis.

The first step of *__anaerobic glycolysis__* is the addition of a phosphate group to the glucose molecule. This is called phosphorylation, and it requires energy. The conversion of ATP to ADP releases energy for this reaction to occur; one molecule of ATP is converted to ADP for each molecule of glucose that is phosphorylated. The resulting molecule is *__glucose-6-phosphate, or G6P__*. The formation of G6P prevents glucose from building up to high concentrations in the cell, which would diffuse out of the cell.

The next step is the isomerization of G6P to *__fructose-6-phosphate (F6P)__*. This step neither requires nor releases energy. Then another phosphate is added to F6P, which requires energy in the form of ATP. The result is *__fructose-1-6-diphosphate, or F-1-6-DiP__*. Glucose and fructose are six carbon compounds. F-1-6-DiP then splits into *__two molecules__* of *__glyceraldehyde phosphate__*, (PGAL), a three carbon compound. Each of the two molecules of glyceraldehyde phosphate adds another phosphate to become *__glyceric acid diphosphate__*. NAD is reduced to NADH+H in this reaction. So far two molecules of ATP have been utilized, and none has been produced.

Fructose → *__Glucose__* (C6H12O6) ←galactose
ATP→ADP ↓ Glucokinase
+ PO4
↓
__G6P (Glucose-6-Phosphate)__ (→ glycogen and fat synthesis)
↓
__F6P (Fructose-6-Phosphate)__
ATP→ ADP ↓
+PO4
↓
__F1.6 diphosphate__
↓
__(2) Glyceraldehyde phosphate__
2 (PO4-CHOH-CHOH-CHO)
↓ 2 (NAD →2 (NADH+H)
+ 2 (PO4)
↓
__(2) 1,3 Glyceric acid diphosphate__
2 (PO4-CHOH-CHOH-CHOH-PO4)
2 ADP→ 2 ATP ↓
__(2) Glyceraldehyde phosphate__ + 2 (PO4)
2 ADP→ 2 ATP ↓ 2 (NAD) → 2 (NADH+H)
↓
__(2) Pyruvic acid__
2 (CH3-CO-COOH)

Above: The reactions of anaerobic glycolysis.

Next, each of the two molecules of glyceric acid diphosphate cleaves off a phosphate, forming two molecules of *__glyceraldehyde phosphate__* (PGAL). This step includes the conversion of ADP to ATP.

Glyceraldehyde phosphate then loses its other phosphate moiety and is converted to *__pyruvic acid__*. In this reaction ADP is converted to ATP and NAD is reduced to NADH+H.

Anaerobic Fermentation

If oxygen is absent, pyruvic acid is converted to *lactic acid*. This step is referred to as *anaerobic fermentation*. In this step NADH+H is oxidized to NAD. The formation of NAD and the conversion of pyruvic acid to lactic acid prevent the build up of NADH+H and pyruvic acid and their diffusion out of the cell. NAD must be present in its oxidized form for glycolysis to take place.

Pyruvic acid (CH3-CO-COOH)
oxygen absent   ↓   NADH+H → NAD
Lactic acid (CH3 -CHOH-COOH)

Lactic acid
oxygen present   ↓   NAD → NADH+H
Pyruvic acid

Lactic acid is utilized and not wasted. It is converted to pyruvic acid or to glucose in the liver when oxygen is available. The kidneys and cardiac muscle cells can also convert lactic acid to pyruvic acid and glucose. Lactic acid is toxic and causes fatigue when in high concentrations in skeletal muscle cells.

A synopsis of the steps of anaerobic glycolysis follows:
1. Glucose ($C_6H_{12}O_6$) enters the cell.
2. Glucose is phosphorylated to glucose-6-phosphate (G-6-P). This reaction utilizes one molecule of ATP, and it keeps glucose from building up to high concentrations and diffusing out of the cell.
3. G-6P is isomerized to fructose-6-phosphate (F-6-P).
4. F-6-P is phosphorylated to fructose-1-6-diphosphate (F1-6-DiP). This reaction utilizes one molecule of ATP.
5. F-1-6-DiP is split into *two* molecules of glyceraldehyde phosphate ($C_3O_3H_5PO_4$, or PGAL).
6. PGAL is phosphorylated to glyceric acid diphosphate. ($C_3O_3H_6[PO_4]_2$). This step converts NAD to NADH+H.
7. Glyceric acid diphosphate is dephosphorylated to PGAL. This step converts ADP to ATP.
8. Each molecule of PGAL is converted to pyruvic Acid (CH3COCOOH). This step converts ADP to ATP.

The anaerobic glycolysis of one molecule of glucose produces the following: **(1)** two molecules of pyruvic acid, **(2)** the utilization of two molecules of ATP, **(3)** the synthesis of four molecules of ATP from ADP, and **(4)** the production of two molecules of NADH+H from NAD.

The Krebs Cycle

In 1937 *Hans Adolph Krebs*, a German pharmacologist, made known his work on the metabolic cycle that bears his name. The *Krebs cycle* is also called the *citric acid cycle* and the *tricarboxylic acid cycle*. In 1953 Krebs won the Nobel Prize for his discovery. The Krebs cycle *requires oxygen*, and it is *aerobic respiration*. Without the presence of oxygen the cycle grinds to a halt because NADH+H and FADH2 cannot be oxidized to NAD and FAD in the absence of oxygen. NAD and FAD are required for the Krebs cycle to continue. The cycle grinds to a halt when all the NAD and FAD molecules have been converted to the reduced forms, NADH+H and FADH2. The Krebs cycle takes place in the *mitochondria* of the cell.

The first step in the Krebs cycle is the entry of *pyruvic acid* into the matrix of the mitochondria where it is converted to *acetic acid* (a *two* carbon compound); this step involves the reduction of NAD to NADH+H. Fats and proteins can be broken down into acetic acid, and they can enter the cycle at this point. Next, a molecule of *coenzyme A* is added to an acetate ion, producing *acetyl CoA*. Acetyl CoA reacts with *oxaloacetic acid* (a *four* carbon compound produced by the Krebs cycle), producing a molecule of *citric* acid (a *six* carbon compound.) The preceding reactions are given below.

```
CH3         CH3           H2C-COOH          H2C-COOH
 |      →    |        +     |          →      |
COOH        CO-CoA        HOC-COOH          OHC-COOH
                                              |
                                            H2C-COOH
```

Acetic acid → Acetyl CoA   +   Oxaloacetic acid →   Citric acid

Citric acid has three carboxyl groups (COOH), and it is, therefore, a tricarboxylic acid, which gives the Krebs cycle its alternate name.

A series of steps in the Krebs cycle converts citric acid to ***cis-aconitic acid***, ***isocitric acid***, and ***oxalosuccinic acid.*** ***Ketoglutaric acid***, a five carbon compound, is produced in the next step, which involves the reduction of NAD to NADH+H. Proteins and fats can enter the cycle by forming ketoglutaric acid.

Another series of steps converts ketoglutaric acid to ***succinic acid***, a four carbon acid. This step reduces NAD to NADH+H, and it converts GDP to ***GTP*** (guanosine triphosphate). GTP contains a high energy phosphate bond similar to ATP, and GTP is converted to ATP.

In the next series of steps, succinic acid is converted to ***fumaric acid***, then to ***malic acid***, and then to ***oxaloacetic acid***, which completes the cycle. The total conversion of one molecule of acetic acid to carbon dioxide and water results in the synthesis of ***one*** molecule of ATP (from GTP), the reduction of ***three*** NAD molecules to ***NADH+H,*** and the reduction of ***one*** FAD molecule to ***FADH2.*** In addition, as mentioned above, ***one*** molecule of NAD was reduced to NADH+H when pyruvic acid was broken down into acetic acid. The oxaloacetic acid produced by the cycle is available to react with another molecule of acetate that comes from the breakdown of pyruvic acid. This forms citric acid, and the cycle begins again.

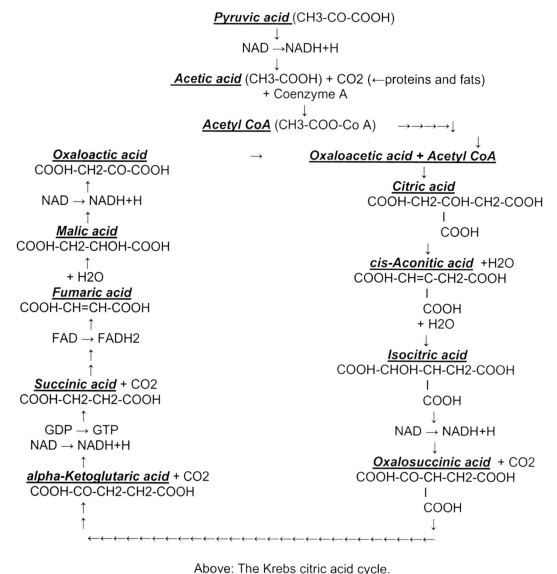

Above: The Krebs citric acid cycle.

Q? What happens to the energy in NADH+H and FADH2?
Answer: It is extracted by sending these reduced coenzymes through the *electron transport chain (cytochrome chain)*. Cytochromes are coenzymes in the chain. They were named from their bright colors.

The Electron Transport Chain

The mitochondrial membrane is a double membrane that encloses the *matrix*. The inner membrane contains folds called *cristae* that increase its surface area. The space between the inner membrane and the outer membrane is called the *intermembranous space.* The electron transport chain consists of *three groups of enzyme complexes* located in tandem fashion *on the inner membrane of mitochondria.* The reactions catalyzed by these enzymes are called *membrane reactions.* The electrons from NADH+H and FADH2 are passed down the chain, and energy is released with each pass. The electron transport chain is aerobic. It *cannot function without oxygen*, nor can it function without the reduced forms of the coenzymes derived from *niacin* (vitamin B3) and *riboflavin* (vitamin B2). When NADH+H (a niacin derivative) and FADH2 (a riboflavin derivative) are oxidized, protons are released as well as electrons. The protons are pumped into the intermembranous space between the outer and the inner membranes of mitochondria. Each of the three enzyme complexes functions as a proton pump. Energy to run the proton pump is provided by the energy extracted from the passage of electrons down the chain. The electrons are passed down the chain to its end. *Cytochrome a3* is the final coenzyme in the chain. There the electrons are picked up by an oxygen atom, which also reacts with two protons to form a molecule of water.

The electron transport chain complexes consist of the following:
Enzyme complex #1
   1. *NADH + H* enters the chain at the first enzyme complex. NADH+H is oxidized; it gives up two electrons and two protons to another nucleotide, flavin mononucleotide, or FMN. The electrons continue to enzyme complex #2. The protons first enter the *matrix,* but then they are pumped into the *intermembranous space*.
   2. Five separate iron-sulfur complexes act as coenzymes in the first enzyme complex.

Enzyme complex #2.
   1. Coenzyme Q is a relatively small molecule that can move about in the membrane; it acts as a shuttle for the electrons between enzyme complex #1 and enzyme complex #2. *FADH2* enters the chain at enzyme complex #2. FADH2 is oxidized and gives up two electrons and two protons to Coenzyme Q. The electrons continue down the chain, giving up energy with each passage. The protons first enter the *matrix*, but then they are pumped into the *intermembranous space*. Because FADH2 enters the chain later than NADH + H, fewer electron passes are made with FADH2 and consequently less energy is made available than with NADH + H.
   2. Cytochrome b, an Fe-S (iron-sulfur) complex and cytochrome c-1 are coenzymes in this complex. (Note: ALL FIVE of the cytochromes utilize Fe (iron ions) as a cofactor in the passage of electrons.)

Enzyme complex #3
   1. Cytochrome c acts as a shuttle for the electrons between enzyme complex #2 and enzyme complex #3. The other coenzymes in this complex include two copper (Cu) ions, cytochrome a and cytochrome a-3. Cyanide inhibits aerobic respiration by binding with the iron ion of cytochrome c oxidase.

At the end of the electron transport chain, *NADH + H has been oxidized to NAD*, and *FADH2 has been oxidized to FAD*. A pair of electrons on cytochrome a-3 and a pair of protons from the matrix are picked up by an oxygen atom to produce a molecule of *H2O.*

NADH + H goes through three complexes, and enough energy is extracted through the passage of its pair of electrons down the chain to produce *three* molecules of ATP from ADP.

FADH2 goes through only the second and third complexes, and only *two* molecules of ADP are phosphorylated to *ATP* for each pair of electrons from FADH2 that go through the chain.

Above: The electron transport chain.

Iron, sulfur and copper serve as cofactors for the oxidation-reduction reactions of the electron passage. Iron has two common valences, +2 and +3. Sulfur, like oxygen, has six electrons in its outer ring and is an effective oxidizing agent. Copper has two common valences, +1 and +2.

Q? O.K., so you've released a lot of energy from the oxidation of NADH + H and FADH2. How does that produce ATP?
Answer: Through the *chemiosmotic mechanism* described below.

The Chemiosmotic Mechanism

As you saw in the electron transport chain, NADH + H and FADH2 are oxidized to NAD and FAD on the inner membrane of mitochondria. This process removes two electrons and two protons from each molecule of NADH+H or FADH2. The electrons are shuttled through the chain to its end where they are picked up by an oxygen atom in the final oxidation reaction. The *protons are initially released into the matrix*, but then they are *pumped into the space between the inner and outer membranes of the mitochondria* (the intermembranous space). Each of the three enzyme complexes of the electron transport chain also functions as a *proton pump.* This pump creates a high concentration of protons (hydrogen ions) and a *low pH* in the intermembranous space. It also creates a steep electrochemical gradient across the inner membrane. Opposite charges attract. A high concentration of protons in the intermembranous space makes it *highly positively charged.* Protons are pumped out of the matrix, making the matrix negatively charged. Also the protons in the intermembranous space have a strong tendency to diffuse down their concentration gradient into the matrix, but the inner mitochondrial membrane is impermeable to protons, so ordinary diffusion does not occur except through *channel ports* in the inner membrane. The diffusion of protons through these channels is a flow of charged particles, which is an *electrical current*. The proteins that make up the channel ports are *enzymes* that catalyze the reaction, ADP + PO4 → ATP, and those enzymes are named *ATP synthase*. The electrical current caused by the *flow of protons* from the intermembranous space to the matrix is what *powers the enzymatic conversion of ADP to ATP.*
ADP + H2PO4- → ATP + H2O
Adenine + ribose = adenosine.
ATP = adenine + ribose + 3(H2PO3 -)

Summary of the electron transport chain
Electrons travel down the chain in pairs.
One molecule of NADH + H produces three molecules of ATP from ADP.
One molecule of FADH2 produces two molecules of ATP from ADP.
NADH + H and FADH2 are oxidized in this process. They lose electrons and protons and they release energy. NAD and FAD are reformed and are used again to accept electrons (and protons) in the Krebs cycle.
The final electron acceptor (oxidizing agent) is oxygen. Without oxygen the whole process grinds to a halt as the electrons stack up with no place to go.

The Maximum Total ATP Production from One Molecule of Glucose:
Glycolysis (from glucose to pyruvic acid).
  2 ATP utilized (subtracted from the total).
  4 ATP produced.
  2 NADH + H produced (producing 6 ATP).
Krebs Cycle (from pyruvic acid to oxaloacetic acid).
  2 ATP produced (from 2 GTP).
  8 NADH + H produced (producing 24 ATP.
  2 FADH2 produced (producing 4 ATP.

The total theoretical maximum energy production from the metabolism of one molecule of glucose is ___38___ *molecules of ATP* (-2, +4, +6, +2, +24, +4 = 38). This process has an efficiency of 40%, not counting the ATP that is utilized to energize the proton pump. The other 60% is given off as heat.

The total of the chemical reactions is C6H12O6 + 6 O2 → 6CO2 + 6H2O.
The products of the metabolism of glucose are ***carbon dioxide and water***. Five percent of the total blood CO2 is dissolved in the plasma and is easily removed by the lungs. Five percent is bound to plasma proteins or hemoglobin in the red blood cells, and is less easily removed. Ninety percent is in the form of carbonic acid (H2CO3) or the bicarbonate ion (HCO3-) and serves as a buffer for the blood. The water is utilized or excreted.

The origin of mitochondria

By now you should have an appreciable respect for the metabolic actions that take place within mitochondria. Mitochondria are necessary for cells to accomplish ***aerobic respiration***. Anaerobes live in oxygen poor environments; they lack aerobic respiration, and mitochondria are absent from the cells of anaerobes.

The origin of mitochondria is just as astounding as are their metabolic activities. ***Eukaryotes*** are organisms with nuclei that contain DNA. Protozoa are the simplest animals; they include amoebae and paramecia, and they are one-celled eukaryotes. Bacteria have DNA, but they do not have nuclei, and they are not eukaryotes. Bacteria and eukaryotes differ in other ways: (1) Exceptions exist, but it is generally true that eukaryotes are considerably larger than bacteria. (2) Bacteria are surrounded by a rigid membrane; eukaryotes have a flexible plasma membrane underlaid by a flexible cytoskeleton that provides movement and allows for phagocytosis. (3) Bacteria often multiply within hours, which is considerably faster than eukaryotes. (4) Bacteria are able to mutate with alacrity. Eukaryotes mutate slowly. The rapid mutation rate and the rapid multiplication rate of bacteria are evidenced by the rapid development of resistance to antibiotics by some bacteria. (5) Bacteria have the ability to share genetic material with their neighbors, including bacteria of different species, which increases the speed of their genetic change.

The membranes of the endoplasmic reticulum, the nuclear membrane, the Golgi body and the plasma membrane are connected and continuous. The membranes of mitochondria are separate, and it is now accepted that mitochondria had a bacterial origin. But the bacterial origin of mitochondria is not unique. Chloroplasts and hydrogenosomes are specialized organelles of bacterial origin that also were inculcated into primordial protozoa. ***Chloroplasts*** contain chlorophyll, which utilizes sunlight and carbon dioxide to synthesize organic molecules, producing oxygen as a byproduct. Chloroplasts are responsible for photosynthesis in all green plants. ***Hydrogenosomes*** are located in some anaerobic protozoa and fungi. They appear to have originated from mitochondria, but hydrogenosomes produce hydrogen and ATP under anaerobic conditions. Much of the original DNA of mitochondria, chloroplasts and hydrogenosomes has been relocated to the nucleus of the eukaryote, but mitochondria and chloroplasts retain some of their original DNA, RNA and ribosomes. That explains why a cell cannot regenerate new chloroplasts or mitochondria from its nuclear DNA alone. The DNA of most hydrogenosomes has been transferred totally to the nuclei of their anaerobic hosts. A ciliated protozoan that inhabits the hind gut of the cockroach is the only species yet found that has hydrogenosomes with DNA. Hydrogenosomes are sometimes found in conjunction with methane producing bacteria ***(methanogens).*** Methanogens utilize carbon dioxide and the hydrogen let off by hydrogenosomes to produce ATP. The atmosphere of the young earth contained an appreciable amount of methane, a large amount of which is thought to have been produced by methanogens.

A rapid mutation rate afforded bacteria the ability to develop photosynthesis, aerobic respiration and methanogenesis. Eukaryotes were able to take advantage of these processes by engulfing bacteria that had those abilities. The incorporation of mitochondria and chloroplasts was a necessary prerequisite for eukaryotes to develop into multicellular organisms.

The bacterial-protozoan relationship that begot mitochondria was symbiotic. Bacteria contributed new metabolic pathways to the larger protozoan. In turn the protozoan supplied pyruvate, carbon dioxide and/or hydrogen for the bacteria to use as fuel. The advantages for bacteria to live within a cell persist today and are illustrated by many pathogenic bacteria. Diseases such as Legionnaires' disease, meningococcal meningitis, gonorrhea, Rocky Mountain spotted fever, typhus and others are caused by microorganisms that live and multiply within human cells. DNA of the AIDS virus has been shown to have the ability to attach itself to nuclear DNA where it becomes part of the cell's genome.

Fat metabolism

Fat is stored primarily as triglycerides, which contain three fatty acids and one glycerol moiety. Adipose tissue releases triglycerides into the blood when needed, and the liver can convert glycerol to ***glyceraldehyde phosphate (PGAL)***. Glucose can be synthesized from PGAL, or PGAL can enter the ***glycolytic pathway***. Fatty acids are broken down in two-carbon segments to ***acetic acid***, which enters the citric acid cycle as ***acetyl Co-A***. If fatty acid breakdown is excessive, ***ketone bodies*** accumulate and can cause ***acidosis***. Ketone bodies accumulate when more acetic acid is produced from fat than can be utilized by the citric acid cycle. The ketone bodies produced are ***acetone, acetoacetic acid and beta hydroxybutyric acid***. The latter two are acidic, and large quantities in the blood will produce a metabolic acidosis known as ***ketosis.*** Diabetics who are not under control do not have the ability to utilize glucose efficiently. They catabolize fats for energy excessively, and they tend to become acidotic from the build up of ketone bodies. People who are ***starving*** do not have adequate glucose available, and they also develop ketosis due to excessive fat catabolism.

Some glycolysis is necessary to prevent ketoacidosis, but a majority of the energy normally produced by the body comes from fat catabolism. Most of the body's stored energy is fat; fat reserves can supply enough energy for 119 hours of running, whereas carbohydrate reserves (glycogen) can only supply enough energy for 1.6 hours of running. One gram of fat produces nine kilocalories of energy, whereas one gram of carbohydrate produces only four kilocalories of energy.

Protein metabolism

Proteins can also be used to produce ATP. First they are broken down into individual amino acids. The amino acids are then stripped of their amino groups by a process known as ***deamination***. The remaining molecule can then be converted to pyruvic acid or to a compound in the Krebs cycle. Amino acids are not stored in the body. The proteins synthesized from amino acids have a function, and when proteins are catabolized for energy, that function is lost.

Following deamination the amino group (NH2) becomes ***ammonia*** (NH3), which is toxic. The liver detoxifies ammonia through the ***ornithine cycle***, in which two molecules of ammonia are combined with one molecule of carbon dioxide to make ***urea,*** (NH2CONH2). Urea is excreted in the urine. ***Bilirubin and ammonia*** will build up in the blood if the liver is diseased and failing; this results in ***jaundice and hepatic coma***. Hepatic coma is due to the build up of ammonia and is usually fatal.

The ***liver*** is essential in the detoxification process. The synthesis of ***urea*** from ammonia and carbon dioxide occurs in the liver as a result of the ***ornithine cycle***. ***Creatine phosphate*** is a compound in muscle that stores a high energy phosphate bond that can be converted to ATP. Creatine is converted into ***creatinine*** in the liver, and creatinine is excreted in the urine. The ***purines*** (adenine and guanine) are broken down to ***uric acid*** by the liver, and uric acid is excreted in the urine. An inability of the kidneys to excrete a sufficient amount of uric acid can result in ***gout***, a painful arthritic disorder that is associated with crystallization of uric acid in the joints. Organ meats (kidneys, liver, and glands) are rich in purines and should be avoided in patients with gout.

Temperature Control

Heat is produced by the breakdown of glucose, proteins, fats and ATP. ***Thyroid hormones*** increase the metabolic rate, which increases the production of heat. Thyroid hormones contain ***iodine***, which makes them unique in the body. Thyroid hormone secretion is controlled by TSH (thyroid stimulating hormone) from the anterior pituitary.

**Sympathetic stimulation** increases the metabolic rate and heat production.

Heat produced by ATP utilization in skeletal muscles accounts for 25% of the heat produced at rest. Vigorous exercise increases muscular heat production by thirty to forty times. _**Shivering**_ is contraction of antagonistic muscle groups as a response to a low body temperature. Shivering produces heat; it is controlled by the hypothalamus.

The normal body temperature is 98.6 degrees F (37 degrees C), but it is not constant. The body temperature is normally lower in the morning and higher following activity.

Body heat is lost from the skin through _**radiation**_ to the air and the _**conduction**_ of heat to clothing and other objects that are being touched. Radiated heat is carried upward and away from the body by _**convection currents**_ in the air. The ability of the body to radiate heat is dependant the _**body mass and surface area.**_ Mass and surface area are reflections of the body weight and shape. Tall, thin, angular individuals with long limbs are classified as _**ectomorphs**_. Corpulent, rounded, heavy individuals with short limbs are classified as _**endomorphs.**_ A _**mesomorph**_ is a muscular individual. Ectomorphs have the greatest ability to dispense with heat, but they are more susceptible to extreme cold. Endomorphs excel in retaining heat, but they are more susceptible to fever and heat stroke. Mesomorphs are intermediate in heat dispensation.

Air is a poor conductor of heat, and fabrics that contain minute air pockets provide the best insulation. Dilation of blood vessels in the skin exposes the inner heat of the body (core temperature) to the outside and leads to heat loss as long as the ambient temperature is not excessive. Body heat is also lost through the respiratory tract, urine and feces. Conversely if the body's core temperature is low, cutaneous vessels will constrict to conserve heat.

The radiation of heat is greatly reduced or eliminated in hot environments because the air temperature is near or above the temperature of the body. In this situation the only effective mechanism for the body to cool itself is through _**evaporation.**_ Sweat glands produce perspiration, which wets the body surface, and the evaporation of sweat takes away substantial amounts of heat. Air movement and low humidity both enhance heat loss by evaporation; evaporation is reduced when the air is humid and still.

Nuclei in the _**hypothalamus**_ sense temperature and control vasoconstriction, vasodilation, sweating and shivering.

**Fever** is an abnormally high body temperature. Common causes of fever include an infectious disease, extensive physical trauma, CNS damage and a neoplasm (cancer). It is incorrect to equate "temperature" with "fever." Everyone has a temperature, be it normal or abnormal; a fever is an abnormally high temperature. Cytokines known as _**pyrogens**_ are released by leukocytes and macrophages that have phagocytized pathogens. Pyrogens trigger the hypothalamus to increase the body's thermostat. Fever is helpful in discouraging the growth of many microorganisms; however, if the body temperature exceeds 106 degrees F, a _**positive feedback**_ mechanism begins. The increased temperature increases the metabolic rate, which further increases the body temperature. Fluid and electrolytes are lost through sweating; heat cramps and heat exhaustion may follow. _**Heat cramps**_ are painful muscle spasms that are due to electrolyte loss. _**Heat exhaustion (heat stroke)**_ is characterized by hypotension, dizziness, fainting, nausea and vomiting. A body temperature of 108 degrees F (42 degrees C) is quite dangerous, and a temperature of 110 degrees F (43 degrees C) is often fatal.

The enzyme systems of our bodies function best at temperatures between 97-100 degrees F. Enzyme activity slows down at lower temperatures, and body temperatures below 90 degrees F may cause death.

Temperatures above 106 degrees F result in some metabolic reactions accelerating out of control. Some enzymes lose their ability to function at high temperatures because proteins become _**"denatured"**_ (change shape and lose their function). Other enzymatic reactions accelerate beyond control, which generates more heat than the body can give off. Cells die, and death ensues unless rapid cooling is initiated. Immersion in cold ice water is the quickest and best way to treat severe hyperthermia. Body heat is transferred much more quickly to water than to air.

Exposure to wind and cold air temperatures without proper protective clothing can lead to an excessive loss of body heat, which is called ***hypothermia.*** Immersion of the body in cold water can quickly cause hypothermia, and clothing is generally of little value in preventing heat loss when submerged (only wool retains any ability to insulate when it is wet). The hypothalamus responds to hypothermia by stimulating vasoconstriction in the skin and by instigating shivering, which increases heat production by skeletal muscles. The breakdown of fat produces more energy than the breakdown of carbohydrate or protein. When one gram of fat is burned, nine kilocalories of heat energy are produced; however, when one gram of carbohydrate or protein is burned, only four kilocalories of heat energy are produced. Most cells in your body have a high water content. When that water freezes, ice crystals form and their jagged ends rip into cell membranes. The cells form leaks, molecules congeal, proteins unwind and become ineffective, and the cells die. Frostbite is cellular death in the skin from hypothermia. Infants and hibernating animals contain stores of ***brown fat,*** which when burned produces very little ATP but produces a great deal of heat. When the core body temperature drops to 91 degrees F (33 degrees C), the metabolic rate drops so low that shivering and cutaneous vasoconstriction cannot keep pace with the loss of heat to a cold environment. A ***positive feedback*** mechanism begins, and the body temperature continues to fall. Ventricular fibrillation and death may occur at temperatures less than 90 degrees F (32 degrees C), but some people have been known to survive despite a body temperature below 84 degrees F (29 degrees C).

Cells with little water or a high fat to water ratio are relatively resistant to hypothermia. Spermatozoa, ova and bone marrow cells can be preserved if they are kept within a carefully controlled temperature range.

Study Guide
1. What is meant by the BMR?
2. In what chemical form is most fat stored?
3. What are the essential fatty acids?
4. What is the difference between an essential and a non essential amino acid?
5. Follow a molecule of glucose in potato starch from your mouth to storage as glycogen in the liver.
6. Review heat exhaustion and hypothermia.
7. Know what the suffixes –ase and –ose signify.
8. Thoroughly review the redox reaction.
9. Know the meaning of the terms enzyme and coenzyme, and give examples.
10. Understand how enzymes and coenzymes function in a redox chemical reaction.
11. Understand what NAD and FAD are, and how they work in metabolic reactions.
12. Know the meaning of the following terms: glycogen, glycogenolysis, glycogenesis, gluconeogenesis, glycolysis, aerobic, anaerobic, cellular respiration and anaerobic fermentation.
13. Appreciate the contributions of Hans Adolph Krebs to science.
14. Be able to recognize the structure and formula of a simple sugar like glucose.
15. Review anaerobic glycolysis (the breakdown of glucose to pyruvic acid) and understand the processes involved.
16. Understand the role of lactic acid formation in anaerobic fermentation.
17. Review the Krebs citric acid cycle; understand how it works and where it takes place.
18. Review the cytochrome chain; understand how it works and where it is located.
19. Recognize the importance of mitochondria, coenzymes and oxygen in the electron transport mechanism.
20. Know that a small amount of DNA is present in mitochondria. Know that mitochondria are considered to be of bacterial origin, and that all mitochondria are inherited from the mother.
21. Know how the chemiosmotic mechanism converts ADP to ATP.
22. Know the structure of ATP, ADP and 3'5'cyclic AMP, including the moieties involved and the locations of the high energy phosphate bonds.
23. Define appetite, anorexia, leptin and cholecystokinin.
24. What are the origins of mitochondria, chloroplasts and hydrogenosomes?

Chapter Twenty-six

Nutrition

Nutrition is the ingestion and digestion of substances needed for life. Those substances include amino acids, fats, carbohydrates, vitamins and minerals. The catabolism of carbohydrates, fats and proteins supplies the energy needs of the body through glycolysis, the Krebs cycle and the electron transport chain.

Dieticians classify carbohydrates as simple or complex. **_Simple carbohydrates_** are monosaccharide and disaccharide sugars. **_Complex carbohydrates_** are long starch polymers (polysaccharides). Unrefined foods contain complex carbohydrates, and they have a significant fiber, protein and micronutrient (vitamins, minerals) component. Simple carbohydrates are rapidly absorbed, and they give a sudden rise in blood sugar. Complex carbohydrates must be broken down before absorption can occur, and they elevate the blood sugar more slowly and to a lesser degree. Diabetics in particular are best advised to consume complex carbohydrates in place of simple carbohydrates.

Carbohydrates are present in glycoproteins, proteoglycans and GAG compounds; they make up the glycocalyx of the cell membrane, and the sugars ribose and deoxyribose are part of the nucleotide structure. **_Lipids_** constitute most of the cell membrane; some lipids function as hormones and prostaglandins, and lipids are an essential part of lipoproteins. **_Proteins_** include enzymes, globulins, albumin, glycoproteins, lipoproteins, muscle proteins and many other compounds. Carbohydrates, lipids and proteins have previously been discussed. This chapter will focus on the effects of vitamins, minerals, fiber, the controversy involving dietary fat, and the effects of alcohol. The cycling of carbon and nitrogen by living things will also be discussed.

Vitamins
Vitamins are chemicals that are necessary for metabolism in some way. Vitamins or their precursors cannot be synthesized by the human body, and most vitamins must be present in the diet. Vitamin K, riboflavin, pantothenic acid (vitamin B5), biotin (a B vitamin), and folic acid (a B vitamin) are produced by **_bacteria in the large intestine_**, but only small quantities are absorbed from this source. Feces contain more biotin than does food. Some animals practice coprophagy, which is the ingestion of one's own feces. It is thought that this is done in order to increase the intake of vitamins and other nutrients.

Fat soluble vitamins
The **_fat soluble vitamins_** are vitamins A, E, D and K. Fat soluble vitamins will not be absorbed from the intestines unless fat is present. The liver has the capacity to store fat soluble vitamins. Water soluble vitamins are not stored in the body, and excessive amounts are rapidly excreted in the urine.

Vitamin A (retinol) is the parent compound of retinal, the photochemical used by photoreceptors of the retina. Vitamin A is also necessary for the health of the skin and other epithelial tissues. Carotene, a vitamin A precursor, is the form that is usually found in the diet. Too much artificial carotene can produce symptoms of toxicity (nausea, vomiting and hepatosplenomegaly), but huge amounts are necessary for toxic symptoms to appear.

Ergosterol is a plant sterol (a lipid with four rings based on the formula for cholesterol). Ergosterol is converted to **_vitamin D-3_** in the skin when it is exposed to ultraviolet light. Vitamin D-3 is converted to **_calcitriol_**, the most active form of vitamin D, by reactions in the liver and kidneys. Vitamin D is necessary for bone formation because calcium absorption from the GI tract and calcium reabsorption from the kidney tubules require vitamin D.

Vitamin K includes a group of similar compounds that are necessary for the synthesis of prothrombin and other clotting factors by the liver.

Vitamin E (tocopherol) is an antioxidant that prevents cellular damage from free radicals. It contributes to wound healing and the detoxification of chemicals by the liver.

Water soluble vitamins

The _**water soluble vitamins**_ are vitamin C and the B complex of vitamins. _**Vitamin C (ascorbic acid)**_ is necessary for collagen synthesis, wound healing, iron absorption and the metabolism of amino acids. Ascorbic acid plays a major role in fighting infections. Most of the animal kingdom is able to synthesize ascorbic acid; the only exceptions are primates, guinea pigs, the red vented bulbul and the East Asian fruit bat. Vitamin C is plentiful in fruits and vegetables, but it is rapidly destroyed by heat. A lack of vitamin C can result in scurvy, a disease in which collagen synthesis and wound healing are derelict, and tissues bleed easily. Before 1753 the diet fed to British sailors was lacking in vitamin C; as a result, scurvy was epidemic on British ships.

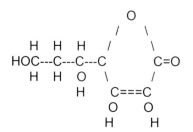

Left: Vitamin C. Most of the animal kingdom can synthesize vitamin C from glucose. Man is one of the exceptions.

The _**B complex**_ of vitamins presently includes about fifteen compounds. They are numbered, but the numbers are not in common usage for all the B vitamins. Some of the numbered B vitamins are vitamin B1, or _**thiamine**_; vitamin B2, or _**riboflavin**_; vitamin B3, or _**niacin;**_ vitamin B5, or _**pantothenic acid**_; vitamin B6, or _**pyridoxine**_, and vitamin B12, or _**cyanocobalamine**_. _**Biotin, folic acid, paraaminobenzoic acid**_ (PABA), _**choline**_ and _**inositol**_ are also members of the B vitamin complex.

The B group of vitamins is necessary for one or more metabolic reactions to take place, and deficiency states are reflected by symptoms. A lack of _**thiamine**_ results in the neurologic disorder known as _**beri beri**_. _**Riboflavin**_ is the basis for the co-enzyme, FAD. A deficiency of riboflavin produces ulcerations in and around the mouth and inflammation and irritation of the eyes. _**Niacin**_ is the basis for the co-enzyme, NAD. The metabolism of niacin is linked with that of the amino acid, _**tryptophan.**_ A deficiency of either niacin or tryptophan results in _**pellagra**_, which is a disease characterized by dermatitis, diarrhea and dementia. The mucous membranes of the mouth are often ulcerated in pellagra. Pellagra was epidemic in the American South following the Civil War because the diet consisted mostly of corn, which is deficient in tryptophan. _**Pantothenic acid**_ is the basis for co-enzyme A, which is necessary for cellular respiration and the metabolism of fats and amino acids. A deficiency of pantothenic acid can result in premature aging. _**Pyridoxine**_ is necessary for the synthesis of proteins and nucleic acids. _**Biotin**_ is required for the synthesis of nucleic acids and for the metabolism of fatty acids and amino acids. _**Folic acid**_ is necessary for red blood cell development and DNA synthesis. _**Choline**_ is an ingredient in phospholipids and acetylcholine. _**Inositol**_ functions as a second messenger. _**Vitamin B12**_ is required for red blood cell production. A deficiency of vitamin B12 leads to pernicious anemia and neurological defects known as combined system disease. Intrinsic factor is a glycoprotein produced by parietal cells in the stomach. Intrinsic factor is necessary for the absorption of vitamin B12. Vitamin B12 is the only necessary substance in the body known to contain _**cobalt.**_

A deficiency of one B vitamin generally reflects a deficient diet and occult deficiencies of multiple B vitamins. Therefore, if a vitamin deficiency is found, multivitamin therapy is recommended. Thiamine, riboflavin and niacin deficiency states are often the first to be symptomatic, and synthetic forms of these vitamins are added to flour and cereals today.

Several of the vitamins, especially vitamins A and D, can be taken in excess, which has rarely led to a condition known as _**hypervitaminosis**_. A _**recommended daily allowance (RDA)**_ for each vitamin has been established by the Federal Government. The RDA values are revised frequently.

Minerals

A mineral is not the same as a metal. A mineral is an inorganic element or compound that can be extracted from the earth. A metal is an element or alloy that is lustrous and conducts heat and electricity. Metals can be melted, and they are malleable. Not all minerals are metals; sulfur and phosphorus are minerals, but they are not metals.

At least twenty-six different elements are required for the human body to function properly. ***Fourteen of those elements are classified as minerals***, but minerals constitute only about 4% of our weight. The four most common elements in the body are not minerals; they are: hydrogen (H), oxygen (O), carbon (C), and nitrogen (N). The minerals in greatest abundance in the body are calcium (Ca), phosphorus (P), sodium (Na), chlorine (Cl), magnesium (Mg), potassium (K), sulfur (S), and iron (Fe).

H, O, C, N, Ca, and P, are classified as ***major elements*** in the body. Some of the uses for the major elements are:

Calcium is necessary for the crystallization of bone salts and formation of the teeth. It is used as a co-enzyme and in muscle contraction.

Phosphorus is necessary for the formation of bones and teeth. It is an ingredient in phospholipids, nucleotides and creatine phosphate.

Na, Cl, Mg, K, S and Fe are classified as the body's ***lesser elements***. Some of the uses of the lesser elements are:

Sodium is the main cation in the blood and extracellular fluid. It is necessary for nerve and muscle impulse propagation.

Chlorine is the main anion in the blood and extracellular fluid. Hydrochloric acid is produced in the stomach.

Magnesium is present in bones and teeth. It is a co-enzyme in the Krebs cycle and in the production of ATP.

Potassium is the main cation in intracellular fluid. It is necessary for nerve and muscle impulse propagation.

Sulfur is a co-enzyme in the cytochrome chain, and it is an ingredient in three amino acids. Disulfide bonds give proteins their structure.

Iron is a necessary ingredient in hemoglobin and myoglobin, and it functions as a coenzyme in the cytochrome chain.

Other elements are required in only minute amounts and are called ***trace elements.***. They include the following:

Zinc is used as a coenzyme and is a component of insulin. Zinc promotes wound healing and red blood cell development.

Manganese is necessary for fatty acid, cholesterol and urea synthesis, and it helps to regulate blood glucose.

Copper is used as a co-enzyme and in the synthesis of hemoglobin and melanin.

Fluorine strengthens teeth and bones.

Iodine is a necessary ingredient in thyroid hormones.

Chromium is necessary for glucose metabolism.

Selenium is an antioxidant and a co-enzyme.

Cobalt is an ingredient in vitamin B12.

Molybdenum promotes aspects of nitrogen metabolism. It is an essential coenzyme for nitrate reductase, a plant enzyme that converts nitrogen into a useful form.

Vanadium is a coenzyme used by the heart, kidneys and reproductive organs.

Silicon helps form healthy bones and connective tissue. It is helpful in preventing cardiovascular disease.

Germanium improves oxygen delivery to the tissues and the removal of toxins from the tissues.

Boron improves brain function and alertness, and it improves calcium absorption.

Trace elements can be toxic when in excess. For example, ***hemochromatosis*** is an inherited disease of ***iron*** metabolism. In this disease iron stores in the form of hemosiderin build up to levels that are fifty to one hundred times normal in organs, especially the liver and pancreas. Liver failure, diabetes mellitus, cardiac failure and testicular atrophy are common in this disease.

Copper can also be toxic. ***Wilson's disease (hepatolenticular degeneration)*** is an uncommon inherited disease of copper metabolism in which copper is first deposited within cells of the liver, cornea and basal ganglia of the brain. Cirrhosis, neurologic symptoms and renal dysfunction are common complications. The copper deposits in the cornea can be seen on ophthalmologic exam. The neurologic symptoms often mimic Parkinson's disease; they include tremor, rigidity, dementia and psychosis. Wilson's disease usually becomes symptomatic around the age of 10-14, and it can be fatal. The defective gene, which is located on chromosome #13, is especially prevalent in Central America. In El Salvador one in 186 suffers from the disease.

Fiber

Fiber adds nothing nutritionally, but it is a necessary ingredient in the diet. Most fiber consists of indigestible polysaccharides and plant gums. Fiber serves to absorb water, soften the stool, and increase the bulk of the stool. Constipation, diverticuli, hemorrhoids and colon cancer result from a lack of fiber in the diet. A bulky stool increases peristalsis and quickens the passage of feces through the colon, which reduces the risk of those disorders. Some fiber is water soluble and some is not. Cellulose, hemicellulose and lignin are **water insoluble** fibers. Water insoluble fibers have no effect on cholesterol elimination, and too much water insoluble fiber can interfere with absorption. **Pectins** are **water soluble fibers** that form a gel that **absorbs bile acids** and prevents their reabsorption; this serves to **lower the blood cholesterol** because cholesterol is used by the liver to synthesize bile acids. Pectins are found in whole grains, legumes (peas and beans), other vegetables and fruits.

The Dietary Fat Controversy

Cholesterol

Coronary artery disease, stroke and peripheral vascular disease are rampant today. They are caused by **atherosclerosis,** the leading killer in the western world. Such has not always been the case. One hundred years ago deaths from pneumonia and tuberculosis far exceeded deaths from atherosclerosis.

Atherosclerosis is the formation of fatty plaques **(atheromas)** in the walls of medium-size and large arteries. Injury to the endothelium allows plasma to seep into the arterial wall. Cholesterol is relatively insoluble, and it precipitates in the arterial wall where it sets up an inflammatory response. Leukocytes invade, and monocytes phagocytize cholesterol and other lipids, becoming fat laden "foam cells" in the process. **Endothelial damage** and the presence of a large **inflamed atheroma** in the wall of an artery increase the risk of **clot formation**, which can totally occlude the artery. Occluded arteries lead to **ischemia** (poor blood perfusion), **hypoxia** (low oxygen) and **necrosis** (cell death). Any tissue can suffer from ischemia due to poor arterial perfusion, but the **coronary arteries** and the **carotid arterial tree** appear to be especially vulnerable. Atherosclerosis in other arteries can lead to serious illness. Blockage of the renal arteries may produce hypertension and renal failure; blockage of a mesenteric artery can infarct a portion of the gut; blockage of an iliac artery can lead to the loss of a lower limb.

It is natural that the search for the cause for the rise in atherosclerotic deaths became prominent in the media as well as scientific circles. That search led to the finding that a high level of cholesterol in the blood (**hypercholesterolemia**) was associated with atherosclerosis. Suddenly cholesterol was the demon, and the rush was on to avoid cholesterol in the diet. Cholesterol is present in animal fat, but it is absent in vegetable fat. Advertising slogans began screaming "No Cholesterol" (in our product), and informed shoppers began to substitute margarine for butter and other animal fats.

But a closer look at cholesterol revealed some contradictory facts. Cholesterol is a necessary compound for the body. It is the parent compound from which bile acids and steroid hormones are synthesized, and it is an essential ingredient in cell membranes. **Eighty percent** of the body's cholesterol is synthesized in the liver from glucose; only **twenty percent** originates in the food we eat. Low cholesterol diets are consistently disappointing in lowering the level of cholesterol in the blood; only a 4% to 13% decline in blood cholesterol can be expected from a low cholesterol diet, and low cholesterol diets have given no improvement in death rates secondary to atherosclerosis. Clearly other factors beside dietary cholesterol are involved in atherosclerosis.

Cholesterol is carried in the blood in **lipoproteins**. Lipoproteins exist as **chylomicrons,** very low density lipoproteins (**VLDL**), low density lipoproteins (**LDL**), and high density lipoproteins (**HDL**). Chylomicrons are fat droplets that are absorbed into lacteals in the small intestine. They consist mostly of triglycerides with a small amount of cholesterol and a thin coating of protein. Chylomicrons are broken down to VLDLs, and VLDLs are converted to LDLs by the liver. LDLs function to transport cholesterol to the tissues. LDLs are 50-60% cholesterol, and the cholesterol in atheromas comes from LDLs. Atheromas occur when plasma LDL levels are high. HDLs contain little cholesterol when they are formed, but they scavenge for cholesterol and they transport cholesterol to the liver. The liver excretes cholesterol into the bile, and it converts cholesterol to bile acids, which are also excreted into the bile.

LDLs are called the "bad cholesterol" because high levels lead to atherosclerosis. **_HDLs are called the "good cholesterol"_** because they reduce atherosclerosis. A high ratio of LDL cholesterol to HDL cholesterol is a paramount predictor for atherosclerosis.

Other factors that increase the risk for atherosclerosis include:
(1) Smoking. The association of smoking with vascular disease is well documented and strong. Smoking increases LDL levels and decreases HDL levels.
(2) Hypertension. High blood pressure is injurious to arterial walls and promotes atheroma formation.
(3) Diabetes. Diabetes is often associated with hypertension, obesity and metabolic imbalances, all of which accentuate the effect of hyperglycemia on the blood cholesterol level.
(4) Homocystinuria is a genetic disease characterized by high levels of the amino acid, homocysteine, in the blood. Homocysteine damages the endothelium of arterial walls, which leads to atheroma formation. Homocysteine also promotes the formation of blood clots.
(5) Familial hypercholesterolemia is a genetic disease characterized by high levels of LDLs in the blood.
(6) Aging. The cholesterol level in the blood is higher in the aged.
(7) Male sex. Men are more susceptible to atherosclerosis than women because male hormones increase the blood cholesterol level.
(8) Obesity. A diet high in calories, high in refined carbohydrates, high in cholesterol and high in total fat will promote atherosclerosis. Weight loss reduces the blood cholesterol level
(9) A sedentary lifestyle. Exercise lowers the blood cholesterol level, and it lowers LDLs in the blood.
(10) A deficiency of several B vitamins including folic acid, vitamin B6 and vitamin B12 will increase the risk for atherosclerosis.

It has been shown that cholesterol-lowering drugs lower the risk of coronary heart disease and stroke. These drugs are effective in hypercholesterolemia of all causes.
The cholesterol brouhaha has moderated, and cholesterol is less frequently regarded as a dietary villain.

Trans fat

Trans fats are not present in nature. They are formed by bubbling hydrogen gas through heated vegetable oils, which contain unsaturated fatty acids. The result is labeled **_"partially hydrogenated"_** vegetable oil. Margarine is partially hydrogenated vegetable oil. Molecules such as fatty acids are three dimensional compounds, and they have a definite shape and structure. Hydrogenation partially saturates the unsaturated fatty acids in the vegetable oil. In the process the remaining **_C=C bonds are distorted_**, which changes the shape of the fatty acid from the natural **_cis_** structure to the **_trans_** structure. Trans fats retain at least one C=C bond, and they are unsaturated fats. Fully hydrogenated oils have no C=C bonds, and they are saturated fats. Fully saturated fats are never trans fats, although both trans fats and saturated fats have similar deleterious effects.

When cholesterol was linked to coronary heart disease, the informed shopper rushed to buy trans fats (margarine) in order to avoid cholesterol. Bakers and confectioners preferred the new product because it was cheap, it made foods stay fresh longer, it had a longer shelf life, and it was less greasy to the touch.

But drawbacks to _trans_ fat have surfaced. It has been found to increase triglyceride levels, increase LDL levels, and decrease HDL levels, all of which **_promote atherosclerosis_**. _Trans_ fat also increases inflammation within atheromas.

The risk of coronary artery disease is not influenced by a low cholesterol diet; however, a diet low in saturated fat and low in _trans_ fat lowers the risk of coronary artery disease. The Federal government requires grocery items to be labeled for the presence of _trans_ fat ("partially hydrogenated" vegetable oil). The cities of New York and Philadelphia have outlawed the addition of _trans_ fats to restaurant food.

Lipids are important components of the diet. They not only serve as a source of calories, they serve as hormones; they **_transport_** and **_store_** fat soluble vitamins and other fat soluble micronutrients, and they are essential ingredients in **_cell membranes_**. **_Trans fats have been deformed to the extent that they do not serve a role in these functions._**

Studies have associated *trans* fats with several disease states, and more may follow. Disorders linked to dietary *trans* fat include

(1) Atherosclerosis, including coronary heart disease and stroke.
(2) Fetal and infant developmental disorders and delayed development.
(3) Diabetic control difficulties have been linked to *trans* fats.
(4) Breast cancer and colon cancer have been linked to *trans* fat.

In summary **_cholesterol_** is a natural and necessary substance in the body. Hypercholesterolemia is indeed a sign of atherosclerosis, but one must look beyond the amount of cholesterol consumed in the diet to find the culprit responsible for hypercholesterolemia. Cholesterol becomes a problem in individuals who have other risk factors such as smoking, diabetes, hypertension, obesity and a sedentary life style.

On the other hand **_trans fats_** are unnatural molecules that have been injected into our food supply. The addition of *trans* fats has been associated with coronary heart disease and other disorders, and the future may prove they are toxic in other ways as well.

Unsaturated Fatty Acids

Three polyunsaturated fatty acids are traditionally regarded as "essential." They are **_arachidonic acid, linoleic acid and linolenic acid_**. Arachidonic acid and linoleic acid are **_omega-6_** fatty acids, and linolenic acid is an **_omega-3_** fatty acid. Two additional omega-3 fatty acids are essential to human physiology -- **_eicosapentaenoic acid (EPA) and docosahexaenoic acid (DHA)._** EPA and DHA can be synthesized from linolenic acid, but that conversion is inefficient, so EPA and DHA should be in the diet.

The carbon atoms in a fatty acid are numbered by chemists beginning at the carboxyl (acidic) end of the molecule. The last carbon atom of the chain is called the "omega" carbon. Physiologists name fatty acids according to the location of carbon double bonds (C=C), beginning with the omega carbon. The omega-3 fatty acids have a C=C bond between the omega-3 and omega-4 carbon. The omega-6 fatty acids have a C=C bond between the omega-6 and the omega-7 carbon.
All of the essential fatty acids have 3, 5, or 6 double carbon bonds, and all have 18, 20 or 22 carbon atoms. All essential fatty acids have the **_cis_** configuration.

The **_omega-6 fatty acids_** are parent compounds to substances that **_promote inflammation and blood clotting_**. These compounds include **_prostaglandins and eicosenoids_** (leukotrienes, thromboxanes and prostacyclins). Omega-6 and omega-3 fatty acids compete for the same enzymes. For that reason **_omega-3 fatty acids will decrease immunity and the inflammatory response._** **_They will also decrease the ability of the blood to clot._** The desired ratio of ometa-6 to omega-3 fatty acids in the diet is about 3:2. The average American diet has a ratio of 10-30 omega-6 fatty acids to one omega-3 fatty acid.

Many scientific articles have recently been published that tout benefits of increasing the amount of omega-3 fatty acids in the diet. When omega-3 fatty acids are added to the diet, they have been found to lower cholesterol levels, lower triglyceride levels, lower blood pressure, raise HDL levels, and improve coronary heart disease. Omega-3 fatty acids have also been found to have a stabilizing effect on the cardiac rhythm in arrhythmic states.

Beta amyloid and tau protein are two substances that are deposited in the brain in dementia. The accumulation of these compounds is reduced when DHA is given. **_DHA and EPA have been found to improve memory and learning capacity_**. Preliminary studies also show beneficial effects from DHA and EPA in autism, hyperactivity, schizophrenia, bipolar disorders, burns, eating disorders, asthma, macular degeneration, Crohn's disease and ulcerative colitis.

High levels of omega-3 fatty acids may produce deleterious effects including a reduced immune response, a decreased ability for the blood to clot and an increased tendency to hemorrhage.

Studies of the effects of omega-3 fatty acids on the brain suggest that DHA improves the structure of the myelin sheath and the neurons, and EPA improves neuronal function. Eight percent of the weight of the human brain is omega-3 fatty acids.

Omega-3 and omega-6 fatty acids are polyunsaturated fatty acids found in many plant foods. They are present in lesser amounts in most meats. The source for supplemental omega-3 fatty acids is generally ***fish oil***. Fatty ocean fish like mackerel and salmon are good sources for omega-3 fatty acids. Fish do not synthesize omega-3 fatty acids; they get them from algae in their diet.

Unsaturated fats are especially vulnerable to ***rancidity.*** Fats become rancid when they undergo hydrolysis and oxidation. ***Hydrolysis*** splits triglycerides into free fatty acids and glycerol. ***Oxidation*** is more complex; it involves the addition of oxygen to carbon atoms with double bonds. This produces ***hydroperoxides and free radicals***, both of which are highly reactive classes of compounds. These chemicals destroy nutrients, and they produce the noxious odors and tastes that occur with rancidity.

Antioxidants retard the rancidification process, and they are often added to foods that contain lipids. Lipid soluble anti-oxidants include vitamin E (tocopherols) and several synthetic compounds including BHA (butylated hydroxyanisole), BHT (butylated hydroxytoluene) and ethoxyquin (propyl gallate). Rancidity is promoted by exposure to oxygen, heat, light, metals, salt, water, bacteria and molds. Snack foods such as potato chips are often packaged in nitrogen-filled bags to reduce oxidation and protect the chips from compression.

Alcohol Compounds

Several alcohol compounds are in common usage today. Ethyl alcohol, methyl alcohol and isopropyl alcohol are toxic to humans, and their metabolism produces even more toxic compounds. Alcohols are soluble in water and in lipids; they are rapidly absorbed when ingested, and they easily penetrate the blood-brain barrier. After ingestion, 20% of ethyl alcohol is absorbed in the stomach and 80% in the upper intestines. Alcohols are oxidized in the liver by the enzyme alcohol dehydrogenase.

Ethyl alcohol

Ethyl alcohol (ethanol or grain alcohol) is an addictive ingredient in the diet of many people; it is the cause of alcoholism. Ethyl alcohol is oxidized to acetaldehyde in the liver. Acetaldehyde is further oxidized to acetic acid, which enters the Krebs cycle as acetyl CoA. Thus, ethyl alcohol is a source of calories and ATP. If the intake of ethanol is excessive, acetaldehyde accumulates to toxic levels, causing inflammation, injury and death to hepatic cells. Acetaldehyde also produces inflammation in the pancreas, which can lead to pancreatitis.

```
    H  H        alcohol dehydrogenase      H  H                        H   OH
    HC--C-OH  ------------------------>  HC-C=O  ------------------>  HC---C=O
    H  H                                    H                           H
    Ethyl alcohol                        Acetaldehyde                 Acetic Acid
```

In chronic alcoholism fat catabolism is largely replaced by ethanol. Fat builds up in liver cells, creating what is called a "fatty liver." The destruction of liver cells by acetaldehyde leads to fibrosis (scarring). The liver attempts to regenerate, which produces the nodular, scarred characteristics of cirrhosis.

Ethanol and its metabolites cause neurons to leak potassium. As a result neurons become hyperpolarized and unresponsive. A blood alcohol level above 400 mg/100cc is often fatal.

Other side effects of ethanol abuse include GI bleeding, delayed clotting, and malnutrition. A thiamine deficiency (vitamin B1) is especially common in alcoholics.

Alcoholics often suffer neurological symptoms when alcohol is withdrawn. They may go into ***delirium tremens (DTs)*** with mental confusion, irritability, tremors, hallucinations and convulsions (seizures). The life span of the alcoholic averages twenty-six years less than the nonalcoholic.

Antabuse (disulfiram) is a drug used to treat alcoholics. Antabuse inhibits enzymes that break down acetaldehyde. Following ethanol ingestion, the individual taking Antabuse rapidly accumulates acetaldehyde, which leads to vomiting, headache, chest pain and tachycardia. These unpleasant symptoms dissuade the alcohol abuser from future ethanol ingestion.

The costs and effects of alcohol upon society are overwhelming. Alcoholism, drunkenness and accidents caused by alcohol are responsible for hundreds of thousands of deaths annually in the United States. The cost that the country pays for alcohol abuse runs into the hundreds of billions of dollars. Ten percent of all Americans have an alcohol problem, and twenty-five percent of all hospitalized patients require treatment for an alcohol induced medical condition. Ethyl alcohol is implicated in 50% of all major trauma cases, 50% of all homicides and 40% of all assaults. Forty to fifty percent of all incarcerated prisoners who have committed violent crimes were under the influence of ethyl alcohol when the crime was committed.

One must ask why people become alcoholics. A genetic component appears to be undeniable. Alcohol has the ability to create a euphoric effect in some people but not others, and this may be a trigger for alcoholism. Alcoholism runs in families who have been found to have a gene variant on the short arm of chromosome #11. A variant on chromosome #4 has also been implicated to a preference for drinking ethyl alcohol. Alcoholism is world wide, but some racial groups and professions are especially susceptible. American Indians, the Keltic Irish, the legal profession, house painters and the male sex have above average levels of alcoholism. Orientals are the least susceptible. Alcoholic American Indians have a high incidence of the variant gene on chromosome #11. Orientals have a tendency to develop unpleasant flushing when they imbibe. Although female alcoholism is less prevalent than male alcoholism, female alcoholism runs a more fulminate course. Female alcoholics develop cirrhosis more commonly and at a younger age, and they die eleven years earlier than their male counterparts.

Two categories of alcoholics are appreciated; they are designated type 1 and type 2. Type 1 alcoholics develop the disease later in life, and there is a greater psychological dependent component present in these people. Type 2 alcoholics are described as thrill seekers. They develop alcoholism at a younger age, and they are more likely to have a genetic component to their disease.

The genetics of alcoholism have been linked to genes on chromosomes #11 and #4. These genes code for enzymes that lead to the synthesis of dopamine, serotonin and receptors for GABA and dopamine. In addition the gene for alcohol dehydrogenase is on the short arm of chromosome 11.

Methyl alcohol

Methyl alcohol (methanol or wood alcohol) is a common industrial byproduct. At one time methanol toxicity was produced by breathing vapor in poorly ventilated factories. Now nearly all methanol toxicity is produced by the unwitting ingestion of methanol.

$$\begin{array}{ccc} \text{H} & & \text{H} & & \text{OH} \\ \text{HC-OH} \xrightarrow{\text{alcohol dehydrogenase}} & \text{HC=O} \longrightarrow & \text{HC=O} \\ \text{H} & & & \\ \text{Methanol} & & \text{Formaldehyde} & & \text{Formic acid} \end{array}$$

Alcohol dehydrogenase converts methanol to formaldehyde, and formaldehyde is further oxidized to formic acid. Due to the highly toxic nature of these metabolites, the ingestion of as little as 20 ml of methanol can be fatal. Methanol toxicity is manifest by extreme acidosis, nausea, vomiting and neurological symptoms. Permanent blindness is a common finding in survivors of methanol poisoning.

Isopropyl alcohol

Isopropyl alcohol (isopropanol) is also known as "rubbing alcohol." It is a constituent of antiseptic solutions, and it may be added to ethyl alcohol to make "denatured alcohol." Isopropyl alcohol produces none of the euphoric effects attributed to ethyl alcohol, but isopropyl alcohol does affect the central nervous system. Isopropyl alcohol is approximately twice as toxic as ethanol. The ingestion of isopropyl alcohol can produce a coma that lasts up to fourteen hours. After awakening, the patient typically has no sequelae if vomiting and aspiration have not occurred.

$$\underset{\text{Isopropyl alcohol}}{HC\underset{H}{\overset{H}{—}}C\underset{H}{\overset{OH}{—}}CH\underset{H}{\overset{H}{}}} \xrightarrow{\text{alcohol dehydrogenase}} \underset{\text{Acetone}}{HC\underset{H}{\overset{H}{—}}C\overset{\overset{O}{\|}}{}CH\underset{H}{\overset{H}{}}}$$

Isopropyl alcohol is oxidized to acetone in the liver. Acetone can be detected in the urine and on the breath following the ingestion of isopropyl alcohol.

The Carbon Cycle

Organic molecules are the molecules of life; they are synthesized by living things. They are complex molecules that are chains and rings of carbon. **_Chlorophyll_** is the substance in green plants and algae that catalyzes the conversion of carbon dioxide in the atmosphere into organic compounds. Oxygen is released into the atmosphere as a byproduct of this reaction. The energy for the conversion of CO_2 to complex organic molecules comes from sunlight. The process is termed **_photosynthesis,_** and photosynthesis is the basis for all life on Earth. The complex carbon molecules synthesized by green plants undergo decay by microorganisms when the plants and animals die. If the plant is eaten by an animal, the organic molecules can be utilized by the animal, or oxygen can be utilized in the breakdown of the organic molecules to produce energy. The breakdown of plants produces carbon dioxide (CO_2), water, nitrates and other waste products. The carbon dioxide enters the atmosphere; it is taken up by plants and recycled into organic molecules. Oxygen is given off in the process. The carbon in living things is but a small percentage of the total carbon on Earth. Most of the Earth's carbon is in the form of carbonates in rock or dissolved in the oceans. Shell fish convert oceanic carbon dioxide to carbonates. When shellfish die, their skeletons eventually settle of the ocean floor and become buried as a layer of carbonate rock. The reserves of oil, coal and other fossil fuels contain organic carbon that has not been broken down completely by microorganisms. Vulcanism releases a great deal of carbon dioxide into the atmosphere. Diamonds and graphite are pure carbon.

The Nitrogen Cycle

Nineteenth century German chemists discovered that nitrogen compounds such as nitrates and ammonia acted as fertilizers for crops. Nitrates and ammonia are not organic compounds. Later in that century, Sir Alfred Howard, an Englishman, was living in India when he noted that native farmers fertilized their fields with residue from previous crops. Howard knew that this residue consisted of organic molecules that were based on carbon.. His work in the field established the concept of organic farming.

Nitrogen is a necessary element for life. The atmosphere is 78.1% nitrogen, but atmospheric nitrogen exists as the dimer, N_2, and nitrogen cannot be utilized by green plants in that form. Nitrogen must first be **_"fixed,"_** meaning that the N-N bond must be broken and the nitrogen atoms must be linked to oxygen, eventually forming **_nitrates (NO3-)._** Nitrogen fixing is accomplished by certain bacteria in the soil and by the effects of lightning in the atmosphere.

Plants utilize nitrates to add nitrogen to carbon compounds forming amino acids and other nitrogen-containing organic molecules. Animals and soil microorganisms utilize or catabolize these compounds, and they give off ammonia (NH_3), urea, uric acid and other nitrogen compounds. Animals convert most of the ammonia to urea [$CO(NH2)2$] prior to excretion. The ammonia and other nitrogen compounds produced by decay and by animal excretion are oxidized to nitrates, which are recycled by plants into amino acids and other complex nitrogen-containing organic compounds.

Study Guide

1. Name three coenzymes that are classified as vitamins.
2. What is a mineral?
3. How does pectin lower the cholesterol level in the blood?
4. What is a vitamin?
5. Be familiar with vitamins A, C, D, E and K.
6. Be familiar with the B complex of vitamins.
7. Recognize the elements that are used in human metabolism.
8. Know how the ingestion of fiber is beneficial.
9. What is a *trans* fat?
10. Where is cholesterol used in the body?
11. What are the omega-3 fatty acids?
12. What are the omega-6 fatty acids?
13. What is rancidity, and which foods are most susceptible to becoming rancid?
14. Describe some of the effects of ethanol, methanol and isopropyl alcohol on the body.
15. Appreciate some of the causes and social costs of alcoholism.
16. Outline the carbon cycle.
17. Outline the nitrogen cycle.

Chapter Twenty-seven

The Respiratory System

**Respiration** refers to the utilization of oxygen by living beings to produce energy, carbon dioxide and water. We have previously discussed cellular respiration, wherein mitochondria utilize oxygen in the production of ATP (energy), carbon dioxide and water. Respiration for the whole organism refers to the inhalation of air and the exchange of gases (oxygen and carbon dioxide) across the thin membranes of the alveoli of the lungs.

The Atmosphere

Today the earth's atmosphere is composed almost entirely of nitrogen and oxygen. Dry air contains about 78.1% nitrogen and about 20.9% oxygen, but that has not always been true. The earth is about four and one half billion years old, but it is only in the last 500 million years that oxygen became abundant in the air. Before then, the atmosphere consisted largely of nitrogen, carbon dioxide, carbon monoxide and methane. The explosion of chlorophyll-containing plant life beginning about 500 million years ago reformed the atmosphere so that it contained an abundant amount of oxygen. The presence of oxygen in the atmosphere allowed large animals to develop, because then the mitochondria in animal cells could effectively produce energy in the form of ATP.

The function of the lungs is to allow the _**diffusion of oxygen**_ into the blood and _**carbon dioxide**_ out of the blood. Dry air in Earth's atmosphere is made up of _**78.084% nitrogen**_ and _**20.946% oxygen**_. The other 1% is made up primarily of argon, which constitutes 0.934% of the dry atmosphere. _**Carbon dioxide constitutes only 0.038%**_ of dry air. Inspired dry air, therefore, contains 78.084% nitrogen, 20.946% oxygen and only 0.038% carbon dioxide. These are percentages for dry air. Water vapor is present and normally constitutes 1-4% of the total volume of air.

Carbon dioxide is constantly being added to the atmosphere by animals, which metabolize carbohydrates, fats and proteins to produce energy, carbon dioxide and water. Carbon dioxide is also produced by the burning of fossil fuels and by decay and decomposition of plants and animals by microorganisms.

Despite the constant addition of CO_2, the volume of carbon dioxide in the atmosphere remains quite low as a percentage of the atmosphere. The reason for that is that CO_2 is effectively being removed from the atmosphere in two ways. First, _**green plants avidly take up carbon dioxide**_ and use it in the synthesis of carbohydrates, fats, proteins and other organic molecules. It has been shown that green plants grow faster when the amount of carbon dioxide in the air is increased.

Second, gases are soluble in water. Fish have no difficulty absorbing dissolved oxygen in adequate amounts through their gills, and carbon dioxide is _**twenty times more soluble**_ in water than is oxygen. The high solubility of CO_2 in water allows the _**oceans to absorb large quantities**_ of the gas. The solubility of carbon dioxide is also the reason carbon dioxide is the gas chosen by soft drink bottlers to give "fizz" to their drinks. The high solubility of CO_2 in water allows plasma to carry the dissolved gas. Inspired air contains only 0.038% CO_2, and so CO_2 readily diffuses down its concentration gradient from plasma to air in the alveoli of the lungs.

Third, the weathering of rocks removes carbon dioxide from the atmosphere. When rain falls, it picks up carbon dioxide from the atmosphere. CO_2 reacts with rainwater to form carbonic acid. Carbonic acid dissolves rock, producing bicarbonate and calcium and other cations that are washed into the ocean. Plankton in the ocean utilize the calcium and bicarbonate to make their shells of calcium carbonate, After the plankton die, their shells fall to the bottom of the sea where they become a stable layer of calcium carbonate (limestone).

There is considerable concern today that atmospheric carbon dioxide is influencing the earth's climate. Carbon dioxide in the atmosphere reflects infrared rays back to Earth, not allowing them to escape into space. This warms the earth, and the earth's temperature is rising. Studies have shown that the level of atmospheric carbon dioxide has doubled in the past 160,000 years. In more recent times the concentration of atmospheric carbon dioxide has increased from 0.03158% in 1959 to 0.0385% today. Carbon dioxide is soluble in water, and today's oceans are showing changes resulting from an increased concentration of carbon dioxide. Carbon dioxide in water exists primarily as carbonic acid and bicarbonate, and the pH of ocean water has decreased by 0.1 units in the past two hundred years. Today the oceans contain about 120 mg/l of dissolved carbon dioxide; however, the solubility of carbon dioxide is 1.45 grams per liter of water, so considerably more carbon dioxide could be taken up by the oceans.

Expired air contains less oxygen and more CO_2 than inspired air. The amounts of these gases in expired air are not constant; they depend on physical activity and the health of the respiratory, circulatory and urinary systems. The oxygen level in expired air is usually about 13.7%, and the CO_2 level averages about 5.3%. Hemoglobin greatly aids oxygen solubility in the blood. Carbon dioxide binds to hemoglobin, but most carbon dioxide in the blood is dissolved in the plasma as carbonic acid or bicarbonate. Carbon dioxide in the blood lowers the pH because of the reaction,

$$CO_2 + H_2O \longleftrightarrow H_2CO_3 \longleftrightarrow H^+ + HCO_3^-.$$

Healthy lungs are necessary to keep the tissues supplied with oxygen and rid the body of the acidity produced by CO_2.

Parts of the Respiratory System

The respiratory system consists of the upper respiratory tract (the nose, pharynx and upper wind pipe), and the lower respiratory tract (the lower air channels and the alveoli of the lungs).

Air enters the **_nose_** where it is **_warmed and humidified_** by the mucosa of the **_turbinates_**. The superior, middle and inferior turbinates increase the surface area of the nasal passages, which aids in warming and humidifying the incoming air. The mucosa of the respiratory tract (including the nose and sinuses) contains goblet cells, which secrete mucus. Mucus collects bacteria and debris, and cilia move the mucus toward the mouth where it is expectorated (spit out) or swallowed.

The inferior turbinates have an extensive venous plexus. Every thirty to sixty minutes the veins of alternate sides of the nose dilate, which swells the mucosa. The swelling restricts the passage of air through that side of the nose, and it replenishes moisture to that side. The mouths of the naso-lacrimal ducts are under the inferior turbinates; they help to moisten the nasal mucosa with tears. Nosebleeds **_(epistaxis)_** are common because of the extensive vascularity of the nose.

The **_pharynx_** is the passageway from the back of the nose to the larynx (voice box). The pharynx is divided into an upper nasopharynx, a central oropharynx and a lower laryngopharynx. The **_nasopharynx_** is the area at the rear of the nose and above the soft palate. It contains the **_adenoids_** (pharyngeal tonsils), which are nodules of lymphatic tissue. The **_Eustachian tubes_** (auditory tubes) open into the nasopharynx and connect the middle ears with the nasopharynx. The **_internal nares_** are the openings into the nose from the nasopharynx. The **_external nares_** are the nostrils.

The **_oropharynx_** is the area at the back of the mouth. The **_palatine tonsils_** are lymph nodules on the lateral walls of the oropharynx. There are also lymph nodules at the base of the tongue, which are **_lingual tonsils_**. The three pairs of tonsils (pharyngeal, palatine and lingual) form a ring of lymphatic tissue around the pharynx. This lymphatic tissue serves to destroy pathogens that penetrate the mucosa. Below the oropharynx is the laryngopharynx, which extends inferiorly to the junction of the windpipe and the esophagus. The pharynx is encircled by striated muscles, which constrict with swallowing and prevent material from entering the nose or the larynx.

The **_larynx_** contains the vocal cords. Vocal sounds are produced by constriction of the cords during exhalation. The upper entrance to the larynx is protected by the epiglottis, which folds over the larynx during swallowing, thereby directing material into the esophagus. Food and drink are also prevented from entering the larynx by vestibular folds in the larynx. During swallowing the following muscular actions direct food and drink into the esophagus and away from the larynx: **(1)** the soft palate elevates, **(2)** the oropharynx and laryngopharynx constrict, **(3)** the larynx is elevated, and **(4)** the epiglottis folds over the larynx.

The larynx occupies a higher position in infant throats; this positioning allows the epiglottis to touch the soft palate, which creates an airway from the nasopharynx to the larynx. The epiglottis reflects milk away from the air stream, which allows an infant to breathe continuously while feeding.

The **_larynx is a cartilaginous case_** consisting mostly of hyaline cartilage; it is significantly larger in adult males than it is in females or preadolescent males. The thyroid cartilage of the larynx is palpable in the neck; it is the largest of nine separate pieces of cartilage in the larynx. The cricoid cartilage is a ring of cartilage in the inferior larynx that connects the larynx to the trachea. The epiglottic cartilage supports the epiglottis; it is the only elastic cartilage in the larynx; the other cartilaginous tissues of the larynx are hyaline cartilage. Three pairs of small cartilages support the vocal cords; they are the arytenoids, the corniculate and the cuneiform cartilages. The intrinsic muscles of the larynx are supplied by the vagus nerves. They rotate the arytenoid, corniculate and cuneiform cartilages and allow for the utterance of different pitched sounds. The extrinsic muscles of the larynx connect the larynx to the hyoid bone, and they elevate the larynx during swallowing.

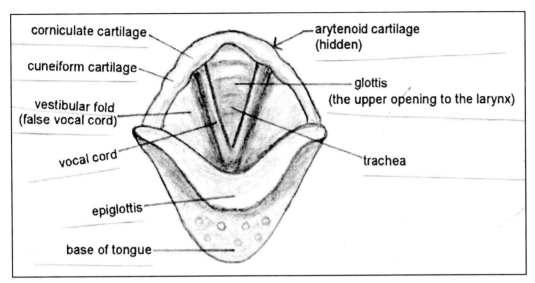

Above: A laryngoscopic view of the vocal cords. This is what every anesthetist hopes to see. The epiglottis and the base of the tongue are at the bottom in this drawing. Cartilaginous rings in the trachea can be seen through the vocal cords.

Inflammation of the larynx is **_laryngitis_**. Laryngitis leads to hoarseness, but it is usually not a serious disorder. However, the epiglottis of young children is subject to an infection by *Hemophilus* bacteria that can lead to marked swelling of the epiglottis and suffocation. Epiglottitis, laryngeal trauma and other causes of upper airway obstruction may require a tracheostomy, which is an incision into the trachea with placement of a breathing tube into the airway below the site of the obstruction.

The muscular actions of the larynx and pharynx are not always successful in keeping food and drink out of the larynx and trachea. When a solid or liquid enters the airway, it is known as **_aspiration._** The trachea may become blocked, and a person can neither breathe nor speak following aspiration of an object of significant size or liquid of a significant quantity. The **_Heimlich maneuver_** may be successful in forcing the object out of the airway and saving a life. In this maneuver the abdomen is compressed forcefully and quickly with the patient bent forward. The diaphragm is forced upward, which creates a pressurized exhalation. When the Heimlich maneuver is successful, the object is dislodged and forced up and out of the airway.

The **_trachea_** is a tube about four to five inches long that leads from the larynx to the right and left mainstem bronchi. The walls of the trachea and major bronchi contain **_cartilaginous rings_** that are shaped like the letter "C" and are incomplete dorsally. These incomplete rings keep the trachea and major bronchi from collapsing. The gaps in the rings allow for expansion of the esophagus and compression of the bronchi during swallowing.

The trachea divides into a right and a left **_mainstem (primary) bronchus_**. The primary bronchi further divide into **_secondary (lobar) bronchi_** that lead to each lobe of the lungs. The right lung has three lobes (upper, middle and lower). The left lung has two lobes (upper and lower). The heart is tilted to the left, and it occupies more space on the left side of the thorax than on the right side. This allows less space for the left lung than the right; consequently the left lung is the smaller of the two lungs. The counterpart to the right middle lobe is the lingula of the left lung, whose bronchus is a branch of the upper lobar bronchus.

Bronchi further divide into short **_tertiary bronchi_**, which then divide into **_bronchioles_**. The walls of bronchioles do not contain cartilage, and when the bronchiolar smooth muscle constricts, the lumen may close almost completely. This condition is called **_bronchospasm._** One common cause of bronchospasm is asthma.

The smallest branches of the bronchioles terminate in tiny air sacs called **_alveoli_**. Gaseous exchange occurs in the alveoli.

The **_lungs_** are located in the chest cavity separated by the **_mediastinum_**, which contains the heart.   They are protected by the ribcage. The base of each lung rests on the diaphragm, whose contractions produce inspiration (inhalation) by increasing the size of the chest cavity. The **_hilum_** of a lung is an indented area on the medial side of each lung where the primary bronchi, pulmonary veins and pulmonary artery enter.

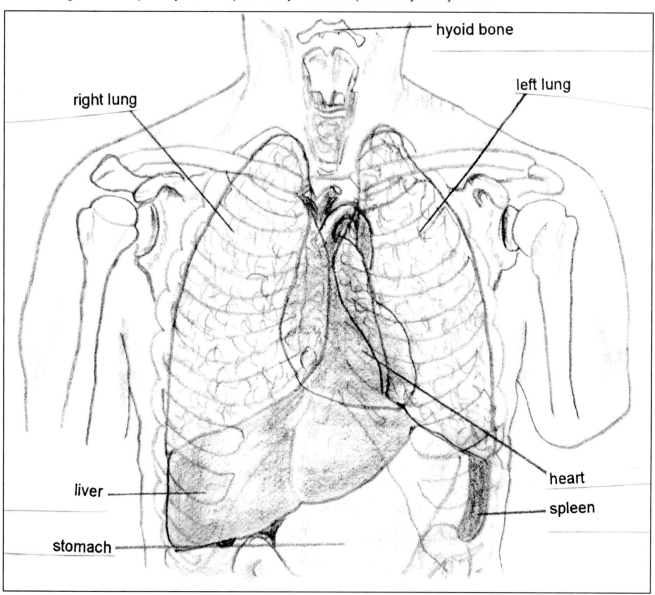

Above: The lungs are situated in the chest cavity. The space between the lungs is the mediastinum.   The lungs are surrounded by visceral pleura, and the chest cavity is lined by parietal pleura. The pleural cavity is the potential space between the visceral pleura and the parietal pleura. A penetrating chest injury or a ruptured alveolus can allow air to enter the pleural cavity, creating a pneumothorax.

The **_pleurae_** are thin connective tissue membranes. The parietal pleura lines the chest wall; the visceral pleura lines the surface of the lungs. The space between the parietal and the visceral pleura is called the pleural cavity. Normally this space is occupied only by a thin film of serous fluid, which serves to prevent friction. During inspiration the atmospheric pressure is greater than the pressure in the pleural cavity. External air can be sucked into the pleural cavity through a penetrating chest wound or a ruptured alveolus. In these situations air can gradually fill the pleural cavity and collapse the lung. Air in the pleural cavity is a **_pneumothorax._** A spontaneous pneumothorax can result from the rupture of an alveolus into the pleural cavity. The treatment of a pneumothorax requires placement of a tube into the pleural cavity, the opposite end of which is placed under water. The natural elasticity of the lungs increases the pressure in the chest cavity during expiration, and a chest tube can slowly remove air during expirations. Air cannot enter the pleural cavity through the tube because its opposite end is submerged.

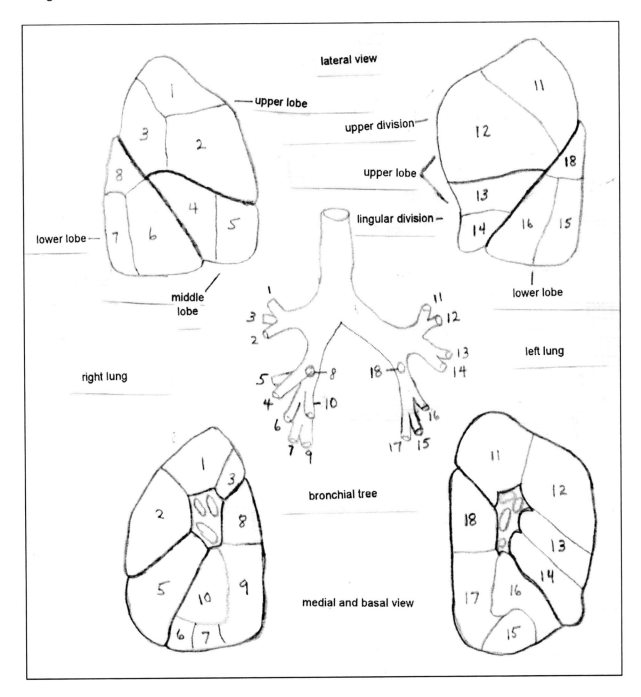

Above: The bronchial tree, showing the lobes and segments (lobules) of the lungs. The right lung has three lobes, an upper, middle and a lower lobe. The left lung has only two lobes, an upper and a lower. The lingula is a division of the left upper lobe that is the counterpart of the middle lobe of the right lung. The numbers of the segments match the numbers of the bronchial branches. Lobar pneumonia fills an entire lobe with infectious fluid (exudate). It was a common cause of death in years past. The causative agent is the pneumococcus.

Right: A histologic section of the lung. The spaces are air-filled alveoli.

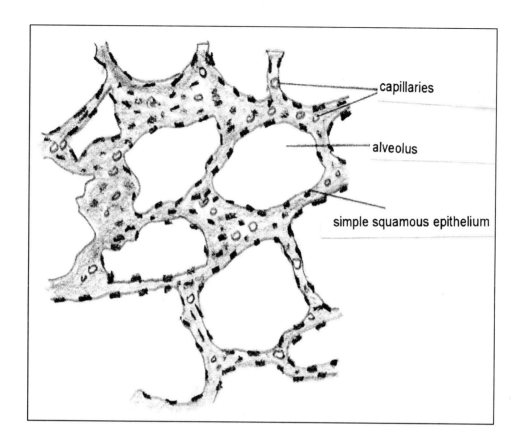

capillaries

alveolus

simple squamous epithelium

Alveoli are lined by a thin layer of ***simple squamous epithelium***. Capillaries fill the spaces between alveoli. Oxygen and carbon dioxide diffuse through the epithelium of the alveoli and the endothelium of the capillaries. Some alveolar cells secrete a lipoprotein with surfactant properties that act like a soap or detergent to decrease the surface tension. The surfactant keeps the alveolar membranes from sticking together, which would close their air sacs. Premature infants often have a deficiency of pulmonary surfactant, which can result in respiratory distress due to collapsed alveoli. The administration of oxygen may not be adequate therapy for these infants; the administration of a surfactant may be necessary.

Aspects of Pulmonary Function

Ventilation is the term for the movement of air in and out of the alveoli. Ventilation involves ***both inhalation (inspiration) and exhalation (expiration).*** The pressure of the atmosphere, the pressure within the pleural cavity and the pressure within the alveoli and bronchial tree are all instrumental in ventilation. Inhalation is produced by contraction of the diaphragm; it is aided by the contraction of the external intercostal muscles, which pull the ribcage upward and outward. The diaphragm and external intercostal muscles relax during exhalation. Contraction of the internal intercostal muscles assists in forced exhalation by pulling the ribs down and inward, which reduces the size of the chest cavity. The abdominal muscles can also help with forced expiration by pushing the relaxed diaphragm upward and decreasing the volume of the chest cavity. Very little or no muscular work is normally required for exhalation because the lungs contain a considerable amount of elastic tissue, which compresses the lungs and produces exhalation.

Contraction of the diaphragm and external intercostal muscles expands the chest cavity, which expands the pleural cavity and, therefore, the lungs as well. With expansion of the lungs the pressure in the alveoli and bronchial tree decreases. Air enters the nose and respiratory passages to equalize this pressure. This fills the alveoli with air.

In exhalation (expiration) the volume of the chest cavity shrinks, which increases the pressure in the pleural cavity and in the lungs; this forces air from the alveoli out the trachea to the nose and mouth. The elasticity of the lungs makes them partially collapse with exhalation. In emphysema the normal elasticity of the lungs is lost, which makes expiration difficult. Muscular contraction by the internal intercostal muscles and the abdominal muscles may become required in order to reduce the volume of the chest and exhale.

A *spirometer* is an instrument used to measure the amount of air that an individual can inhale and exhale. This instrument is used in *pulmonary function tests*. When being tested with a spirometer, the individual breathes into a tube, and the amount of exhaled air is measured in a canister.

The *tidal volume* is that amount of air that moves in and out of the respiratory system during one average inhalation and exhalation cycle. Shallow breathing results in a low tidal volume; deep breathing results in a high tidal volume. The average tidal volume is 500 cc.

The *vital capacity* is the amount of air in a maximum exhalation that follows the deepest possible inhalation. The average is 3500-5000 cc. To produce the maximum inhalation, accessory respiratory muscles are brought into action to assist the diaphragm and the external intercostal muscles. The accessory muscles of respiration include the sternocleidomastoid, serratus anterior, pectoralis minor, and the scalenes. These muscles serve to elevate and expand the chest and enlarge the chest cavity.

The *inspiratory reserve* is the maximum amount of air that can be taken in minus the tidal volume. The average is 2000-3000 cc.

The *expiratory reserve* is the maximum amount of air that can be exhaled after a normal inhalation minus the tidal volume. The average is 1000-1500 cc. The abdominal muscles (rectus abdominis, internal and external obliques and the transversus abdominis) are brought into play to assist the internal intercostal muscles during forced expiration.

The *minute respiratory volume* is the amount of air normally moved in and out of the lungs in one minute. It is the same as the tidal volume multiplied by the number of respirations per minute.

Residual air is the amount of air remaining in the lungs following the most forceful exhalation. An average is 1000-1500 cc. Residual air in the alveoli allows gaseous exchange to continue between breaths.

Oxygen and carbon dioxide are the two most important gases that diffuse across the alveolar membrane. *Nitrogen* (N2) is the most abundant gas in the atmosphere, and nitrogen gas is dissolved in the blood stream, but dissolved nitrogen gas in the blood is normally in balance with nitrogen in the atmosphere, and nitrogen does not usually play a physiologic or pathologic (disease causing) role. An exception is in *deep sea diving*, where the air breathed is under greater pressure, forcing more nitrogen to be dissolved into the blood. If the pressure of the air breathed is suddenly reduced, as may occur during ascent, the pressure of dissolved nitrogen in the blood can greatly exceed the pressure of nitrogen in atmosphere. This can cause bubbles of nitrogen in the blood to come out of solution. This condition is known as *decompression sickness*, and it results in painful joints, which causes the victim to curl up, hence the common name, *"the bends."* Nitrogen bubbles in the blood of those with decompression sickness can cause emboli, which can be fatal.

Gaseous *diffusion* involves the movement of molecules from an area of greater concentration to an area of lesser concentration. *Each gas moves according to its own pressure gradient*, which is called its *partial pressure* or "P". The atmospheric pressure at sea level is about 760 mmHg. That means that the pressure produced by the earth's atmosphere at sea level is capable of raising a column of mercury 760 mm. Air is about 21% oxygen, so the P of oxygen (PO_2) at sea level is 0.21 x 760, or 160 mmHg. An individual breathing air at sea level could not possibly raise his blood PO_2 above 160 mmHg. To do so would mean that oxygen would have to diffuse from an area of lesser to an area of greater concentration, and no gas or molecule in a liquid solution will do that.

The concentration of CO_2 in the air is only about 0.04%, so the PCO_2 in air is 0.0004 x 760, or 0.3 mmHg. This contrasts to an average PCO_2 level of about 40 mmHg in the pulmonary artery. Because there is so little CO_2 in the air relative to the amount of CO_2 in the body, carbon dioxide is always diffusing down gradient from the pulmonary capillaries to the alveolar air.

Several natural laws govern the diffusion of oxygen and carbon dioxide.

(1) **_Boyle's law_** states that the pressure exerted by a given quantity of gas decreases when the gas is allowed to expand and occupy a larger area. This law reflects the pressure changes that occur with expansion and contraction of the chest cavity.

(2) **_Charles' law_** states that the volume of a gas is directly proportional to its temperature. Air that enters the alveoli has been warmed to 98.6 degrees F (37 degrees C). This warmer air occupies more space and helps to expand the lungs.

(3) **_Henry's law_** states that the ability of a gas to dissolve in water depends on the water solubility constant of the gas and the partial pressure of that gas in the air above the water level. This law is significant when one considers that CO_2 is quite soluble in water and has a low partial pressure in the air. In contrast oxygen is plentiful in the air (has a high partial pressure), but its solubility in water is only one-twentieth that of CO_2, which is why hemoglobin is necessary for oxygen to be carried in the blood.

(4) **_Dalton's law_** states that the total pressure of a gas mixture (such as air) is equal to the sum of the partial pressures of all of the gases in the mixture. The total atmospheric pressure is, therefore, the total air pressure; however, it is the partial pressures of the individual gases that govern their diffusion.

Only 1.5% of the oxygen in the blood is dissolved in the plasma, and if oxygen transport depended solely on dissolved oxygen in the plasma, very little oxygen could reach the tissues, and one would die of hypoxia. **_98.5%_** of the oxygen in the blood is bound to **_hemoglobin_** in the erythrocytes, and hemoglobin is effectively responsible for oxygen transport. Each molecule of hemoglobin is capable of carrying up to four molecules of O2. Oxygen binds to the **_ferrous ion in the heme moiety_** of hemoglobin. The linkage between oxygen and heme is weak, and heme gives up oxygen and lets it diffuse into the tissues wherever the PO2 is low. Hemoglobin carrying oxygen is **_oxyhemoglobin_**. **_Deoxyhemoglobin_** is hemoglobin with no oxygen molecules attached. When each hemoglobin molecule has four oxygen molecules bound to it, it is said to be 100% saturated. The uptake of an oxygen molecule by hemoglobin is facilitated by the presence of other oxygen molecules attached to the heme moiety, as long as the heme is not saturated. The presence of one oxygen molecule changes the shape of the hemoglobin molecule in a way that makes it easier for the second, third and fourth oxygen molecule to bind.

Deoxyhemoglobin is a dark maroon-purple color, especially when carbon dioxide is bound to it (carbaminohemoglobin). That accounts for the blue skin hue (cyanosis) of patients with poorly oxygenated blood.

An arterial puncture is used to withdraw arterial blood for **_blood gas analyses_**, which are tests that measure the **_PO2, PCO2, and pH_** of arterial blood. These tests reflect the ability of the respiratory system to function and the efficacy of treatment. An arterial blood gas analysis includes a measurement of the amount of dissolved oxygen in the plasma of an artery (PaO2). This level is normally 70-100 mm of Hg (mercury). Oxygen that is dissolved in the plasma and oxygen that is bound to hemoglobin are measured separately. Breathing pure oxygen or being placed in a hyperbaric chamber will dramatically increase the amount of oxygen dissolved in the plasma, but it will normally have little or no effect on the level of oxygen bound to hemoglobin. That is because arterial hemoglobin should be already saturated with oxygen or nearly so. The amount of oxygen carried by hemoglobin is directly related to the amount of hemoglobin in the blood. Arterial hemoglobin that is less than 97% **_saturated_** (with oxygen) reflects deficient gaseous exchange in the alveoli or a right to left cardiac shunt.

Oxygen bound to hemoglobin and dissolved oxygen in the plasma are separate stores for oxygen, but oxygen molecules move freely between these stores. Alveolar oxygen enters the plasma as dissolved oxygen, which then becomes bound to hemoglobin in the RBCs. Oxyhemoglobin gives up oxygen, which then becomes dissolved oxygen in the plasma before leaving the capillaries and entering tissue cells. If the level of dissolved oxygen in the plasma is high, oxygen will move from the plasma into the red cells to bind with hemoglobin until the hemoglobin saturation approaches 100%.

Carbon monoxide (CO) is produced by the incomplete combustion of organic molecules in poorly ventilated areas where the oxygen content is low. Carbon monoxide competes with oxygen for the four binding sites on heme, and carbon monoxide binds **_250 times more tightly_** than oxygen. Hemoglobin is called **_carboxyhemoglobin_** if it has one or more molecules of carbon monoxide bound to it. When 50% of the hemoglobin has been converted to carboxyhemoglobin, even the administration of pure oxygen to the patient may not be effective in raising his arterial PO2 and saving his life. That is due to the propensity for carboxyhemoglobin to more tightly bind oxygen and not release it to the tissues. Oxygen administered in a hyperbaric chamber increases the amount of oxygen dissolved in the plasma, and it hastens the separation of carbon monoxide from hemoglobin. However, in the most severe cases, a complete exchange transfusion of erythrocytes may be necessary. It takes an atmospheric concentration of only 0.2% carbon monoxide to be quickly lethal, in which case most of the hemoglobin has been converted to carboxyhemoglobin and cannot deliver oxygen to the tissues. Lesser atmospheric concentrations of carbon monoxide may not be lethal, but they can result in brain damage due to a temporary lack of oxygen getting to the brain and direct toxic effects of carbon monoxide. The toxic effects of carbon monoxide include inhibition of enzymes on the mitochondrial membrane and oxidization, demyelination and inflammation of the brain. The globus pallidus (of the basal ganglia) is especially vulnerable to carbon monoxide. Methylene chloride is an industrial chemical that can cause carbon monoxide toxicity because it is partially metabolized to carbon monoxide in the liver.

Carbon dioxide is twenty times more soluble in water than is oxygen, and five percent of all carbon dioxide is transported in the plasma as a dissolved gas. Another five percent is bound to hemoglobin or plasma proteins. Hemoglobin containing bound carbon dioxide is called **carbaminohemoglobin**. Unlike carbon monoxide, carbon dioxide does not compete with oxygen when it binds to hemoglobin because the two gases bind to different sites on the hemoglobin molecule – the **oxygen to the heme** portion, and **carbon dioxide to the globin** (protein) portion. Hemoglobin can, therefore, transport both oxygen and carbon dioxide simultaneously. However, carbaminohemoglobin tends to off load oxygen (the Bohr effect), and oxyhemoglobin has less ability to bind CO_2 (the Haldane effect). **Ninety percent** of all carbon dioxide is transported in the blood as **carbonic acid** (H_2CO_3) or the **bicarbonate ion** (HCO_3-). Carbon dioxide reacts with a molecule of water to form carbonic acid. Carbonic acid is a weak acid and one of the major buffers in the blood. Some carbonic acid molecules dissociate into the bicarbonate ion and a hydrogen ion according to the following formula

$$CO_2 + H_2O \longleftrightarrow H_2CO_3 \longleftrightarrow HCO_3- + H+$$

This reaction is catalyzed by the enzyme, **carbonic anhydrase**. The amount of carbonic acid in the blood is proportional to the amount of carbon dioxide in the blood; thus **the pH of the blood reflects the amount of carbon dioxide in the blood.**

Respiration is controlled by input from the central nervous system. The **medulla** and the **pons** contain centers that **regulate inspiration and expiration**, and these centers alternate in activity. Sensory impulses to the respiratory centers determine the respiratory rate and the tidal volume. **Baroreceptors in the lungs** detect stretching (inhalation) and initiate exhalation by depressing the inspiration center. Inflation is detected by stretch receptors in the naturally elastic bronchial tree, which then initiates exhalation. This is called the **Hering-Breuer reflex**.

The respiration rate and the degree of inflation are generally controlled by the brain stem. The cerebral cortex can override the regulatory centers in the medulla and pons with voluntary breathing, but there are limits to this override. You can hold your breath until you turn blue and lose consciousness, but you will not die because the cerebrum relinquishes control in the unconscious state, and the brain stem will take over.

The **aortic bodies and the carotid bodies** are small vascular nodules located in the aortic arch and near the bifurcation of the carotid arteries. They contain **sensors** that respond to the blood **pH, PCO2, and PO2**. The **vagus** nerves carry signals from these sensors to the brain stem where they influence the respiratory rate and tidal volume. When either the pH falls, the PCO2 rises, or the PO2 falls, impulses from these sensors stimulate centers in the brain stem to increase ventilation. The normal blood pH is 7.4, and it is imperative that the pH does not vary much from that level. The **blood pH** is the most important parameter governing respiration.

Disorders of Pulmonary Function

Acidosis refers to too many hydrogen ions in solution and a low pH in the blood. Acidosis stimulates the brain stem to increase the respiratory rate and tidal volume. This leads to the loss of CO_2 and, therefore, a loss of carbonic acid (H_2CO_3), which leads to a correction in the pH. Acidosis may be due to a respiratory problem **(respiratory acidosis)** resulting in a high H_2CO_3 level because the lungs fail to remove CO_2 at the normal rate. Or acidosis may be of metabolic origin **(metabolic acidosis)**, which is characterized by a low CO_2 because the lungs are hyperventilating in an attempt to raise the pH of the blood by reducing the level of carbonic acid. Causes of metabolic acidosis include **(1)** untreated diabetes mellitus. These patients metabolize fatty acids and amino acids in great quantities because glucose cannot enter skeletal muscle cells without insulin, which is lacking in juvenile type diabetics. The skeletal muscle cells and the plasma become overwhelmed with acids and the products of fatty acid metabolism called **_ketone bodies_**, and the blood pH is lowered. **_Starvation_** also leads to **_ketoacidosis_** secondary to excessive fat catabolism. **(2)** Some patients with kidney disease will develop acidosis because the sodium pumps in their kidneys function poorly. Acidosis develops because sodium pumps also excrete hydrogen ions. **(3)** Patients with severe diarrhea may develop acidosis because they lose large amounts of sodium, and a deficiency of sodium impairs hydrogen ion excretion in the urine. **(4)** A build up of lactic acid can produce metabolic acidosis. Lactic acidosis occurs in hypoxia and from exposure to some toxins and drugs that inhibit aerobic respiration.

The ingestion of too many antacid medications can produce a **_metabolic alkalosis_**. Another cause of metabolic alkalosis is excessive vomiting, which removes the normal acidity of the stomach. In these situations the lungs have a limited ability to compensate by decreasing the respiratory rate because oxygen must continue to be supplied to the tissues by pulmonary ventilation. Patients with **_bulimia_** habitually vomit after eating, and these patients are subject to a metabolic alkalosis due to hydrogen ion loss. They also may develop hypokalemia and hyponatremia due to excessive potassium and sodium loss. Most bulimic deaths appear to be due to cardiac arrest associated with hypokalemia.

Patients with **_respiratory alkalosis_** have a high blood pH and a low pCO2. Respiratory alkalosis results from hyperventilation (breathing too deep and too fast). This is most often the result of hysteria, anxiety or emotional trauma. In these cases breathing air with a higher than normal pCO2 will increase the blood carbonic acid level and lower the pH. These patients are often told to breathe in and out of a paper bag.

The normal level of CO2 dissolved in arterial blood is 37-43 mmHg. A level below 37 mmHg is called **_hypocapnia_**, and a level above 43 mmHg is called **_hypercapnia_**. The blood levels of dissolved carbon dioxide, carbonic acid and bicarbonate are largely controlled by the lungs.

Hypercapnia can result from any pulmonary disorder that interferes with the removal of CO2. This is the situation in **_respiratory acidosis_**, and it is accompanied by hypoxia.

Hypocapnia results from hyperventilation, which may be an attempt by the lungs to correct a **_metabolic acidosis._** A metabolic acidosis results from an abnormally excessive production of acids; diabetic ketoacidosis is an example. The rapid and deep respiratory pattern of one suffering from metabolic acidosis is called **_Kussmaul_** respiration; it is an attempt to raise the pH of the blood by ridding the body of CO2.

A low blood oxygen level will affect the respiratory rate only when the arterial PO2 drops **_below 60 mmHg_**. (Remember that the atmosphere has a PO2 of 160 mmHg). This is called the **_hypoxic drive_**, and it is most commonly seen in mountain climbers above 10,000 feet who have a malady called **_altitude sickness or mountain sickness_**. Severe cases develop headache and disorientation. Fatal pulmonary edema and cerebral edema may follow.

Pneumonia is an inflammation involving at least part of a lung. Pneumonia is typically caused by pathogenic bacteria, viruses or fungi. In **_lobar pneumonia_** at least one lobe of a lung becomes filled with a purulent exudate (the thick yellow fluid commonly called pus, which contains pathogenic microorganisms and phagocytes). The alveoli of an affected lobe or lobes are filled with a purulent exudate and cannot function in gaseous exchange. Lobar pneumonia is usually caused by bacteria known as pneumococci (*Streptococcus pneumoniae*).
Bronchopneumonia is the term used for inflammation that is primarily in the bronchial tree. The etiology of bronchopneumonia is often viral.
Pneumonitis is a nonspecific term used for pulmonary (lung) inflammations with various etiologies including idiopathic (of unknown cause).

Tuberculosis has been a scourge of mankind for many centuries. A century ago it was one of the major causes of death in the United States. Tuberculosis attacks the lungs more than any other organ, but tuberculosis of the urinary tract and GI tract are not uncommon, and tuberculosis is also a cause of meningitis. Tuberculosis can spread from the lungs to the GI tract by habitually swallowing sputum rather than spitting it out. Tuberculosis is usually spread from person to person by airborne contact with the causative organism, *Mycobacterium tuberculae*. In tubercular lung infections an area becomes necrotic and can only heal by forming a fibrotic scar. Untreated tuberculosis can be chronic and progressive, but it often has periods of inactivity and recrudescence. People who are exposed to tuberculosis commonly develop an asymptomatic infection that is only detected at a later date by a positive skin test. Even these cases may develop an active infection after many years if resistance wanes and the bacillus has not been eradicated. A great step forward in the treatment of tuberculosis occurred in 1947 with the release of streptomycin, the first antibiotic effective against the tubercle bacillus. Unfortunately the tubercle bacillus has developed resistance to streptomycin as well as other antibiotics. In spite of bacterial resistance, control of tuberculosis was steadily improving in this country due to isolation of active cases and careful disposal of potentially infectious material. But the recent surge of uncontrolled immigration has seen many cases of active, untreated and contagious tuberculosis and other infectious diseases cross our borders, and the incidence of tuberculosis is now rising.

Leprosy is caused by a Mycobacterium of the same genus as tuberculosis (*Mycobacterium leprae*). Leprosy, like tuberculosis, tends to be chronic and progressive with periods of inactivity and recrudescence.

A *pulmonary embolus* is a solid object, a liquid bolus or a gaseous bubble that travels from the systemic venous circulation to the pulmonary artery. Emboli tend to occlude a branch of the pulmonary arterial tree. They can cause bleeding and infarction (tissue death due to lack of blood supply) in a section of a lung. A *thrombus* (blood clot) in a vein of a lower extremity is the most common source of a pulmonary embolus. Small emboli typically cause *atelectasis* (alveolar collapse), which may be permanent. A large embolus can block the right or left pulmonary artery, which would put great pressure on the right ventricle, and possibly cause it to go into failure.

Chronic obstructive pulmonary disease, or COPD, is obstruction of airflow due to pathologic changes in the lungs. One cause of COPD is allergic asthma, which involves constriction of the bronchioles secondary to the release of histamine. Frequent exposure to chemicals or irritants in the air can cause chronic bronchitis, which can lead to COPD. *Emphysema* is the loss of normal lung elasticity; it is the eventual and permanent result of chronic over-inflation of the lungs produced by chronic COPD. Emphysema is characterized by the gradual expansion of individual alveoli. Adjacent alveoli then merge to form large, poorly functional air spaces that are surrounded by fibrous tissue.

Cigarette smoking injects irritants and carcinogenic (carcinoma causing) chemicals into the lungs. Breathing second hand cigarette smoke also exposes one to these carcinogens. Cigarette smoking is the primary cause (but not the only cause) of *chronic bronchitis, emphysema and lung cancer*. Lung cancer is also linked to *radon* gas exposure. Radon is a radioactive product of uranium decay; it has been found in the air of uranium and cobalt mines, and it may be in the air of basements in areas where there is uranium in the soil. Neoplasms (cancers) that arise in the lungs are typically aggressive, and cures are uncommon; only seven percent will survive longer than five years after they are diagnosed. Most lung cancers arise in the large bronchi. Squamous cell carcinomas and adenocarcinomas are the most common cell types, and they are both related to cigarette smoking. The squamous cell type arises from basal cells of pseudostratified epithelium in the bronchi; the adenocarcinomas arise from glands in the lamina propria (submucosa) of the bronchi. Less common is the small cell or "oat cell" carcinoma, which is very aggressive and metastasizes quickly. Oat cell carcinomas are highly malignant, but they are probably not related to cigarette smoking. They are much less common than squamous cell carcinomas or adenocarcinomas of the lung. A mesothelioma is a tumor of the pleural mesothelium that is related to both cigarette smoking and asbestos exposure. More Americans die from lung cancer than from any other type of cancer, and the incidence of lung cancer has been doubling every fifteen years.

Bronchiectasis is a pathologic segmental dilation of the bronchioles. It is usually the result of chronic bronchitis in an individual with a genetic susceptibility to bronchiectasis. Frequent coughing causes intermittent excessive pressure inside the bronchioles, which gradually dilate. Cilia cannot remove mucus and bacteria effectively from the dilated bronchioles, and recurrent infections are common.

The primary and secondary bronchi can be visualized by placing an observation tube into the trachea of an anesthetized patient, and a biopsy can be taken through this tube. This is procedure is called *bronchoscopy;* it is often used to diagnose a bronchogenic carcinoma or a lung lesion of unknown etiology that is found on x-ray. A *bronchogram* is a radiologic procedure involving the injection of an absorbable radio opaque substance into the bronchial tree. Bronchiectasis is usually diagnosed by a bronchogram.

Cystic fibrosis, or *mucoviscidosis*, is an autosomal recessive inherited disease that affects one newborn in every 2500. It is most common in Caucasians of northern European descent. The saline layer that normally underlies the mucus is defective in cystic fibrosis, and mucus is too dense and viscous for cilia to transport without the saline layer. Repeated and chronic lung infections with the gradual loss of pulmonary function results. Bronchiectasis and emphysema are common side effects. Another sign of cystic fibrosis is malabsorption, which results from blockage of the pancreatic duct and bile ducts by thick mucus.

Study Guide

1. Define respiration.
2. Define ventilation.
3. How does the nose affect inspired air?
4. Describe the three pairs of tonsils.
5. Review the anatomy of the larynx
6. Name the passageways of the respiratory system between the pharynx and the alveoli.
7. What is a pneumothorax? What is its relationship to the pleural cavity?
8. Know what is meant by vital capacity and tidal volume.
9. Understand the cause of decompression sickness.
10. List the natural laws that govern the diffusion of gases.
11. Know the following terms: oxyhemoglobin, deoxyhemoglobin, carbaminohemoglobin and carboxyhemoglobin.
12. Review the bicarbonate buffer system, and understand how it is affected by the lungs.
13. What is the Hering-Breuer reflex?
14. What is Kussmaul breathing?
15. What is ketoacidosis?
16. Understand the causes and effects of metabolic acidosis, respiratory acidosis, metabolic alkalosis and respiratory alkalosis.
17. Know what is meant by pneumonia, pneumonitis, bronchitis, bronchiectasis, COPD, and emphysema.

Chapter Twenty-eight

The Urinary System

The urinary system encompasses ***two kidneys, two ureters, the urinary bladder and the urethra.*** The kidneys remove wastes and water from the blood and create urine, which travels through the ureters to the bladder. The urethra is a tube connecting the bladder to an external orifice where urine is eliminated.

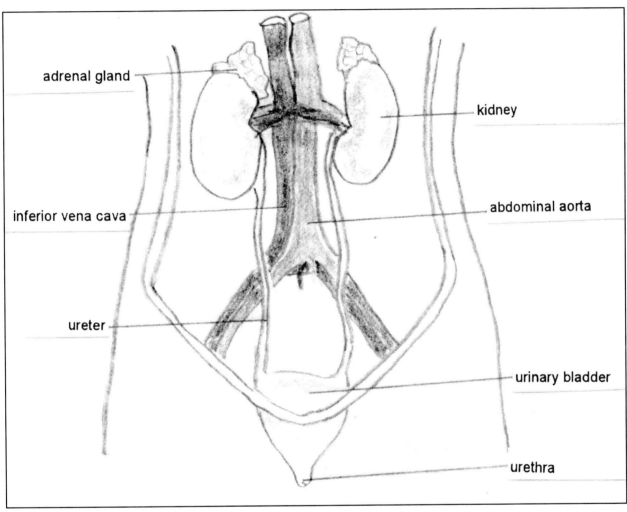

Above: The female urinary system and nearby structures are outlined. The aorta and inferior vena cave have been cut away above the renal arteries.

Urethra

The ***urethra*** is about 18-cm. long in ***males***. It exits the bladder and immediately passes through the ***internal urethral sphincter***, a ring of involuntary smooth muscle. It then passes through the prostate gland and the muscles of the pelvic floor where it is surrounded by the ***external urethral sphincter***, a ring of striated muscle that is under voluntary control. The urethra then passes into the ***penis***. The external urethral orifice is at the tip of the penis.

The urethra is about four cm. in length in ***females***. It leaves the bladder and is surrounded by smooth muscle of the ***internal urethral sphincter***. It then passes through the muscles of the pelvic floor where it is surrounded by striated muscle of the ***external urethral sphincter*** before it reaches the external urethral orifice. The vagina is posterior to the urethral orifice; the clitoris is anterior to the urethral orifice. Young girls should be taught never to wipe the anus in a forward direction because that practice could introduce fecal bacteria into the urethra and cause a urinary tract infection.

Voiding, or micturition, is the act of urinating. Infants and young children do not have control over their external urethral sphincters; when their bladders are stretched, the sphincters open by a reflex action from the spinal cord. Around age three a ***micturition center in the pons*** takes over. The cerebral cortex and other centers in the brain connect to the micturition center in the pons and can affect or control urination. Voiding can be enhanced by a Valsalva maneuver (contraction of the abdominal muscles while holding the breath). In males contraction of the bulbocavernosus muscle in the floor of the pelvis expels the last few drops of urine from the urethra.

Bladder

The urinary ***bladder*** is located in the pelvis posterior to the pubic symphysis. It is a muscular sac that is largely made up of the ***detrusor muscle***, a muscle that contains three layers of smooth muscle. The maximum capacity of the bladder is about 700-800 ml. Contraction of the detrusor muscle expels urine through the urethra when the urethral sphincters are relaxed. ***Sympathetic stimulation*** relaxes the bladder and constricts the internal urinary sphincter. It can subdue a stretch reflex of the bladder and inhibit urination. Parasympathetic stimulation from the sacral nerves causes the bladder to contract. The micturition center in the pons receives signals from the amygdala and the cerebrum that can cause unwanted micturition in times of fear or crisis.

The ***transitional epithelium*** of the bladder forms wrinkles called ***rugae*** when the bladder is empty. Transitional epithelium also lines the ureters and the proximal urethra. Most of the urethra has pseudostratified columnar epithelium with mucous glands (goblet cells). The urethra has stratified squamous epithelium near the external urethral orifice.

The ***trigone*** is a triangular area in the bladder floor that lacks rugae. The points of the trigone are the right and left ureteral orifices and the internal urethral orifice.

Ureters

The ***ureters*** are retroperitoneal tubes leading from the kidneys to the bladder. They have transitional epithelium and a layer of smooth muscle. Contractions of the smooth muscle in the ureters propel the urine to the bladder even when the individual is supine. The ureters pass dorsal to the bladder and enter the lower part of the bladder. A filled bladder compresses the ureters against the vertebral column, which prevents retrograde urine flow.

Kidneys

The ***kidneys*** are two bean shaped organs that are located deeply in each side of the abdomen. They lie in the lumbar areas between ***T-12 and L-3***. The kidneys are ***retroperitoneal***. The right kidney is usually slightly lower than the left because the liver occupies more space on the right. An adrenal gland lies on top of each kidney. ***Rene*** is another word for kidney, and ***"renal"*** refers to the kidneys.

The kidney is surrounded by a fibrous sac called the ***renal capsule***. The renal capsule is anchored at the hilum, and it serves a protective function. Adipose tissue and fascia surround the renal capsule and provide further protection from trauma. Disruption of these protective tissues can result in ***nephroptosis,*** or a ***floating kidney***, which can result in a blocked ureter.

The ***hilum*** of a kidney is an indented area on the medial surface where renal vessels and the ureter connect to the kidney. The hilum occupies a space called the ***renal sinus***. Urine drains into collecting channels called ***calyces*** in the renal sinus. A sagittal section of a kidney reveals the ***parenchyma*** (glandular tissue) encircling the ***renal sinus***. Two or three smaller minor calyces open into a major calyx, and the major calyces converge to form the ***renal pelvis***, a funnel-shaped structure that is continuous with the ureter.

The ***parenchyma*** is divided into a peripheral area called the ***cortex*** and a central area called the ***medulla***. The medulla is made up of six to ten ***pyramids*** that project into the renal sinus. Each pyramid is pointed toward the renal sinus by a blunt point called a ***renal papilla.***

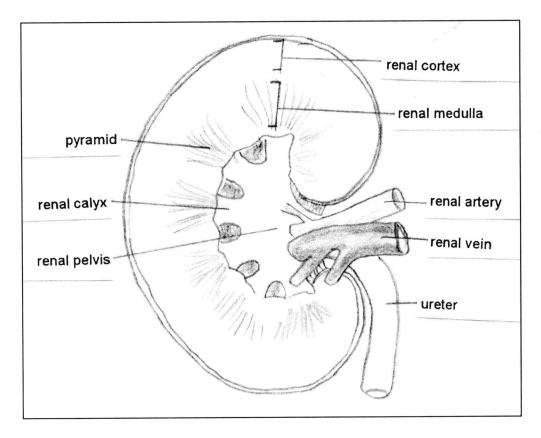

Right:
A sagittal
section of
a kidney.

renal cortex

renal medulla

pyramid

renal artery

renal calyx

renal vein

renal pelvis

ureter

The Nephron

Secretion is the release of a substance from a cell or organ. _Excretion_ is the process of eliminating wastes from the body. The kidneys remove substances from the blood and place them in the urine by _secretion_. Urine and feces are expelled from the body by _excretion_. _Reabsorption_ by the kidneys is the process by which a substance moves from the tubular fluid back into a tubular cell, tissue fluid or the blood.

An individual kidney weighs less than six ounces, yet the two kidneys receive 21% of the resting cardiac output. The renal arteries branch directly from the abdominal aorta and enter the kidneys at the hilum. The renal arteries branch into segmental arteries, and further branching eventually leads to an _afferent arteriole_ of a _glomerulus_. A glomerulus is a tuft of about 50 intertwined capillaries where the glomerular filtration of blood occurs. Blood leaves the glomerulus via an _efferent arteriole_. The glomerulus is the first of several structures that make up the _nephron_, a long microscopic tube that is the working unit of the kidney. The other structures of the nephron are the _proximal convoluted tubule (PCT), the loop of Henle_ (nephron loop), the _distal convoluted tubule (DCT),_ and a _collecting duct_ that empties into a minor calyx. The _glomerular filtrate_ undergoes a series of changes between the glomerulus and the end of the collecting duct, which results in the formation of _urine_. The nephron accomplishes these changes by making use of _filtration, diffusion, active transport, passive transport and semipermeable membranes with different porosities._

The kidneys contain about one million glomeruli. Each _glomerulus_ is surrounded by two layers of a membrane (Bowman's membrane). Between the inner and outer layers of this membrane is a space that is continuous with the nephron tube. Bowman's membrane is folded over the glomerulus like the letter "C;" the glomerulus fits inside the "C." The glomerulus and its surrounding membrane are called the _renal corpuscle_. The inner layer of Bowman's membrane is in contact with the glomerulus, and it surrounds capillaries of the glomerulus with _podocytes_. Podocytes are cells with special pores that allow all substances except cells and large molecules such as proteins to be _filtered into the lumen of the nephron tube_. This passage is called _glomerular filtration_, and the fluid produced is the _glomerular filtrate_. Glomerular filtration _(GF)_ is enhanced by the large blood supply to the kidneys and a relatively high capillary pressure in the glomeruli. This high pressure is created partially by a relatively large afferent arteriole and a relatively small efferent arteriole. The high capillary pressure makes glomeruli particularly susceptible to damage from hypertension.

As a consequence of the glomerular filtration pressure, water and solutes enter the nephron tube at the rate of about **_150-180 liters per day_**. This is an amount equal to 50-60 times the volume of plasma in the body. 99% of the volume of the GF is reabsorbed, and the normal urine output is about 1-2 liters per day.

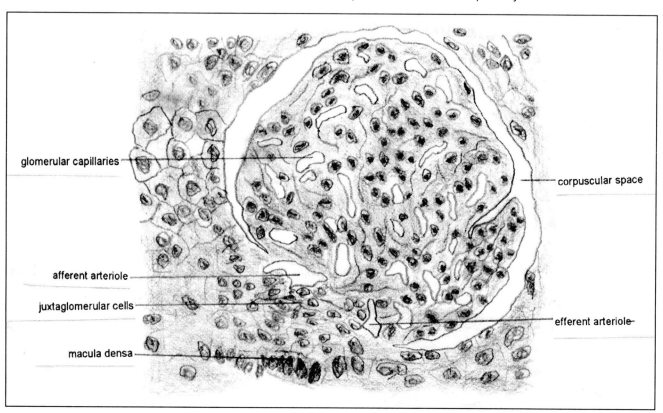

Above: A drawing of a glomerulus, also known as a renal corpuscle.

Glomerular filtration (GF) is controlled by several factors:
(1) Smooth muscle in the afferent and the efferent arterioles controls the diameters of these vessels. To increase the GF rate, the afferent arterioles dilate and the efferent arterioles constrict. This increases the GF pressure. To decrease the GF rate the afferent arterioles constrict and the efferent arterioles dilate.
(2) **_Renin_** is an enzyme released by the **_juxtaglomerular apparatus._** Juxtaglomerular cells are special cells around the afferent and efferent arterioles of the glomeruli that are sensitive to blood pressure. Juxtaglomerular cells are influenced by tightly packed cells of the **_macula densa_**, which is an area of the DCT (distal convoluted tubule) adjacent to the juxtaglomerular cells. **_Renin_** converts angiotensinogen (a plasma protein) to angiotensin I. Angiotensin converting enzyme (ACE) in the lungs and in the kidneys converts angiotensin I to angiotensin II. **_Angiotensin II_** is a powerful vasoconstrictor that stimulates aldosterone release by the adrenal cortex, ADH release by the posterior pituitary, and sodium reabsorption from the kidney tubules. Angiotensin II acts to decrease GF, increase water and sodium reabsorption, increase the blood volume, and increase the blood pressure.
(3) The **_sympathetic nervous system_** innervates arterioles in the kidneys and causes them to constrict. This reduces blood flow through the kidneys, and it decreases the GF rate. Prolonged sympathetic stimulation occurs in marathon runners, and these athletes can develop injury to their glomeruli due to hypoxia that results from prolonged vasoconstriction. **_Hematuria_** (blood in the urine) is present in 18% of all runners following a marathon, and a few have developed renal failure as a result.

Venous blood flowing from the efferent arterioles of a glomerulus enters **_another capillary bed_** that surrounds the PCT (proximal convoluted tubule), the loop of Henle and the DCT (distal convoluted tubule). The PCT is a convoluted tubule in the cortex that receives tubular fluid from the renal corpuscle. Tubular fluid from the PCT drains into the loop of Henle, which is a straight section of the nephron that loops into the medulla and then back into the cortex. Tubular fluid from the loop of Henle drains into the DCT, another long convoluted section, but not as long as the PCT. Tubular fluid from the DCT drains into a collecting duct, then into a minor calyx.

A **_proximal convoluted tubule_** (PCT) is a tiny tubule lined by simple cuboidal epithelial cells that have **_microvilli_** on their inner surfaces. 150-180 liters of glomerular filtrate enter the proximal convoluted tubules every day. The **_reabsorption_** of water, sodium, glucose, chloride, bicarbonate, potassium, magnesium, phosphate, calcium, some peptides and other substances occurs in the PCT. Reabsorption is carried out by active transport, secondary active transport, passive transport and diffusion.

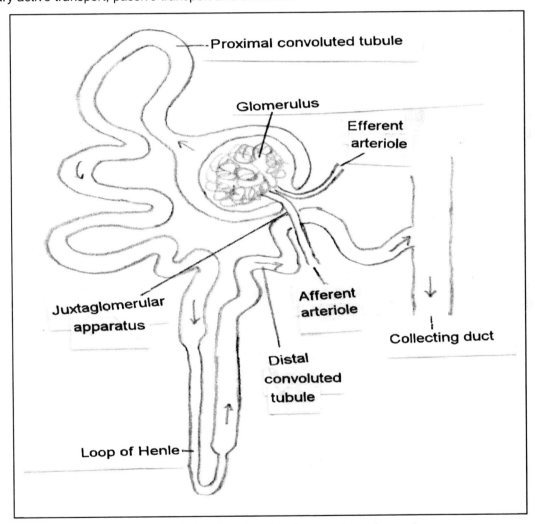

Above: A drawing showing the structure of a nephron.

Substances that are filtered into the tubular fluid of the PCT are handled differently by the nephron. **_Sodium_** is the primary cation in the extracellular fluid, and it must be conserved. Sodium is reabsorbed from the tubular fluid of the PCT through channels that also admit glucose. Cuboidal cells of the PCT then pump sodium into the interstitial fluid. This maintains a high salinity and a high osmolarity in the tissue fluid, especially in the medulla. **_Chloride_** ions accompany the reabsorption of sodium ions because of the attraction between cations and anions.

150-180 liters of _**water**_ are filtered through the renal corpuscle into the tubular fluid of the PCT daily, but water is reabsorbed throughout the nephron, and only 1-2 liters of water are excreted in the urine in a twenty-four hour period. Two-thirds of the water filtered is reabsorbed in the PCT. The nephron loop of Henle is also of primary importance in the _**reabsorption of water.**_ Desert animals have long nephron loops that are extremely efficient in water reabsorption. Fish and amphibians lack nephron loops.

The descending limb or first segment of the _**nephron loop of Henle**_ leaves the cortex and dives into the medulla. The ascending limb or second segment rises back into the cortex. The _**descending limb is permeable to water,**_ but it is impermeable to sodium and other solutes. The intercellular fluid in the medulla is quite salty and has a high osmolarity. This causes water to leave the tubular fluid of the descending limb and enter the tissue fluid by osmosis. The ascending segment of the loop of Henle is relatively impermeable to water and sodium, however, sodium is pumped out of the tubule and into the tissue fluid by active transport in this segment. This maintains high salinity in the interstitial fluid of the medulla. The result of the flow of tubular fluid through the loop of Henle is reabsorption of both water and sodium.

A _**collecting duct**_ receives tubular fluid from multiple nephrons. The collecting ducts begin in the cortex and pass into the medulla where water is reabsorbed. Plasma and the GF fluid have an osmolarity of _**300 mOsmoles**_ per liter. Tubular fluid leaving the collecting ducts (now called urine) may have an osmolarity of up to _**1200 mOsmoles**_ per liter.

**Glucose** is reabsorbed along with sodium in the PCT by active transport; it leaves the tubular cells and enters the interstitial fluid and the blood by passive transport.

**Potassium** is the major intracellular cation and must be conserved. The concentration of potassium in the blood and the glomerular filtrate is low, which limits its potential for loss. The loss of potassium, magnesium and phosphate ions is further reduced by reabsorption of these ions from the tubular fluid by diffusion. However, aldosterone stimulates cells of the DCT to reabsorb sodium and secrete potassium, and some diuretic agents cause a loss of significant amounts of potassium, which can result in life threatening hypokalemia. Although a significant amount of potassium is present in most foods, supplemental oral or IV potassium is indicated when the blood potassium level falls below normal.

**Bicarbonate** ions are present in significant amounts in the glomerular filtrate. Cells of the PCT and DCT generate bicarbonate and _**hydrogen ions**_ from carbon dioxide and water. The hydrogen ions are pumped into the tubular fluid where they neutralize the bicarbonate ions of the glomerular filtrate. Urine is usually mildly acidic due to the active pumping of hydrogen ions into the tubular fluid.

Amino acids, small peptides and lactic acid are reabsorbed in the PCT by active transport.

Wastes

Most of the _**secretion**_ of wastes into the tubule occurs at the _**PCT**_ level. This includes the secretion of urea, uric acid, hydrogen ions, bicarbonate ions, bile acids, ammonia, catecholamines, and many pharmaceutical drugs including penicillin, morphine and aspirin.

**Urea, uric acid, creatinine and ammonia** are nitrogenous wastes that must be removed from the body. A _**cardiac arrhythmia**_ may occur in renal failure that is associated with an excess of urea, ammonia, uric acid and creatinine in the blood and an accompanying electrolyte imbalance ($Na+$, $K+$, $Cl-$ and $HCO3-$).

**Urea** [$CO(NH2)2$] is filtered into the GF along with water and other solutes, but it is partially reabsorbed by diffusion in the PCT, the loop of Henle and the DCT. The net result is an average decrease in the blood urea from 20 mg/100cc in the renal artery to 10.4 mg/100cc in the renal vein. _**Azotemia**_ is a term for an elevated _**blood urea nitrogen level (BUN).**_ _**Uremia**_ is the term for azotemia that is symptomatic. Symptoms of uremia may include diarrhea, vomiting, and dyspnea.

**Uric acid** is a nitrogenous breakdown product of _**purines**_ (adenine and guanine). Uric acid is filtered into the tubular fluid at the renal corpuscle, but it is almost entirely reabsorbed in the PCT. It is then secreted back into the tubular fluid in the loop of Henle, the DCT and the collecting duct. ***Gout*** may result when uric acid levels in the blood become elevated. Gout is a painful joint disorder that is characterized by the crystallization of uric acid in the tissues.

Creatinine is a breakdown product of ***creatine phosphate***, a nitrogenous base in muscle tissue that stores high energy phosphate bonds. Creatinine is filtered into the tubular fluid at the glomerulus. It is a large molecule that does not diffuse back into the tubular cells. An insignificant amount of creatinine is secreted by the DCT.

Ammonia (NH_3) is a product of amino acid (protein) catabolism. It is created by deamination of amino acids and nitrogenous bases. Ammonia is quite toxic and must be detoxified. The ***liver*** accomplishes that by the ***ornithine cycle***, whereby two ammonia molecules are combined with one molecule of carbon dioxide to create urea. Arginine and citrulline are amino acids that are part of the cycle. The steps involved in the ornithine cycle are below.

$$NH_2CH_2CH_2CH_2CHCOOH + CO_2 \quad + \quad NH_3 \quad \rightarrow NHCH_2CH_2CH_2CHCOOH \quad + \quad H_2O$$
$$\qquad\qquad\qquad | \qquad\qquad\qquad\qquad\qquad\qquad\qquad\qquad | \qquad\qquad\qquad |$$
$$\qquad\qquad NH_2 \qquad\qquad\qquad\qquad\qquad\qquad\qquad O{=}CNH_2 \qquad\quad NH_2$$

Ornithine + Carbon Dioxide + Ammonia → **Citrulline**   **+ Water**

$$NHCH_2CH_2CH_2CHCOOH + \quad NH_3 \quad \rightarrow NHCH_2CH_2CH_2CHCOOH \quad + H_2O$$
$$| \qquad\qquad\qquad\qquad | \qquad\qquad\qquad\qquad\qquad\qquad\qquad\qquad | \qquad\qquad\qquad |$$
$$O{=}CNH_2 \qquad\quad NH_2 \qquad\qquad\qquad\qquad HN{=}CNH_2 \qquad\quad NH_2$$

Citrulline   **+   Ammonia →** **Arginine**   **+ Water**

$$NHCH_2CH_2CH_2CHCOOH + H_2O \rightarrow \quad NH_2CH_2CH_2CH_2CHCOOH \quad + \quad H_2N{-}C{-}NH_2$$
$$| \qquad\qquad\qquad\qquad | \qquad\qquad\qquad\qquad\qquad\qquad\qquad\qquad\qquad | \qquad\qquad\qquad\quad \|$$
$$HN{=}CNH_2 \qquad\quad NH_2 \qquad\qquad\qquad\qquad\qquad\qquad NH_2 \qquad\qquad\qquad O$$

Arginine   **+ Water →**   **Ornithine**   **+**   **Urea**

The net result of the ornithine cycle is to convert two molecules of ammonia and one molecule of carbon dioxide into urea. This is the body's most effective way of ridding itself of ammonia, which is toxic. Urea is excreted in the urine.

Hormonal effects

About 36 liters a day of tubular fluid reaches the ***DCT*** where water, sodium, and potassium are reabsorbed and hydrogen ions are secreted. The hormones ***aldosterone, antidiuretic hormone (ADH) and atrial natriuretic hormone (ANH)*** affect the cells of the DCT.

Aldosterone increases sodium reabsorption, which is followed by the reabsorption of water and chloride. Potassium secretion is increased by aldosterone.

ADH increases the permeability of the collecting ducts (in the medulla) to water, and it thereby increases water reabsorption.

ANH opposes the effects of aldosterone and ADH by increasing salt and water secretion. It accomplishes this by **(1)** inhibiting aldosterone secretion by the adrenal cortex, **(2)** inhibiting ADH secretion by the posterior pituitary, **(3)** inhibiting renin secretion by the JG cells, **(4)** inhibiting sodium and chloride reabsorption by the cells of the collecting ducts, and **(5)** increasing the GF rate by dilating the afferent arteriole and constricting the efferent arteriole. This increases filtration pressure.

Parathyroid hormone (PTH) affects the nephron in several ways. **(1)** It promotes calcium reabsorption by the ascending segment of the nephron loop. **(2)** It inhibits phosphate reabsorption by the PCT. This lowers plasma phosphate levels and prevents phosphate from binding with calcium in the blood. **(3)** PTH promotes magnesium reabsorption, and **(4)** it stimulates the kidney to complete the activation of vitamin D to calcitriol.

Laboratory, Medical and Surgical Procedures

Your kidneys can adjust to your degree of hydration. If you drink an excessive amount of water, your urine may have a concentration as low as 50 mOsmoles/liter. If you are dehydrated, your kidneys will conserve water, and your urine may have a concentration of 1200 mOsmoles/liter. The concentration of urine is measured in the laboratory as the urine's specific gravity. A specific gravity of 1.001 is quite low, and it indicates dilute urine. A specific gravity of 1.028 is quite high and indicates a concentrated urine and dehydration.

A **urinalysis** measures the specific gravity; it also measures **(1)** the pH. The normal pH of urine varies between 4.5 and 8.2, but it is most often mildly acidic with an average pH of 6.0. **(2)** The color of urine is examined grossly. It is usually amber due to the presence of urobilinogens, which are breakdown products of bilirubin. **(3)** Proteins are normally absent in the urine. Their presence indicates damage to the glomeruli. Erythrocytes and hemoglobin are absent from the urine except in disease. **(4)** Normal urine does not contain glucose, and its presence indicates a blood glucose level over 300 mg/100cc, which is the highest level that the tubules can completely reabsorb. Glucose in the urine implies diabetes mellitus. **(5)** The urine is examined microscopically for the presence of cells, cell casts (rows of connected cells), bacteria and crystals, any of which can be an indicator of an abnormality.

Blood tests for renal function include measurements of the blood level of **urea (BUN)** and **creatinine**. Some laboratories will report the serum urea level (SUN) instead of the BUN. The **uric acid** level is elevated in renal failure and gout. A **creatinine clearance test** is a measure of how much creatinine is filtered by the glomeruli during a period of time. To perform this test, the blood creatinine level must be known and a 24 hour urine sample must be collected. To calculate the creatinine clearance you multiply the urine creatinine concentration (U) by the urine volume (V) in 24 hours. That tells you the amount of creatinine that has been excreted in a 24 hour period. This figure is then divided by the plasma creatinine level, and the quotient gives a value for the renal clearance of creatinine. Creatinine clearance is a more accurate reflection of glomerular filtration than is urea clearance because creatinine is not reabsorbed or secreted in the tubules to any extent.

An **intravenous pyelogram** (IVP) is a radiographic study that outlines the urinary tract. In this study a radio-opaque dye is injected into a vein, and x-rays are performed as the dye traverses the urinary system. The kidneys, ureters and bladder can all be visualized. The time taken to eliminate the dye is a reflection of the glomerular filtration rate.

Urinary Tract Disorders

Urinary tract infections may be brought about by contamination of the urethra or the blood stream. **Cystitis** is the term for inflammation of the bladder. **Nephritis** means inflammation of the kidneys, and **pyelonephritis** refers to a kidney infection.

Glomerulonephritis signifies an autoimmune disease that affects the glomeruli. One cause of glomerulonephritis is an infection (in the throat or elsewhere) of a specific strain of streptococci. Most individuals recover fully, but some progress to renal failure. (Another strain of streptococci is responsible for rheumatic fever, an autoimmune disease that often results in damaged heart valves.)

The **nephrotic syndrome** involves injury to the glomeruli. It is characterized by massive protein loss in the urine, which causes severe generalized edema. This syndrome has numerous etiologies including infection, diabetes, an autoimmune disorder, drug toxicity, trauma and cancer.

Nephrolithiasis is the formation of stones (calculi) in the urinary tract due to the crystallization of minerals. Renal stones typically contain calcium, phosphate, uric acid and protein, and they may have other ingredients as well. The passage of calculi through the ureters is excruciatingly painful. Staghorn calculi are stones that are lodged in the renal pelvis and are too large to pass. A staghorn calculus may block the renal pelvis and cause failure of that kidney. Kidney stones that are not passed may be approached surgically, or they may be pulverized by an ultrasound beam emission from a lithotripsy unit. Fragments from a shattered stone may then pass through the ureters, bladder and urethra.

Prostatitis is inflammation of the prostate gland that is usually due to an infection. ***Benign prostatic hypertrophy*** (BPH) is an enlarged prostate, a condition that is exceedingly common in elderly men. BPH can result in kidney damage due to the blockage of urine flow. Advanced prostatic hypertrophy is treated by surgical resection of the prostate.

Diuresis is the production of a large amount of urine. ***Diuretic drugs*** are useful when excessive tissue fluid (edema) and excessive blood volume need to be reduced. Therefore, diuretics are useful in hypertension, congestive heart failure and renal failure. Most diuretic drugs act on the cells of the kidney tubules. For example, furosemide (Lasix) inhibits sodium reabsorption throughout the nephron, and chlorothiazide (Diuril) inhibits sodium reabsorption by the DCT cells. ***Caffeine*** acts as a diuretic by dilating the afferent arterioles of the glomerulus. ***Ethyl alcohol*** is a diuretic because it inhibits ADH secretion. (But the large volume of urine excreted by beer drinking college students is due more to the volume of liquid consumed than the inhibition of ADH). ***Mannitol*** is a sugar that is not metabolized, and it is excreted wholly in the urine. When given IV, mannitol increases the blood osmolarity, it increases the blood volume, and it increases the osmolarity in the tubular fluid. These changes result in a diuresis.

Polyuria means "frequent urination," but it generally is used to mean diuresis or excessive urine output. ***Oliguria*** is a term for low urine output. ***Anuria*** is a term for a very low (less than 50 cc per day) urine output.

Primary neoplasms of the kidney are ***Wilm's tumors*** in children and ***hypernephromas*** in adults. Wilm's tumors typically appear in young childhood, and they constitute from 20 to 25 percent of all malignant tumors of childhood. Hypertension is a frequent symptom of Wilm's tumors. Hypernephromas are malignant primary tumors of adult kidneys. Hypernephromas are sometimes associated with obscure fever, polycythemia and lung metastases. About twenty-five percent of patients with untreated hypernephromas will survive more than ten years.

Renal failure affects an increasing number of Americans each year. The patient with renal failure must watch his diet carefully to balance his intake with what his limited kidney function can remove. Proteins in the diet must be severely restricted because the nitrogenous wastes they generate cannot be effectively removed. Water, sodium and potassium also must be restricted in most renal failure patients.

The causes of renal failure include severe hypertension (nephrosclerosis), glomerulonephritis, a urinary tract obstruction, the nephrotic syndrome, renal stones, chronic pyelonephritis, and stenosis (narrowing) of the renal arteries. Toxins such as lead, mercury, carbon tetrachloride, acetone and paint thinners can cause renal failure by killing cells of the tubules. Glomerulonephritis and the nephrotic syndrome involve injury to the glomeruli. In the nephrotic syndrome, glomerular damage produces massive proteinuria, which results in profound edema.

Stenosis of a renal artery and coarctation of the aorta are two causes of hypertension. These disorders lead to low blood flow through one or both kidneys, which results in high renin secretion by the juxtaglomerular cells. Surgical correction leads to a cure for the hypertension produced by these vascular lesions, unless the glomeruli have been irreversibly damaged. Stenosis of one renal artery is a potential cause for severe hypertension, which may severely damage the opposite kidney. Paradoxically, following surgery to repair the stenotic artery, the kidney that had the renal artery stenosis may prove to be the only healthy kidney; the stenosis could have protected it from permanent damage to the glomeruli caused by hypertension.

One treatment option for patients with renal failure is ***hemodialysis***. This treatment requires the patient to spend 4-8 hours three times a week undergoing dialysis. The procedure utilizes diffusion through a semi permeable membrane to accomplish what the patient's kidneys cannot do. A frequent requirement for dialysis is the surgical placement of an AV shunt in the patient's forearm. During the dialysis procedure, blood flows from an artery to the dialysis chamber and then back to a vein of the patient. The AV shunt facilitates the placement of tubes into the blood vessels. The dialysis fluid contains electrolytes and glucose. Urea, creatinine, uric acid, phosphate and sulfate are the primary materials removed by diffusion from the patient's blood.

Peritoneal dialysis is a procedure that involves injecting dialysis fluid into the peritoneal cavity. Waste materials diffuse into the peritoneal fluid, which is later removed.

The first successful organ transplant was performed in 1953; this was a kidney transplant between identical twins. Renal transplantation is no longer a rare procedure because the incidence of chronic renal failure has increased. Dialysis centers across the country are full, and the waiting times for a renal transplant are growing longer.

Study Guide
1. What makes up the urinary system?
2. Describe the ureters.
3. Describe the male urethra and the female urethra.
4. Understand the relationship between the urethra and the prostate gland in the male.
5. What is micturition?
6. Describe the epithelium of the bladder, ureters and urethra.
7. Acquaint yourself with the following landmarks of the kidney: hilum, renal pelvis, parenchyma, cortex, medulla, renal sinus, calyces, pyramids, renal papilla.
8. Understand the nephron and its parts including the glomerulus, PCT, nephron loop of Henle, DCT and collecting duct.
9. Understand the physiology behind water reabsorption by the nephron loop of Henle.
10. Understand the steps and the effects of the renin-angiotensin mechanism.
11. What is urea? How is it synthesized? What function does it serve?
12. What is the precursor of uric acid? What is the precursor of creatinine?
13. How do the following hormones affect the nephron: aldosterone, ADH, ANH, and parathyroid hormone?
14. What blood constituents are normally absent from the glomerular filtrate? ...from the urine?
15. Describe the creatinine clearance test.
16. Define diuresis, polyuria, anuria and oliguria.
17. Understand pyelonephritis, glomerulonephritis and the nephrotic syndrome.

Chapter Twenty-nine

Homeostasis

Homeostasis is the ability of the body to maintain a stable environment. Homeostasis is achieved through negative feedback mechanisms.

Water Balance

The amount of water in the human body varies with the age and fat content of the individual. Elderly and obese people have a lower percentage of their body weight as water. Young, muscular individuals have a higher water content.

Water is constantly being lost in the urine, skin, feces and breath. About two and one-half liters of water is lost daily, and this water must be replaced. **_Water is a by product of metabolism_**, and some water is replaced from the oxidation of carbohydrates, fats and proteins. **_Carbohydrate catabolism produces more metabolic_** water than does the catabolism of fats or proteins, but most water replacement comes from liquids and foods that are ingested.

Hydration and the concentrations of Na+, K+, Cl-, HCO3-, and H+ are inextricably linked by several negative feedback mechanisms.

The **_hypothalamus_** has a thirst center that signals that you are thirsty when it detects a low blood pressure and a high blood osmolarity. The posterior pituitary responds by secreting **_ADH_** (antidiuretic hormone), which stimulates the reuptake of water in the collecting ducts of the kidneys. In dehydration the thirst center will send signals via the sympathetic nervous system to decrease salivation and create a dry mouth, which is an impetus to drink fluids.

Water loss is curbed by a reduction in urine volume. ADH, aldosterone and the renin mechanism serve to decrease urine output. **_Renin_** is an enzyme secreted by the kidneys in response to low blood pressure. Renin begins a cascade of reactions that result in the formation of **_angiotensin II_**, a powerful vasoconstrictor. Angiotensin II raises the blood pressure and stimulates the secretion of ADH from the posterior pituitary and aldosterone by the adrenal cortex. Angiotensin II also stimulates the kidneys to reabsorb more sodium, which is followed by the reabsorption of chloride and water.

Dehydration occurs whenever a sufficient amount of water is not taken in to balance the water that is lost in the urine, sweat, breath and feces. Excessive water loss can be produced by disorders that cause diarrhea or vomiting and by physical activity, especially in hot, humid environments. Cholera is a severe infectious diarrhea that is caused by bacteria of the genus *Vibrio*. The diarrhea associated with cholera is so severe, and water is lost so rapidly that fluid replacement becomes difficult. Most choleric deaths occur from dehydration; infants and young children are especially susceptible. Dehydration with a reduction of blood volume is manifest by hypotension and tachycardia, and it is often associated with electrolyte imbalances. The concentrations of electrolytes in dehydration will vary depending upon whether the loss of water was associated with the loss of sodium and other ions.

Excessive extracellular fluid in the tissues is called **_edema_**. Pulmonary edema is excess fluid in the lungs, which can lead to ventilation failure. Excess fluid within the abdominal cavity is called **_ascites_**; a pericardial effusion is fluid in the pericardial sac; a pleural effusion is fluid in the chest cavity outside the lungs. When water is in excess in the body, and the electrolytes are not in excess, the electrolytes (sodium, potassium, chloride and bicarbonate) will be overly diluted. Sodium is the major cation in the blood, and **_water intoxication_** is characterized by **_hyponatremia_**. It can result from the sudden excessive intake of water from low sodium intravenous fluids or by quickly ingesting large amounts of water. Another cause of excessive bodily water is an excessive secretion of ADH (called inappropriate ADH), which can result from the overzealous use of positive pressure respirators. In water intoxication the plasma sodium concentration may dip to a level low enough to cause pulmonary edema and cerebral edema.

Plasma proteins, especially albumin, are instrumental in creating the osmotic pressure that maintains blood volume. Albumin and other plasma proteins are lost in the urine in the nephrotic syndrome. Massive edema occurs in this order because protein loss reduces the osmolarity of the plasma to the extent that fluid escapes the blood and enters the tissue fluid.

Electrolyte Balance

The major *cations* in plasma are *sodium, potassium and calcium*. Concentrations of these ions must be kept within a narrow range (*Na+, 140-145 mEq/L; K+, 3.5-5.0 mEq/L; and Ca++, 4.5-5.5 mEq/L or 9-11 mg/L*). The most abundant cation in the plasma is *sodium*, and sodium is responsible for 90-95% of the osmolarity of the extracellular fluid. The American diet contains an overabundance of sodium, so the primary concern is getting rid of it; that is a job for the kidneys.
Hypernatremia exists if the plasma sodium concentration exceeds 145 mEq/L. Water retention, increased blood volume, edema and hypertension are side effects of hypernatremia.

As mentioned, *aldosterone* stimulates sodium reuptake by the kidney tubules, and aldosterone secretion is stimulated by the renin–angiotensin mechanism. *Addison's disease* is a condition in which the adrenal cortices become atrophic, and steroid hormone production is low or lacking. Addison's disease is characterized by sodium wasting, water loss and hyperkalemia. *Cushing's disease* involves excessive glucocorticoid production by the adrenal glands. Glucocorticoids have some mineralocorticoid activity, and sodium retention, hypertension and hypokalemia are signs of Cushing's disease.

ANP (atrial natriuretic peptide) is a hormone secreted by the atria of the heart. It causes sodium to be excreted in the urine by inhibiting sodium and water resorption by the nephron. It also inhibits renin and ADH secretion.

Potassium is the most abundant cation in the intracellular fluid (ICF). The amount of potassium in the extracellular fluid (ECF) is small (3.5-5.0 mEq/L), but its concentration must be kept within this narrow range. Potassium is filtered through the glomeruli of the kidneys, and it is secreted into the tubular fluid of the DCT. Aldosterone stimulates potassium secretion and sodium resorption in the nephrons.

Hyperkalemia (> 5.0 mEq/L) and *hypokalemia* (< 3.5 mEq/L) are sometimes associated with diuretic therapy, depending on the drug used. Hyperkalemia occurs *suddenly* in hemolytic states and following a crushing injury. In these situations hyperkalemia results from the sudden lysis of cells, which release intracellular potassium into the blood. When hyperkalemia develops suddenly, reflexes become hyperactive.
Hyperkalemia comes on *slowly* in renal failure or Addison's disease. *(Addison's disease* is atrophy of the adrenal cortex with an associated lack of aldosterone.) Symptoms of hyperkalemia of slow onset include sluggish reflexes and less excitable nerve and muscle tissue.
Cardiac arrhythmias may occur in hyperkalemia, and they can be fatal. Some states in the U.S. carry out the death penalty by injecting potassium chloride into a vein.

Hypokalemia can result from an adrenal tumor that secretes large amounts of *aldosterone* or other steroids with mineralocorticoid activity. *Diuretic therapy, diarrhea and vomiting* can also produce hypokalemia. In *acute hypokalemia* nerve cells and muscle cells become hyperpolarized and less excitable. In *chronic hypokalemia* sodium channels are activated, and cells become hyperexcitable. Muscle weakness, abnormal reflexes and cardiac arrhythmias can result from hypokalemia.

Chloride is the most common anion in the plasma. Chloride ions generally follow sodium ions in and out of the plasma membrane due to ionic attraction, and the chloride concentration generally mimics the sodium concentration. Stomach acidity is produced by *hydrochloric acid* (HCL), and prolonged vomiting can produce a hypochloremic alkalosis.

Calcium is a necessary cation for nerve conduction and muscle contraction, but it must be kept at a low concentration to prevent it from crystallizing with phosphate. Cells contain a protein called _calsequestrin_ that binds with calcium and keeps it from crystallizing. _Parathyroid hormone_ increases serum calcium levels by increasing bone resorption and increasing calcium resorption in the kidney tubules. _Calcitriol_ (active vitamin D) regulates blood calcium levels by increasing bone dissolution, increasing intestinal absorption of calcium, and by decreasing urinary excretion of calcium. Parathyroid hormone is opposed by _calcitonin_, a hormone secreted by the thyroid gland during childhood. Calcitonin decreases the serum calcium level by stimulating osteoblasts and bone growth. _Hypercalcemia_ (> 5.8 mEq/L or > 11.6 mg/100 cc) can result from a parathyroid tumor that secretes excessive amounts of parathyroid hormone, or it can result from hypothyroidism. (Thyroid hormone and calcitonin stimulate bone growth and lower the blood calcium level; these hormones are lacking in hypothyroidism.) Hypercalcemia causes weakness, weak and slow reflexes and cardiac arrhythmias. _Hypocalcemia_ (< 4.5 mEq/L or < 9 mg/100 cc) can result from low dietary calcium, a lack of vitamin D, lactation, acidosis, or hypoparathyroidism. It causes muscles and nerves to be overly excitable; tetany can result. Hypocalcemia is much more common than hypercalcemia.

Phosphorus exists in the blood as the dihydrogen phosphate ion, H_2PO_4-, and the monohydrogen phosphate ion, $HPO_4=$. Phosphates are abundant in foods, and the blood concentration of phosphate is less critical than that of other ions. Phosphate ions are in a state of flux due to the constant production and breakdown of _nucleotides_, and they are important _buffers_ inside the cell and in the plasma. Lowering the phosphate concentration serves to reduce the tendency calcium phosphate to crystallize. This is beneficial in urine because it reduces the incidence of _kidney stones_. A chronically low blood phosphate is potentially harmful because it reduces bone formation.

Acid and Base Balance

The normal _pH_ of blood falls within a narrow range between 7.35 and 7.45. Metabolism produces acids that decrease the pH. Those acids include lactic acid, phosphoric acids, fatty acids, carbonic acid and many others. Acids must be _buffered,_ and the _primary buffers in the blood are phosphates, bicarbonate and proteins._
A buffer acts as a weak acid and a weak base; therefore, buffers can accept H+ ions and remove them from solution, which raises the pH. Buffers can also give up H+ ions (protons) to solution, which would make a solution more acidic and lower its pH.

The _phosphate buffer system_ involves monohydrogen phosphate (_$HPO_4=$_) and dihydrogen phosphate (_H_2PO_4-_). The former is a weak base, and it will remove H+ from solution. The later is a weak acid, and it will give up H+ ions. Phosphates are important buffers in the blood, the renal tubules and inside the cells.

The _bicarbonate buffer system_ involves carbon dioxide (CO_2), which reacts with water (H_2O) to form _carbonic acid_ (H_2CO_3). Carbonic acid is a weak acid that ionizes to H+ and HCO_3- (_bicarbonate)_. Bicarbonate in the blood exists as sodium bicarbonate ($NaHCO_3$). Sodium bicarbonate is ionized in solution and exists as Na+ and HCO_3-. $NaHCO_3$ is a weak base because the bicarbonate ion (HCO_3-) will bind with H+ ions, form carbonic acid, and thereby remove hydrogen ions from solution.

$$H_2O \; + \; CO_2 \; \longleftrightarrow \; H_2CO_3 \; \longleftrightarrow \; H+ \; + \; HCO_2-$$

The bicarbonate buffer system is extremely useful because the _lungs_ exert control over pH through that system. The lungs can exhale CO_2, and by so doing they get rid of acidity. Increased ventilation lowers the amount of CO_2 in the blood, and therefore, raises the pH by lowering the plasma concentration of carbonic acid. Decreased ventilation increases the blood CO_2 and lowers the blood pH.

The _kidneys_ also have a major role in stabilizing the pH of the blood because they can excrete hydrogen ions into the tubular fluid by a process that utilizes CO_2 and bicarbonate. This action reduces the H+ ion concentration and raises the blood pH. _Carbonic anhydrase_ is an enzyme that catalyzes the formation of carbonic acid from CO_2 and water. This enzyme is instrumental in H+ excretion in the urine. _Phosphate buffers_ are present in the glomerular filtrate, and they buffer some of the acidity of the urine. Renal tubular cells release _ammonia_ into the tubular fluid. Ammonia (NH_3) is a highly toxic basic compound. Most ammonia is detoxified in the liver by the synthesis of urea (NH2CONH2). Residual ammonia is secreted into the renal tubular fluid of the kidneys where it reacts with hydrogen ions and chloride ions, forming ammonium chloride, (NH4Cl), a weak acid.

Proteins are the most abundant buffers in the blood. Proteins are made up of amino acids, and each amino acid has one or more carboxyl groups and one or more amino groups. The buffering capacity of proteins is due to **exposure** of their **carboxyl (COOH) groups, which are acidic,** and **amino (NH2) groups, which are basic.** The carboxyl groups are weak acids and give up H+ ions; the amino groups are weak bases and take up H+ ions. The amino acids, aspartic acid and glutamic acid, contain two carboxyl groups, and they are acidic. The amino acids, arginine and lysine, contain two amino groups, and they are basic.

Acidosis is the term for a low blood pH. The normal metabolic activity of the body produces many acidic compounds that would overwhelm the buffering ability to maintain homeostasis if other methods of compensation were not present. Both the lungs and the kidneys function in their own way to balance the pH of the blood through the bicarbonate buffer system. The lungs respond to a low pH by increasing ventilation and exhaling CO_2; the kidneys respond by secreting more hydrogen ions into the tubular fluid. Hydrogen ions in the urine are buffered by the secretion of bicarbonate and ammonia into the tubular fluid. **Respiratory acidosis** is the term used for a low blood pH accompanied by a high CO_2 (and H_2CO_3) in the blood. In this condition the lungs do not function adequately, and CO_2 cannot be properly vented out of the body. **Metabolic acidosis** is the term used for a low blood pH accompanied by a low blood CO_2. In this condition, the lungs are breathing off high amounts of CO_2 in an attempt to compensate for the presence of an excessive amount of acidity produced elsewhere in the body.

Alkalosis signifies an elevated blood pH. In **respiratory alkalosis** a high pH is accompanied by a low CO_2. Respiratory alkalosis is caused by hyperventilation, which is usually caused by acute anxiety. **Metabolic alkalosis** is a high blood pH accompanied by a high blood CO_2. It is uncommon, but it can be caused by an over consumption of antacids (orally or IV) or from the excessive loss of stomach acid by prolonged vomiting.

Alkalosis is usually accompanied by hypokalemia. Hydrogen ions and potassium ions tend to move across the cell membrane in opposite directions. Consequently, alkalosis causes a compensatory movement of hydrogen out of the cell, which in turn is compensated by the movement of potassium ions into the cell, which lowers the blood potassium level.

Acidosis is usually associated with hyperkalemia. In acidosis the excessive H+ in the blood enters the cells, and K+ leaves the cells causing hyperkalemia. (Paradoxically potassium chloride will typically cause acidosis when it is given quickly IV. This occurs because the excess chloride in the blood attracts hydrogen ions from the cells.)

A careful consideration of the status of hydration, pH and electrolyte concentrations is necessary when giving supplemental IV or oral therapy. **Normal saline or 0.9% NaCl is isotonic to plasma**, but it lacks other electrolytes and nutrients.

A **one half normal saline solution** is hypotonic to plasma but will not cause hemolysis. It is especially useful as a slow drip when IV medications are being given, and sodium needs to be restricted.

Ringer's lactate solution contains **glucose and potassium ions, and it is buffered with lactate ions**, but it is not always appropriate because it may cause alkalosis or hyperkalemia, especially in patients with renal failure.

Isotonic glucose (dextrose or D5W) affords water replacement and limited nutrition, but it lacks electrolytes, and it is not indicated in diabetics with high blood sugar levels.

Plasma volume expanders include **hypertonic solutions** of various sugars including **mannitol.** Mannitol is not metabolized, and it remains in the blood until it filters through the kidneys where it acts as an **osmotic diuretic.** Mannitol increases the blood volume, and it cannot be given in congestive heart failure or in renal insufficiency because it may lead to pulmonary edema in those situations.

Study Guide

1. What is metabolic water? Which foodstuffs would you take to the desert because they produce the most metabolic water?
2. How does the hypothalamus affect water balance?
3. Describe the effects of ADH, aldosterone and ANH on water balance.
4. Define edema.
5. Define ascites.
6. What are the major cations in plasma?
7. What are the major anions in plasma?
8. What are the normal values for the serum electrolytes (Na+, K+, Cl-, HCO3-, and Ca++)?
9. How do aldosterone, ADH and ANH affect electrolyte balance?
10. How do plasma proteins affect the blood volume?
11. Understand the causes and effects of hyperkalemia and hypokalemia.
12. Understand the causes and effects of hypercalcemia and hypocalcemia.
13. Define a buffer.
14. What is the normal pH range in the blood?
15. Review the bicarbonate buffer system.
16. Review the phosphate buffer system.
17. Review the protein buffer system.
18. Understand metabolic acidosis, respiratory acidosis, metabolic alkalosis and respiratory alkalosis.
19. Review the following IV fluids: normal saline, one half normal saline, D5W, and Ringer's lactate.
20. How does the intravenous administration of mannitol affect the body?
21. How are acidosis and hyperkalemia related?
22. How are alkalosis and hypokalemia related?

References

Adler, Francis Heed, *Textbook of Ophthalmology*.

Amerman, Erin C., *Exercises for the Anatomy and Physiology Laboratory*.

Cantarow, Abraham and Schepartz, Bernard, *Biochemistry*.

Duke-Elder, Sir Stewart, *System of Ophthalmology*.

Eastman, Nicholson J., and Hellman, Louis M., *Williams Obstetrics*.

Gibson, Glen C., and Harley, Robison D., *Anomalies of Binocular Position, Visual Perception and Ocular Motility in Strabismus*.

Goodman, Louis S., and Gilman, Alfred, *The Pharmacological Basis of Therapeutics*.

Gray, Henry, *Gray's Anatomy*.

Gunstream, Stanley E., *Anatomy and Physiology Laboratory Textbook, Essentials Version*.

Guyton, Arthur C., *Textbook of Medical Physiology*.

Harrison, Tinsley R., *Principles of Internal Medicine*.

Hole, John W., Jr., *Essentials of Human Anatomy and Physiology*.

Johnson, Leonard R., *Essential Medical Physiology*.

Knoll, Andrew H., *Life on a Young Planet, The First Three Billion Years of Evolution on Earth*.

Le Vay, David, *Human Anatomy and Physiology*.

Martin, Lawrence, *All You Really Need to Know to Interpret Arterial Blood Gases*.

Martini, Frederic H., *Fundamentals of Anatomy and Physiology*.

Mader, Sylvia S., *Understanding Human Anatomy and Physiology*.

Pansky, Ben, *Review of Gross Anatomy*.

Ranson, Stephen W., and Clark, Sam L., *The Anatomy of the Nervous System*.

Rizzo, Donald C., *Delmar's Fundamentals of Anatomy and Physiology*.

Saladin, Kenneth S., *Anatomy and Physiology*.

Scanlon, Valerie and Sanders, Tina, *Understanding Human Structure and Function*.

Tortora, Gerard J., *Introduction to the Human Body*.

Van De Graaf, Kent M., and Crawley, John L., *A photographic Atlas for the Anatomy and Physiology Laboratory*.

References

Walker, Gabrielle, *Snowball Earth.*

Williams, Robert H., *Textbook of Endocrinology.*

Williams, J. Whitridge, *Williams Obstetrics,* edited by Nicholas J. Eastman and Louis M. Hellman.

Wintrobe, Maxwell M., *Clinical Hematology.*

Wise, Eric, *Anatomy and Physiology Laboratory Manual.*

Wolff, Eugene, *Anatomy of the Eye and Orbit.*

Woodburne, Russell T., *Essentials of Human Anatomy.*

INDEX

Index

Ventricle, continued,
  right, 219, 227, 231-240, 258, 317
  third, 157, 160, 163, 164, 169
Venule, 219, 222, 225, 279
Vertex position, 249, 259
Vesalius, Andreas, 9
Vesicle, 8, 35, 39, 106, 133, 135, 137, 267
Vestibular apparatus, 166, 188-190
Vestibular ganglion, 190
Viagra, 246
Vibrio, 283, 329
Vibrissae, 70
Vitamin A, see retinol
Vitamin B1, see thiamine
Vitamin B2, see riboflavin
Vitamin B3, see niacin
Vitamin B5, see pantothenic acid
Vitamin B6, see pyridoxine
Vitamin B12, see cyanocolbalamine
Vitamin C, see ascorbic acid
Vitamin D, see calcitriol
Vitamin E, see tocopherol
Vitamin K, 211, 212, 279-281, 297
Vitreous humor, 57, 184, 186
Voltage gated channel, 37, 107, 135, 136
Von Recklinghausen's disease (see neurofibromatosis)
Von Economo's lethargica, 143
Von Willebrand's disease, 211
Vulva, 247

Water balance, 329
Watson, James, 12, 41, 52
Wernicke's area, 162, 168-170
Whipple's disease, 283
Wilm's tumor, 327
Wilson, Woodrow, 142
Wilson's disease, 299

X-ray, 20, 75, 181, 238, 317, 326

Yolk Sac, 258

Zeiss, Karl, 10
Zinc, 16, 26, 299
Zoloft, 179
Zona pellucida, 247, 255-257
Zonules, 182, 183
Zygote, 41, 51, 55, 247, 249, 254-257

Printed in the United States
127226LV00001B/1-82/P